Library of
Davidson College

Diseases of the Reptilia

Diseases of the Reptilia
Volume 1

Edited by

JOHN E. COOPER

*Royal College of Surgeons of England,
Lincoln's Inn Fields, London*

and

OLIPHANT F. JACKSON

*Royal Free Hospital School of Medicine,
Pond Street, London*

1981

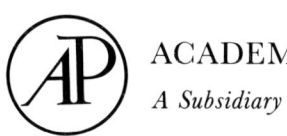

ACADEMIC PRESS

A Subsidiary of Harcourt Brace Jovanovich, Publishers

London · New York · Toronto · Sydney · San Francisco

ACADEMIC PRESS INC. (LONDON) LTD.
24/28 Oval Road,
London NW1 7DX

United States Edition published by
ACADEMIC PRESS INC.
111 Fifth Avenue
New York, New York 10003

Copyright © 1981 by
ACADEMIC PRESS INC. (LONDON) LTD.

All Rights Reserved
No part of this book may be reproduced in any form by photostat, microfilm, or any other means, without written permission from the publishers

British Library Cataloguing in Publication Data
Diseases of the reptilia.
　Vol. 1
　1. Reptiles–Physiology
　I. Cooper, J. E.　II. Jackson, O. F.
　636.089　　　QL641

ISBN 0-12-187901-1
LCCCN 81-66390

Printed in Great Britain by
The Pitman Press, Bath BA2 3BL

Contributors

P.K.C. AUSTWICK, *Nuffield Institute of Comparative Medicine, Zoological Society of London, Regent's Park, London, England. Present address: Aerobiology Unit, Cardiothoracic Institute, Brompton Hospital, Frimley, Surrey GU16 5QE, England*

H F. CLARK, *The Wistar Institute of Anatomy and Biology, 36th Street at Spruce, Philadelphia, PA 19104, USA*

J.E. COOPER, *Royal College of Surgeons of England, Lincoln's Inn Fields, London WC2A 3PN, England*

P.M.C. DAVIES, *Department of Zoology, The University, University Park, Nottingham NG7 2RD, England*

E. ELKAN, *Department of Histopathology, Mount Vernon Hospital, Northwood, Middlesex HA6 2RN, England*

W. FRANK, *Universität Hohenheim, Abteilung Parasitologie, D7000 Stuttgart 70, Emil-Wolff Strasse 34, West Germany*

O.F. JACKSON, *Royal Free Hospital School of Medicine, Pond Street, London NW3 2QG, England*

I.F. KEYMER, *Zoological Society of London, Regent's Park, London, England. Present address: Veterinary Investigation Centre, Norwich, Norfolk NR6 6ST, England*

P.D. LUNGER, *University of Delaware, Newark, DE 19711, USA*

J.R. NEEDHAM, *Division of Comparative Medicine, Clinical Research Centre, Watford Road, Harrow, Middlesex HA1 3UJ, England*

Man with all his noble qualities, with sympathy that feels for the most debased, with benevolence which extends not only to other men but to the humblest living creature, with his god-like intellect which has penetrated into the movements and constitution of the solar system – with all these exalted powers – still bears in his bodily frame the indelible stamp of his lowly origin.

> Charles Darwin *The Descent of Man.*

Preface

The aims of this two-volume book are discussed in Chapter 1. Basically it is intended as an up-to-date guide to the diseases of reptiles with particular, but not exclusive, reference to those in captivity. In this first volume the anatomical and physiological features of the Reptilia are outlined and attention drawn to methods available for laboratory investigation of their diseases and pathology; the succeeding chapters deal with those conditions caused by infectious or parasitic agents. The contributors include clinicians, pathologists, microbiologists, parasitologists and zoologists and we are grateful to them for writing their chapters and for their co-operation in compiling this volume. The staff of Academic Press have been most helpful throughout and guided us in the preparation of the book. Our special thanks are due to Dr. Carl Gans who has not only shown much personal interest but has also commented in detail upon several manuscripts.

The study of diseases of reptiles is still in its infancy and it is inevitable that there should be differences of opinion over a number of subjects. Such disagreement is often an encouraging sign, since it prompts further research, and we have therefore been careful not to edit too severely. It must also be apparent that volumes of this size cannot deal with all aspects of disease in detail; the reader will, therefore, find that some topics are covered more thoroughly than others. This may be indicative of the author's own interests but often it reflects the relative significance of such conditions in captive or free-living populations. Sometimes a paucity of information is due to a lack of available data and it is to be hoped that these gaps in our knowledge will be filled in the next few years.

Originally this book was intended as a single volume. However, it soon became apparent that a two-volume work would be necessary in order to do the subject justice. An unfortunate consequence was that we were asked to condense the references, in particular by omitting the titles of articles and by abbreviating the names of journals. It was with considerable reluctance that we acceded to this request but it seemed preferable to make such a sacrifice rather than to reduce the amount of factual text. We appreciate that as a result, the references may prove less comprehensive than readers might have liked and for this we apologize.

Some of the illustrations in the book are reproduced, in whole or in part, from other publications. Acknowledgements are given in the text but we should like to thank the authors, journals and publishers involved.

We are also indebted to the Trustees of the British Museum (Natural History) for permission to reproduce the photograph of a fracture in an *Iguanodon* (Chapter 1) and to Dr. Alan Charig for permitting one of us (JEC) to see the specimen.

We must express our appreciation to the following who very kindly read and commented upon sections of the book: E. Allen, R.A. Avery, A. d'A Bellairs, R.J. Berry, J.M. Bradley, J.A. Champneys, E.V. Cock, J.F.D. Frazer, C. Gans, A.G. Greenwood, G. Hoff, D.M. Jones, J. Kirkwood, D.H. Molyneux, M.A. Peirce, C. Perkin, R. Richards, M. Rweyemamu, P. Sanderson and P. Zwart.

Our thanks are also due to Mrs. J. Bulman, Miss S. Chamberlain, Miss S. Dowsett, Miss M.E. Ohlsson, Mrs. C. Sandison and Mrs. D. Suttie for assistance with the typing. Miss Sally Dowsett has also given us invaluable help in the compilation of the index. Staff at the libraries of Huntingdon Research Centre, the Royal Free Hospital, the Royal College of Veterinary Surgeons and the Royal College of Surgeons of England have been most helpful in our quest for references.

Last, but not least, we are indebted to our wives and families for their support and encouragement in this work.

London J.E. Cooper
January 1981 O.F. Jackson

Contents

Contributors . . . v
Preface . . . vii

Background

1 Introduction . . . 3
   J.E. COOPER AND O.F. JACKSON

2 Anatomy and Physiology
   P.M.C. DAVIES
       Classification of Reptiles . . . 9
     I Diagnostic features . . . 9
     II Integument . . . 10
     III Musculo-skeletal system . . . 15
     IV Visceral organization and homeostasis . . . 24
     V Metabolism . . . 50
     VI Neuro-endocrine system . . . 61
       References . . . 67

3 Pathology and Histopathological Techniques
   E. ELKAN
     I Introduction . . . 75
     II Pathological examination . . . 77
     III The preparation of sections . . . 79
     IV Photography of pathological material . . . 82
     V Pathological responses in reptiles . . . 82
     VI Some pathological conditions in reptiles . . . 83
       References . . . 91

4 Microbiology and Laboratory Techniques
   J.R. NEEDHAM
     I Introduction . . . 93
     II Equipment and techniques for bacteriology . . . 93
     III Parasitological techniques . . . 126
     IV Haematological techniques . . . 128
     V Biochemical techniques . . . 129

VI Conclusions . . . 130
    References . . . 130

Infectious Diseases

5 Viruses
    H F. CLARK AND P.D. LUNGER
      I Introduction . . . 135
      II Viruses circumstantially associated with reptilian disease . . . 136
      III Viruses associated with reptilian tumours . . . 142
      IV Viruses non-pathogenic for reptiles, in which reptiles may play a reservoir role . . . 152
      V Viruses restricted to reptiles, of unknown disease-producing potential . . . 156
      VI Summary . . . 160
        References . . . 161

6 Bacteria
    J.E. COOPER
      I Introduction . . . 165
      II Normal flora . . . 165
      III Pathogenicity . . . 167
      IV Types of bacterial disease . . . 170
      V Zoonoses . . . 187
        References . . . 188

7 Fungi and Actinomycetes
    P.K.C. AUSTWICK AND I.F. KEYMER
      I Introduction . . . 193
      II Historical . . . 194
      III Mycotic infections . . . 195
      IV Pathogenesis and pathogenicity . . . 203
      V Experimental fungal infection . . . 206
      VI Environmental aspects . . . 207
      VII Discussion . . . 209
        References . . . 228

8 Protozoa
    I.F. KEYMER
      I Subphylum Sarcomastigophora . . . 235
      II Subphylum Sporozoa . . . 254
      III Subphylum Cnidospora . . . 279
      IV Subphylum Ciliophora . . . 283

V Protozoa of doubtful taxonomic position and pathological significance . . . 284
Acknowledgements . . . 285
References . . . 286

9 Endoparasites
   W. FRANK
   I Introduction . . . 291
   II Main sites for parasites in reptiles . . . 293
   III Zoonoses . . . 294
   IV–V Groups of endoparasites . . . 295–350
      IV Phylum Parenchymia . . . 295
      V Phylum Arthropoda . . . 341
         References . . . 350

10 Ectoparasites
   W. FRANK
   I Phylum Parenchymia (Parenchymatic worms) . . . 359
   II Phylum Annelida . . . 360
   III Phylum Arthropoda . . . 362
      References . . . 379

Index . . . i–xxxii

Contents of Volume 2

Non-infectious Diseases

Traumatic and Physical Diseases by Fredric L. Frye
Nutritional Diseases by O.F. Jackson and J.E. Cooper
Neoplastic Diseases by Elliott R. Jacobson
Congenital and Developmental Diseases by A.d'A. Bellairs
Miscellaneous Diseases by J.E. Cooper and O.F. Jackson

Clinical Aspects

Diagnosis and Treatment by O.F. Jackson
Anaesthesia and Surgery by O.F. Jackson and J.E. Cooper
Drugs and Doses by P.E. Holt
Index

Background

1 Introduction

J. E. COOPER

Royal College of Surgeons of England, Lincoln's Inn Fields, London, England.

O. F. JACKSON

Royal Free Hospital School of Medicine, Pond Street, London, England

> The serpent that tempted Eve may be saved, but not Faustus
> Christopher Marlowe, *Dr Faustus*

There are approximately 6000 species of reptile alive today. These poikilothermic vertebrates trace their ancestry back to the Upper Palaeozoic when they evolved from semi-aquatic amphibians. By the end of the Pennsylvanian era there were at least two distinct phylogenetic lines of reptiles; the Pelycosauria, the stem line for the mammals, and the Captorhinomorpha which gave rise to the other reptile groups, and eventually the birds.

The Mesozoic was dominated by 17 orders of reptiles (Romer, 1966) and has been termed "The Age of Reptiles". Their predominance came to an abrupt end about 65 million years ago with the puzzling extinction of all but a few of the major reptilian groups (Carroll, 1969). Today only four orders survive: the Squamata (lizards, amphisbaenids and snakes: 5400 species), Testudines* or Chelonia (tortoises, terrapins and turtles: 219 species), Crocodilia (crocodiles and alligators: 21 species) and Rhynchocephalia (the tuatara, *Sphenodon punctatus*: one species). Of these, only one—the order Squamata—could reasonably be described as progressive and successful at the present time.

---

* referred to as "chelonians" in this book

Reptiles occupy a key role in vertebrate evolution. The primitive reptiles probably differed from their amphibian ancestors in the type of egg produced; in the former it was amniotic, with a tough protective shell, and consisted of an embryo surrounded by embryonic membranes, while amphibian eggs lacked such membranes and were anamniotic. As a result the reptilian egg was more resistant to desiccation and could be laid on land—an important evolutionary step. This, coupled with a keratinized epidermis, strong supportive limbs and probably the development of water insoluble urates as the primary nitrogenous waste product, permitted reptiles relative independence from an aquatic environment.

These and other features of the Reptilia are discussed in some detail in Chapter 2. Although this book is concerned primarily with *diseases* of reptiles, it is important to have an understanding of the anatomy and physiology of the animals in question. Such features as ectothermy radically influence the host–parasite relationship and any attempt at disease diagnosis, treatment or prevention must take them into account.

In this book the terms "ectothermic" and "endothermic" are used in preference to "poikilothermic" and "homoiothermic" ("homeothermic") when matters relating to body temperature regulation are being discussed. As explained in Chapter 2, reptiles are able to exercise some control over their body temperature, but by exploiting external sources of heat rather than their own metabolism. They are thus better termed "ectothermic" (Gk. "external heat") rather than "poikilothermic" (Gk. "variable heat") in this context.

Although professional interest in reptilian diseases and pathology is a relatively recent trend, they appear to have played a part in the life of the order from the earliest times. For example, there has long been interest in pathological lesions found in reptilian fossils, particularly skeletal diseases of dinosaurs (Moodie, 1929). Although these were primarily traumatic in origin (Fig. 1.1), inflammatory and neoplastic lesions have also been diagnosed, and it has been postulated (Campbell, 1966) that viral infections may also have been involved. Although, for obvious reasons, our knowledge of diseases of extinct reptiles must be almost entirely confined to conditions that affected the skeleton, it has been suggested that, amongst other factors, infectious diseases might have played a part in the disappearance of the dinosaurs (Cloudsley-Thompson and Butt, 1977).

An interest in, and knowledge of, diseases of a group or species of animal usually result from a close relationship between those animals and man. In the case of reptiles, the relationship is an incongruous

1   INTRODUCTION   5

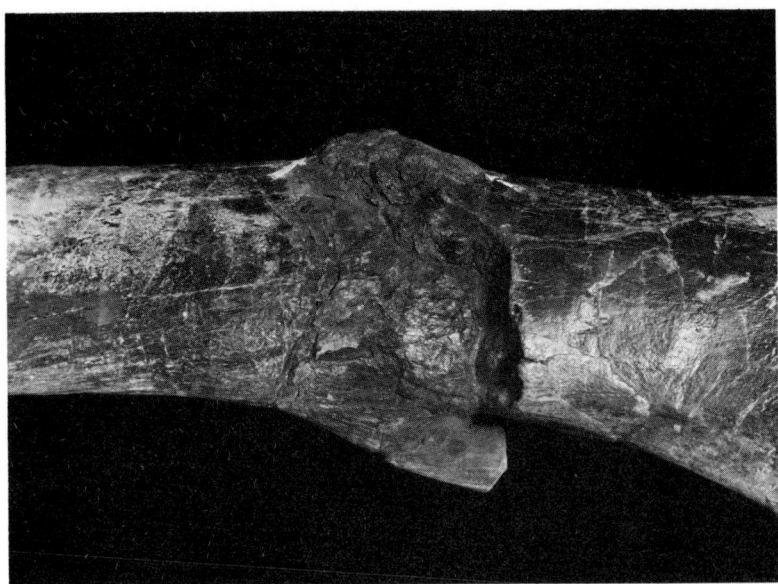

Fig. 1.1. Part of the ischium of an *Iguanodon*, showing a healed fracture (courtesy of British Museum (Natural History)).

one. Reptiles feature extensively in early writings, for example, in the Bible (Leonard and Glenn, 1974), but the link with man in this and other religious texts is usually one of hate or suspicion. The nefarious role of the serpent in the Garden of Eden did much to ensure that man's relations with reptiles (and snakes in particular) would for a long time be largely based on hostility. Nevertheless, as has been pointed out by a number of authors (Elkan, 1977; Morris and Morris, 1965), reptiles have featured in the art, architecture and culture of many races.

Insofar as disease of reptiles is concerned, interest was probably only aroused once man began to carry out scientific experiments on living animals. Although the amphibians, particularly frogs, were mainly used in such work, reptiles also played a part. A spurt of interest also followed the extensive exhibition of reptiles in zoological collections, since the owners of these establishments quickly found that reptiles were no less likely to fall foul to disease than the rest of their charges. There was also some work on reptiles by pioneers of comparative anatomy and pathology; for example, John Hunter described lesions in chameleons and other reptiles (Proger, 1972). Nevertheless, there remained for a long time a tendency for scientists to concentrate upon mammalian and avian diseases and, as a result, study of reptilian pathology lagged sadly behind other disciplines. This situation continues; reptiles have been neglected, particularly in comparison with fish—where, in recent years, there have been great advances in our understanding of disease processes. The reason for this is obvious; both mammals and birds include domesticated species which are of great economic importance. In the case of fish, these too are important sources of food and, in addition, far more fish (often of considerable value) are kept in captivity. Even amphibians have, in many ways, fared better than reptiles, largely because of their use in physiological research and diagnostic tests, e.g. for pregnancy.

What, then, are the justifications for a volume devoted to diseases of reptiles? There are many. First (and possibly foremost), many of the world's species are threatened by habitat destruction and other factors. Disease may play a part and in this context it is worthy of note that very little work has been done on morbidity and mortality in the wild other than surveys of parasites and occasional reports of predation. Research is long overdue and might throw some light on the possible role of disease in free-living populations as well as providing data on potential reservoirs of diseases of man and other animals. For example, the part played by reptiles in the carriage of certain viral infections is discussed in Chapter 5; further work of that calibre is needed.

Because of the decline in numbers of reptiles in many parts of the world, coupled with legislation to prevent their capture and/or importation, those in captivity become more valuable and it is important that they should not die unnecessarily from disease. Great concern has been expressed over the mortality of reptiles in transit and soon after arrival in the importing country and it has been suggested that veterinary examination, including laboratory tests, should be performed on such animals (Honnegger, 1974). Subsequent attention to health is, of course, of importance. This is particularly so now that attempts are being made, often successfully, to breed certain species in captivity. Veterinarians are increasingly being approached for advice on such reptiles and, at present, have few data to which they can refer.

Reptiles are also kept in large numbers for scientific research. Here the maintenance of health is of great importance since diseases and injuries can quickly render scientific investigations useless. There is particular interest in the use of reptiles in biomedical research (Cooper, 1977), including studies on biochemistry and endocrinology (Coulson and Hernandez, 1971) and physiology (Dawson, 1971).

Under such circumstances it is vital to have background data on such parameters as haematology and microbiology; diseases in the stock can again prove disastrous. Reptiles have even played a part in space programmes (Gaidamakin *et al*, 1969): detailed examination of the tissues of these animals was carried out *post mortem*.

A third reason for work on diseases of reptiles is that some infectious conditions are zoonoses; that is, transmissible to man. The classical example is *Salmonella* but other conditions, including certain parasites, may also be a hazard (Cooper, 1973). As a result it is important to obtain information on the carriage of such organisms in both captive and free-living reptiles.

It is hoped that this book will help to provide accessible data on diseases of reptiles. The approach is multidisciplinary and such topics as anaesthesia and surgery are discussed as well as the more clearly defined groups of diseases. The whole field of reptilian disease is expanding rapidly and some probable developments are discussed in this book. It is, for example, likely that changes in disease patterns will be seen as a result of more intensive methods of management, while neoplasia may prove to be a feature of increased longevity. Reproductive disorders and developmental abnormalities are likely to be increasingly recognized as a result of captive breeding. On the other hand, the availability of captive-bred reptiles should help to ensure that animals of known health status are used in research work.

Experimental studies on diseases are particularly needed (Fowler, 1980); there is a dearth of such investigations in reptile work as compared with, for example, fish diseases. New methods of combating disease are likely to be pursued and, hopefully implemented; an example is vaccination against bacterial infections which could, potentially, be of immense value.

The reptiles are vertebrates of great historical and evolutionary importance. They have long fascinated man and are likely to continue to do so. Despite a considerable volume of work on their anatomy, physiology and, in recent years, ecology and ethology, there remains a paucity of data on their diseases and pathology. It is hoped that this book will go some way towards remedying this situation.

References

Campbell, J. G. (1966). *Jl. R. microsc. Soc.* **85**, 163–174.
Carroll, R. L. (1969). *In* "Biology of the Reptilia". (C. Gans, A. d'A. Bellairs and T. S. Parsons, eds), Vol. 1, pp. 1–44. Academic Press, New York and London.

Cloudsley-Thompson, J. L. and Butt, D. K. (1977). *Br. J. Herpet.* **5,** 641–647.
Cooper, J. E. (1973). *Br. J. Herpet.* **5,** 368–374.
Cooper, J. E. (1977). *Lab. Anim.* **11,** 119–123.
Coulson, R. A. and Hernandez, T. (1971). *J. Am. vet. med. Ass.* **159,** 1672–1677.
Dawson, W. R. (1971). *J. Am. vet. med. Ass.* **159,** 1653–1661.
Elkan, E. (1977). *Report of the Cotswold Herpetological Symposium,* 1977, 9–20.
Fowler, M. E. (1980). *In* "Reproductive Biology and Diseases of Captive Reptiles", (J. B. Murphy and J. T. Collins, eds), pp. 267–268. Society for the Study of Amphibians and Reptiles, Ohio.
Gaidamakin, N. A., Parfenov, G. P., Petrukhin, V. G., Antipov, V. V., Saksonov, P. P. and Smirnova A. V. (1969). Patho-morphological and histochemical changes in the organs of turtles on board the 'Zond-5' probe. Paper presented at the 18th IAF Conference, La Plata, Argentina (Translated by M. D. Friedman). Smithsonian Herpetological Information Services, 1970.
Honnegger, R. E. (1974). *Int. Zoo. Yb.* **14,** 47–52.
Leonard, P. M. and Glenn, J. L. (1974). *Utah Herpetologists' League Journal* **1,** 1–8.
Moodie, R. L. (1921). *Bull. geol. Soc. Am.* **32,** 321–326.
Morris, R. and Morris, D. (1965). "Men and Snakes". Hutchinson, London.
Proger, L. W. (1972). "Descriptive Catalogue of the Pathological Series in the Hunterian Museum of the Royal College of Surgeons of England". Part II. E. and S. Livingstone, Edinburgh and London.
Romer, A. S. (1966). "Vertebrate Paleontology" 3rd edition. University of Chicago Press, Chicago.

2 Anatomy and Physiology

P. M. C. DAVIES

Department of Zoology, University of Nottingham, Nottingham, England

Classification of Reptiles

The detailed classification of reptiles is still a matter of disagreement among taxonomists, but in this chapter only the major subdivisions of the group (on which there is wide agreement) need be listed. Further details of the scheme outlined below can be found in Bellairs (1969):

CLASS REPTILIA
   Subclass Anapsida
      Order Testudines (Chelonia) (tortoises, terrapins, turtles)
   Subclass Lepidosauria
      Order Rhynchocephalia (tuatara)
      Order Squamata (lizards and snakes)
   Subclass Archosauria
      Order Crocodilia (crocodiles, alligators, caimans and gharials)

I. Diagnostic Features

Unlike birds and mammals, which can be distinguished from all other vertebrates on the basis of a single visible attribute (feathers and fur respectively), no single external feature serves to distinguish the reptiles. Collectively, however, the following external and internal characteristics amount to a sufficient definition of the group as a whole, in the sense that they enable all its various members to be distinguished from other kinds of vertebrate: (i) reptiles are (primitively) terrestrial and four-legged, aquatic and limbless forms being secondary derivatives of primitively terrestrial and four-legged forms;

(ii) they are covered with horny scales; (iii) they produce amniote eggs or reproductive structures derived from them; (iv) they are "ectothermic" (poikilothermic) relying on external sources of heat for the purposes of body temperature regulation; (v) they possess an incompletely divided heart; (vi) they lack any kind of larval stage in their life-cycles. Diagnosis at subclass level within the Reptilia is based primarily on features of the cranial skeleton, in particular on the presence or absence of openings in the temporal region of the skull ("fenestration", Fig. 2.2 A–E) (see Romer, 1966; Bellairs, 1969; Romer and Parsons, 1977), though some writers have questioned the validity of this basis of classification (Halstead, 1969).

II. Integument

A. General

Compared with the soft, permeable skin of the amphibians, the reptilian integument is hard and impervious, designed to resist the dry, abrasive conditions of terrestrial life, though the degree of physical toughness and physiological impermeability actually attained by the skin varies considerably from group to group. Crocodilians, for example, have tougher exteriors than lizards, but their skins are considerably more permeable to water (Bentley and Schmidt-Nielsen, 1966). But even the most pervious reptile skin is usually considerably less so than that of an amphibian and no amphibian has acquired a skin with the physical toughness provided by the horny epidermal scales of reptiles.

But the reptilian integument is more than simply a protection against dehydration and physical abrasion. The skin of reptiles is an organ-system of considerable complexity with a variety of different functions, ranging from the physical (protection against abrasion and U-V radiation), through the physiological (control of water, gas and heat exchanges), to the behavioural (enhancement of anti-predator defence through cryptic or warning colouration, or of social communication through sexual or threat displays). These are all functions commonly associated with morphological elaborations of the integument into structures such as spines, crests, dewlaps, rattles, armour plating (Fig. 2.3), and less commonly (in reptiles) with the physiological capacity to change colour rapidly. This latter is a visually mediated neuro-endocrinologically controlled response largely confined to four families of lizard (Iguanidae, Agamidae, Chamaeleonidae and Gekkonidae). In addition, the skin functions as a sense organ, being well innervated and equipped in different species with a variety of sensory thickenings, tubercles, pits and bristles (see Section VI below).

B. Epidermis

In its general structure, the skin of reptiles is typically vertebrate, and consists of two main tissue layers: the outer epidermis, which is derived developmentally from the embryonic ectoderm and produces the characteristic surface scales, and the inner dermis, derived from the embryonic mesoderm, which nourishes and supports the epidermis and gives the skin its colour (Fig. 2.9F). However, in its detailed organization the reptilian integument can boast a number of unique features, as well as a considerable degree of within-group variation (Maderson, 1972). The epidermis, in particular, is variable between the different groups, and appears to be more complex in the squamate reptiles than in any other group of terrestrial vertebrates (Flaxman, 1972).

The squamate epidermis differs principally in four ways from that of other vertebrates (Maderson and Chiu, 1970; Flaxman, 1972): (i) at least six different cell types make up the epidermis; (ii) these cells are organized into distinct "epidermal generations" which are successively and periodically shed by the animal; (iii) the processes of cell proliferation and differentiation within the epidermis are synchronized over the entire body surface; and (iv) both types of keratin filament (α- and β-keratin), as distinguished by X-ray diffraction analysis (Rudall, 1947) and staining responses (Maderson, 1964, 1965), are found together within the epidermis, rather than separately at different epidermal locations of the body, as they are in crocodilians and chelonians. As the squamate epidermis has been studied more extensively than the epidermis of any other reptile group, only this sloughing cycle (ecdysis) will be discussed here.

C. Sloughing Cycle

Since the squamate sloughing cycle has been described and summarized by a number of authors (Bellairs, 1969; Maderson 1964, 1965) only an outline need be given here. Immediately after a slough, in the so-called "resting phase" of the cycle, three regions of the epidermis can be distinguished (Fig. 2.1A): (i) an outer, heavily keratinized, acellular zone forming the stratum corneum or "horny layer", in which α- and β-keratin filaments occupy distinct layers, with the latter external to the former and having a serrated outer margin, the *Oberhäutchen*; (ii) an inner, living zone composed of a single layer of cuboidal cells lying directly against the uppermost cells of the dermis and responsible for producing all the other cells of the epidermis in waves of synchronised and cyclical proliferative activity—this is the stratum germinativum; and (iii) an intermediate zone made up of the daughter cells of the stratum germinativum in varying stages of differentiation. In the resting phase, the cells in this zone are relatively little differentiated and few in number, and the outer and intermediate zones together form the "outer epidermal generation".

As the sloughing cycle enters the "renewal phase" (Fig. 2.1B) synchronized mitosis in the stratum germinativum produces successive waves of new daughter cells, which displace the "outer generation" and become progressively differentiated to form the new "inner epidermal generation" (Fig. 2.1C). This latter generation replaces the outer generation at the next slough, but until then both are present in the squamate epidermis, a fact which adds appreciably to its already considerable complexity when examined in section under the microscope (Fig. 2.1D). Sloughing eventually occurs when the two epidermal generations become physically separated by the enzyme-induced breakdown of the innermost cell layer of the outer generation (Fig. 2.1D) and diffusion of lymphatic fluid into the intervening space. Additional help appears to be given by vascular adjustments in the head which cause blood vessels and sinuses underlying the cranial

---

Fig. 2.1. Diagrammatic summary of the sloughing cycle of snakes, showing the sequence of epidermal changes referred to in the text and their correspondence with the six stages described by Maderson (1965). (A) Resting phase. This occurs immediately after the snake has sloughed. (B) Beginning of the renewal phase. Active proliferation by the sg forms a new pIEG, which causes a dulling of the animal's colouration and a slight cloudiness of the eye. (C) Later in the renewal phase. Skin colour very dull and eyes completely cloudy due to the elaboration of the sio. The IEG now well developed. (D) Conclusion of the renewal phase. Colouration brightens with the breakdown of the lto and the formation of a cleavage zone (CZ). The OEG is shed, and the resting phase (A) is resumed (Redrawn after Maderson, 1965).

Note. The prefix p and the suffixes i and o mean 'presumptive', 'belonging to the inner epidermal generation' and 'belonging to the outer epidermal generation' respectively. The legend below excludes these prefixes and suffixes.

A, α-keratin layer; β, β-keratin layer; cl, clear layer of the si; CZ, cleavage zone; IEG, inner epidermal generation; ilc, innermost living cells; iz, intermediate zone (not precisely equivalent to the si); lt, lacunar tissue of the si; Ob, Oberhäutchen; OEG, outer epidermal generation; sc, stratum corneum; sg, stratum germinativum; si, stratum intermedium.

epidermis to swell and so fracture the cleavage plane between the two epidermal generations. As this cleavage process occurs more or less simultaneously over the whole body in squamates, the skin is shed in relatively large—or, in the case of healthy snakes, entire—pieces, in contrast to the piecemeal and unco-ordinated shedding of skin fragments which occurs in the crocodilians and chelonians, in which

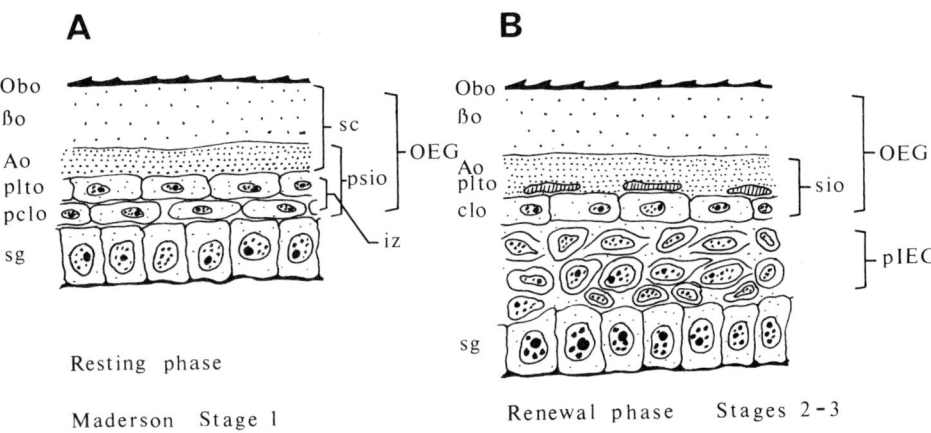

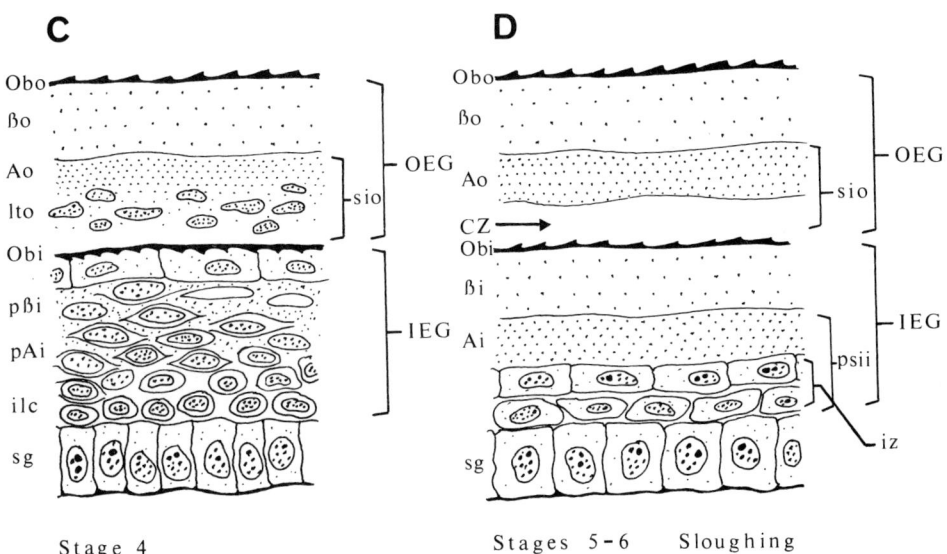

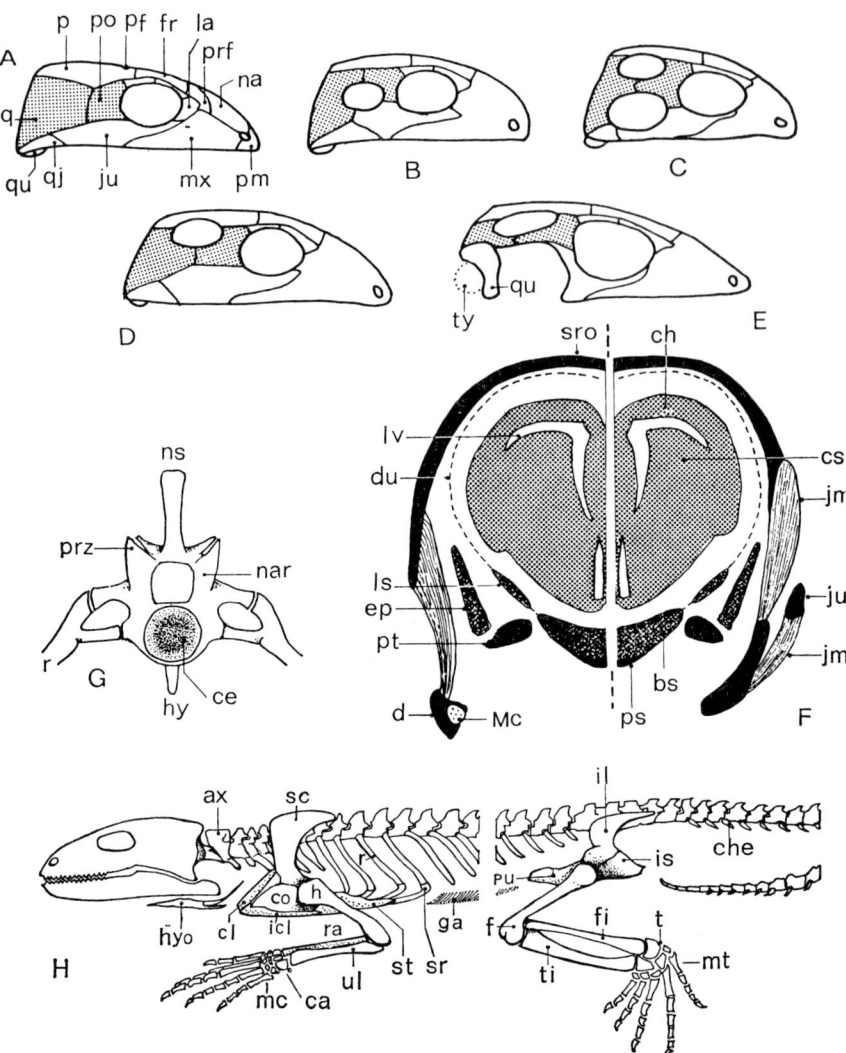

Fig. 2.2. (A–E) Diagrams showing the bones of the temporal region of various reptilian skulls, living and extinct. A, anapsid; B, synapsid; C, diapsid; D, euryapsid; E, modified diapsid (lizard). (F) Transverse section through temporal region of skull showing anapsid condition on left, synapsid on right. Dermal bones shown in black, cartilage in dark stipple. (G) Anterior thoracic vertebra of crocodile with part of a two-headed rib, seen from in front. (H) Skeleton of a 'typical' reptile. Parts of the mid-body and tail regions are missing. (From Bellairs and Attridge, "Reptiles")

ax, axis; bs, basisphenoid; c, canal for spinal cord; ca, carpals; ce, centrum of procoelous vertebra (hollowed in front); ch, cerebral hemisphere; che, chevron; cl,

keratinization and proliferation are continuous rather than cyclical processes. Indeed, shedding in these groups tends to be restricted to the more flexible parts of the integument, such as around the neck and limb joints. Elsewhere on the body, particularly under and around the larger scales, keratin is retained to produce the familiar concentric growth rings of the chelonian integument and the prominent scutes of crocodilians. In certain chelonians, notably the soft-shelled turtles and the leathery turtle (Fig. 2.3A), horny scales are completely absent and the epidermis is uniform and "leathery".

D. Dermis

The dermal-epidermal boundary is marked by the basement membrane of the epidermis. Generally thicker than the epidermis, the dermis consists largely of connective tissue interlaced with collagen fibres, blood and lymphatic vessels, smooth muscle fibres, nerves forming dermal plexuses from which sensory extensions penetrate the epidermis, numerous chromatophores and, in certain lizards, all crocodiles and chelonians, a variety of bony structures forming the 'dermal skeleton' (see later). In contrast to the amphibians, reptiles possess very little in the way of skin glands, the most notable exceptions being the musk glands of crocodiles, the femoral glands of certain lizards and the dorsonuchal glands of some snakes, all of which appear to have a chemosensory function in inter- or intraspecific recognition.

III. Musculo—Skeletal System

Few structures are as revealing on the subject of vertebrate evolution as the skeleton. The reasons for its usefulness in this regard are threefold: bones make better fossils than other parts of the body;

---

clavicle; co, coracoid; cs, corpus striatum; d, dentary; du, dura mater; ep, epipterygoid; f, femur; fi, fibula; fr, frontal; ga, gastralia (abdominal ribs); h, humerus; hy, hypapophysis; hyo, hyoid; icl, interclavicle; il, ilium; is, ischium; im, jaw muscles; ju, jugal; la, lachrymal; ls, laterosphenoid; lv, lateral ventricle of brain; mc, metarcarpal; Mc, Meckel's cartilage; mt, metatarsal; mx, maxilla; na, nasal; nar, neural arch; ns, neural spine; p, parietal; pf, pineal foramen; pm, premaxilla; po, postorbital; prf, prefrontal; prz, pre-zygapophysis; ps, parasphenoid; pt, pterygoid; pu, pubis; qj, quadratojugal; qu, quadrate; r, rib (dorsal segment); ra, radius; sc, scapula; sq, squamosal; sr, sternal rib; sro, skull roof; st, sternum; t, tarsals; ti, tibia; ty, tympanic membrane; ul, ulna.

skeletal organization and adaptive behaviour (e.g. style of locomotion) are functionally inter-dependent, making the former a good predictor of the latter and thus a useful guide to the diversity (past and present) of vertebrate life; skeletal elements (as distinct from skeletal organization and overall design) have changed relatively little during the course of vertebrate evolution, with the result that homologous skeletal units can be readily identified in different groups and used to delineate phylogenetic relationships. Nowhere have these attributes of the vertebrate skeleton been used to greater effect in the analysis of evolutionary histories than in the case of reptiles, and recent efforts to reassess something as elusive as the physiology of extinct reptiles on the basis of largely anatomical evidence (e.g. Bakker, 1971, 1972) reveal just how subtle and potentially illuminating skeletal data can be. The nature and evolution of reptilian bone were discussed by Enlow (1969).

For our present purposes, it is possible to reduce the impressive morphological diversity of living reptiles to basically three patterns of anatomical design (Bellairs, 1969): the "newt-like" pattern of "typical" reptiles, as exemplified by most lizards, the tuatara and crocodilians; the limbless pattern exhibited by some lizards and all snakes; and the "squat pancake" pattern of the chelonians. Some aspects of the skeletal organization of a "typical" reptile are shown in Fig. 2.2H, and of a chelonian in Fig. 2.3. The "typical" pattern will be the basis of the summary which follows. Fuller accounts of reptilian functional anatomy will be found in a range of standard and popular texts on the subject (e.g. Romer, 1956; Bellairs, 1969; Porter, 1972;

Fig. 2.3. Chelonians: (A) leathery turtle (*Dermochelys*); (B) matamata (*Chelys*); (C) mating of tortoises (*Gopherus*); (D) courtship of red-eared terrapin (*Pseudemys scripta elegans*); (E) diagrammatic cross section of chelonian through hind-limb pocket. The rib, shown slightly separated from bony plates, is in fact fused to them; (F) diagrammatic longitudinal section through chelonian; (G) skull of green turtle (*Chelonia*); (H) bony shell and parts of skeleton of terrapin (*Emys*). The plastron is seen from above and the extremities are not shown. (From Bellairs and Attridge, "Reptiles")

asc, acromion process of scapula; bc, body cavity; bm, back muscles; br, bridge (cut) joining carapace with plastron; co, coracoid; em, emargination of skull roof; f, femur; fr, frontal; h, humerus; il, ilium; is, ischium; ju, jugal; lu, lung; mx, maxilla; obm, oblique abdominal muscle; p, parietal; pla, plastron; pm, premaxilla; pp, postorbital; prf, prefrontal; pu, pubis; qj quadratojugal; qu, quadrate (forms a kind of otic notch); r, rib; sc, scapula; sq, squamosal; trm, transverse abdominal muscle. Epidermal scutes or laminae (in black): c, centrals; l, laterals; ma, marginals. Bony plates: e, entoplastron; epl, epiplastron; hyo, hyoplastron; hyp, hypoplastron; ne, neurals; nu, nuchal (proneural); pe, peripherals; pl, pleurals; xp, xiphiplastron.

2 ANATOMY AND PHYSIOLOGY 17

Bellairs and Attridge, 1975; Webb *et al*, 1978) as well as in general texts of comparative vertebrate anatomy (e.g. Baer, 1964; Romer and Parsons, 1977).

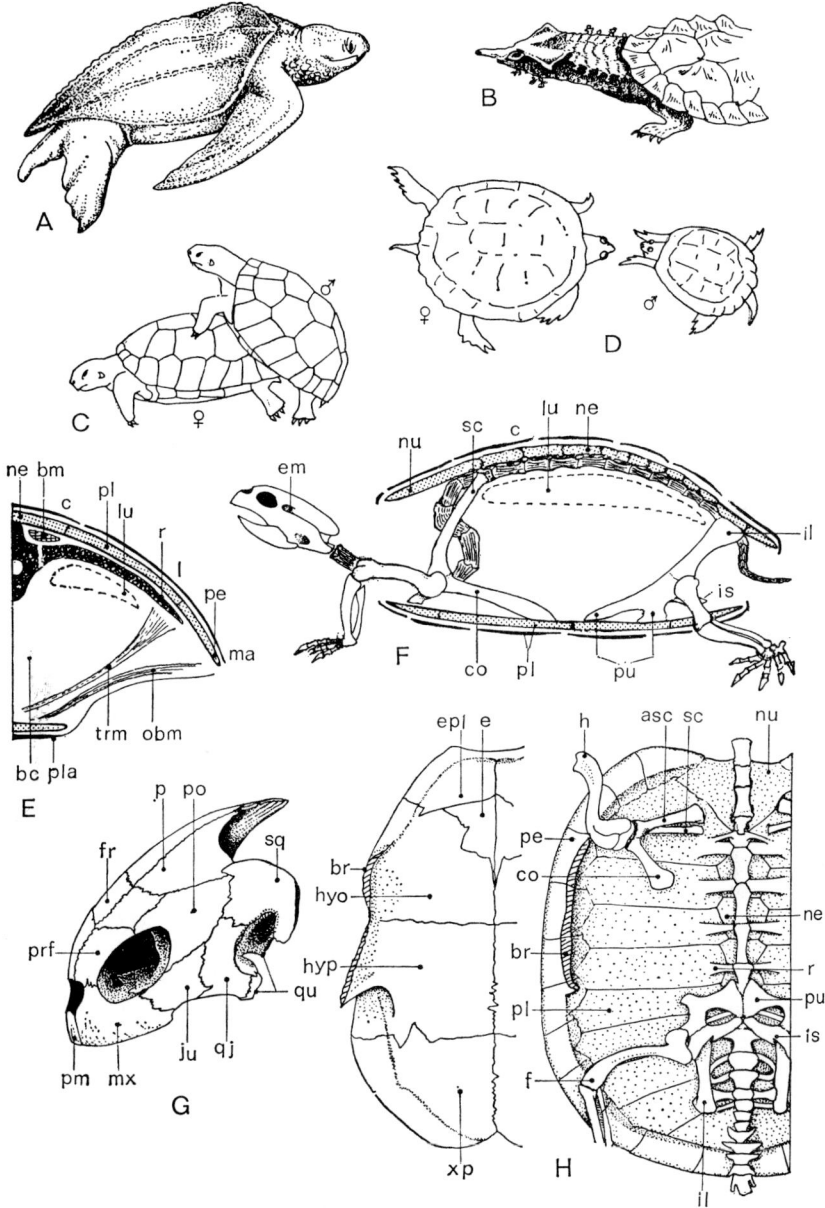

A. Axial Skeleton

There are many ways in which the vertebrate skeletal system can be subdivided for analytical purposes, the most convenient in the present context being that which distinguishes between the "axial" and "appendicular" skeletons. The axial skeleton is made up of the vertebral column, ribs and cranium; the appendicular skeleton of the limbs and girdles.

Vertebral column Individual reptilian vertebrae are not unlike other vertebrae in most basic respects (Fig. 2.2G) though the subdivision of the vertebral column into five distinct regions only one of which bears ribs is not strictly possible, since any of the regions, from cervical to caudal, may bear ribs. Nevertheless some regional differentiation within the vertebral column does occur in reptiles, and even approaches mammalian levels in the crocodilians. It is least well defined in the snakes, where the only unequivocal differentiation is that between caudal and "pre-caudal" vertebrae (Hoffstetter and Gasc, 1969).

Inter-vertebral articulation occurs at three points in most reptiles—between the faces of adjacent centra, which are mostly procoelous, and between pairs of zygopophyses. However, in snakes and a few lizards, an additional pair of articulations occurs between zygosphenes (anteriorly projecting processes of the neural arch) and zygantra, recesses on the back of the preceding neural arch which receive the zygosphenes. These extra articulations serve to prevent inter-vertebral rotation about the longitudinal axis of the vertebral column. In the tortoises and turtles, no articulation occurs at all between the majority of trunk vertebrae because the vertebral column in the trunk region and the ribs, are fused to the bones of the dermal carapace (Fig. 2.3F, H).

The chelonian "shell" illustrates very well the important distinction in vertebrates between the "dermal skeleton" (composed of dermal or "membrane" bone, which is usually not preformed in cartilage), and the "endoskeleton", composed of bone and cartilage, the former always preformed in the latter (hence "replacement bone"). In most terrestrial vertebrates, dermal bones are retained only in the construction of the cranium and shoulder, but in some (e.g. the chelonians) the dermal body armour so characteristic of ancient fishes has also been retained.

The chelonian shell (Fig. 2.3F) consists of two main components, the dome-shaped carapace, and the ventral plastron, both of which have the same basic composition: an outer covering of keratinized scales or scutes derived from the epidermis (see earlier), and an inner layer of bony plates produced in the dermis. The trunk region of the vertebral column is fused to the inner surface of the carapace. The cervical vertebrae of tortoises and turtles, in contrast to the rigid trunk vertebrae, are very loosely articulated with one another allowing the neck-bending necessary when the head is withdrawn into the shell.

With the exception of a few burrowing forms, reptiles have well developed tails, and the caudal vertebrae show a number of structural modifications associated with different functions. Small intervertebral chevron bones extending from the underside of the caudal vertebral column (Fig. 2.2H) are greatly extended in some aquatic reptiles to produce support for the flattened, paddle-like tails which provide them with their locomotive power. The same is true of the neural spines of the caudal vertebrae in these animals. In the tuatara, many lizards and possibly a very few snakes (Wilson, 1968), a variable number of caudal vertebrae, starting usually at about the fifth caudal vertebra in lizards, possess an unossified fracture-plane or septum in the mid-region of the centrum which enables these animals to shed their tails (autotomy) as a defence against predators. The wound quickly heals, and eventually (in most species) a new, though morphologically less perfect tail develops; precisely how the open wound so effectively resists infection remains an intriguing and as yet unresolved question.

Ribs Most pre-caudal vertebrae have ribs of one kind or another in typical reptiles, the exceptions being the atlas and axis, which only bear ribs in the crocodilians and some snakes. Vertebrae in the neck region have ribs, but these do not connect with the sternum. The longer, anterior trunk ribs have cartilaginous extremities ("sternal ribs"—Fig. 2.2H) by which they connect (except in the snakes many lizards, amphisbaenids and chelonians) with the mostly cartilaginous sternum. Snakes and chelonians have no sternum. Another set of cartilaginous "ribs"—the so-called abdominal or parasternal ribs ("gastralia")— may be embedded in the abdominal musculature of some lizards behind the sternum (Fig. 2.2H), uniting in many cases to form a mid-ventral series of "chevrons" connected by ligaments to the ends of the posterior truncal ribs. Despite the use by some authors' of the same name, these structures do not correspond to the bony, dermal "gastralia" of crocodilians (Bellairs, 1969). Snake ribs are generally robust and lacking in cartilaginous segments, and are attached at their distal ends to the ventral scales.

Apart from the limbless forms, most living reptiles have two sacral vertebrae the ribs of which have become fused to form prominent, wing-like processes which are attached to the ilium, thus providing the pelvis with additional support and stability.

Cranium The cranial skeleton is highly complex and variable (Figs. 2.3G and 2.4), for which reason a detailed description of it is beyond the scope of this review. For analytical purposes, it is useful to consider the skull as consisting of two incomplete shells (Fig. 2.2F), one inside the other, and each having a distinct evolutionary and ontogenetic history. The outer shell consists of dermal bones (Fig. 2.4A) forming a protective framework for the skull, and openings (or the lack of them) in the temporal region of this shell have long been important in the classification of reptiles (Fig. 2.2A–E). Most of the bones of the upper and lower jaws are also dermal in origin (Fig. 2.2F). The inner shell consists of a mixture of cartilage and replacement bone which arises developmentally by the partial ossification of the embryonic chondrocranium and, to varying degrees, encloses the

---

Fig. 2.4. (A) Skull of skink, *Mabuya carinata*. Cartilaginous regions shown in machine stipple. (B) Diagram showing cranial kinesis in lizard. Directions of movement of upper and lower jaws shown by arrows. The fixed occipital segment is shown in cross-hatching and the cartilaginous parts of the skull are stippled. The numbers 1–4 indicate the positions of the main kinetic joints; at 3 a cartilaginous peg from the supra-occipital projects into the back of the parietal in the midline. (C) Skull of the viper, *Cerastes aegyptiacus*. Arrows show direction of movement of jaw bones during fang erection. (D) Ventral view of the skull (less mandible) of *Python sebae* showing a few of the numerous jaw muscles, mainly on left. (E) Skull of *Amphisbaena manni*, showing extra-stapes. (F, G, H) Transvere sections through skull at mid-eye level in lizard (F), burrowing lizard (G) and snake (H). (I) Egg tooth (et) of *Natrix natrix* attached to premaxilla, from left. (J) Pleurodont tooth of the adult herbivorous marine iguana (*Amblyrhynchus*) from inner side. (From Bellairs and Attridge, "Reptiles")

ang. angular; ar, articular; b, brain; bo, basioccipital; bp, basipterygoid process of basisphenoid; cor, coronoid; d, dentary; ec, ectopterygoid; ep, epipterygoid; est, extra-stapes (= extra-columella); f, fang; fr, frontal; ios, interorbital septum (calcified region shown in darker stipple in A); ju, jugal; la, lacrimal; lp, levator pterygoidei muscle (cut); mx, maxilla; na, nasal; oj, opening for duct of Jacobson's organ; os, orbitosphenoid; p, parietal; pa, palatine; pg, pterygoideus muscle; pga, accessory pg; pm, premaxilla; po, postorbital; pp, protractor pterygoidei muscle; pr, prootic; prf, prefrontal; ps, parasphenoid; pt, pterygoid; ptf, postfrontal; qu, quadrate; rp, retractor pterygoidei muscle; rv, retractor vomeris muscle; s, basisphenoid; san, surangular; smx, septomaxilla; so, supraoccipital; sq, squamosal; st, stapes (= columella auris); ste, supratemporal; stf, superior temporal fenestra; tr, trabecula; vo, vomer:.

2 ANATOMY AND PHYSIOLOGY

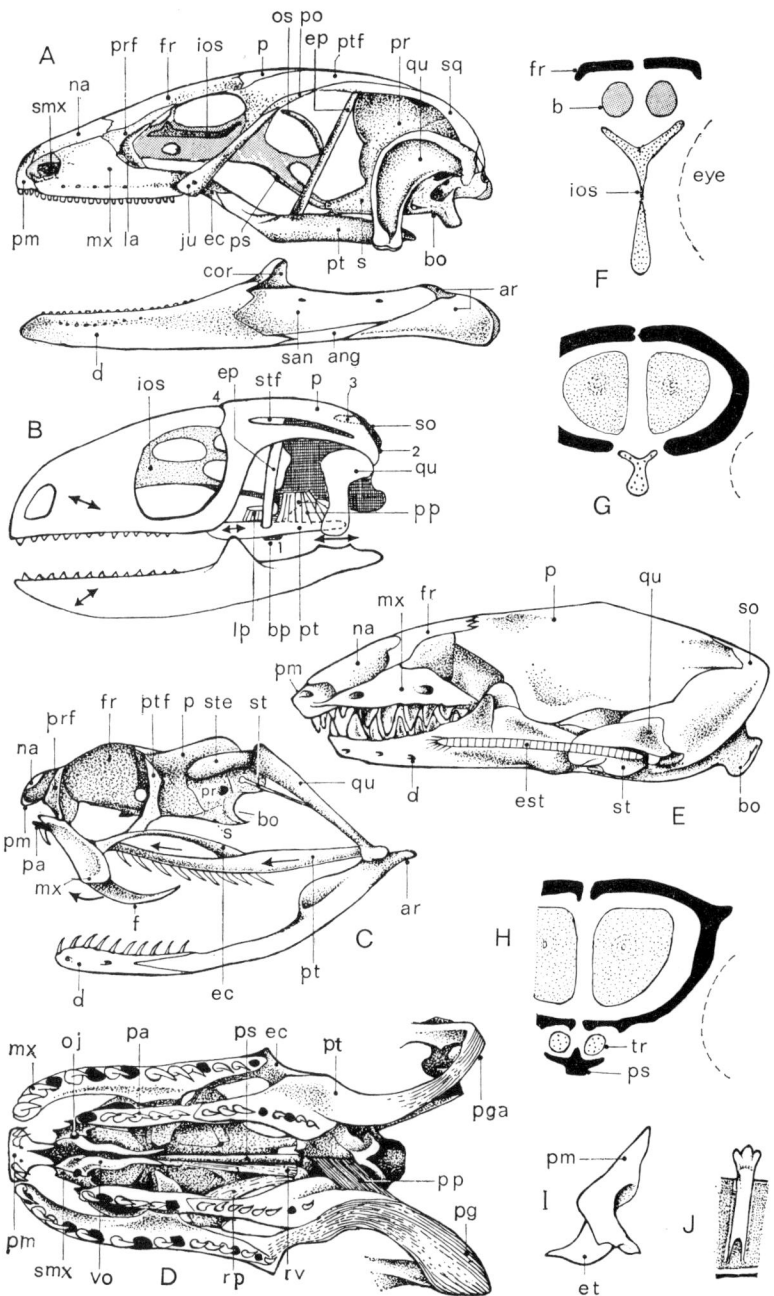

brain. At the rear of the braincase, just below the foramen magnum, is the single occipital condyle characteristic of reptiles, by means of which the skull articulates with the vertebral column.

The skulls of chelonians and crocodilians are solid and inflexible structures, with the bones of the upper jaw firmly welded to the remainder of the cranium (Fig. 2.3G). But in the squamates, the skull is more lightly and flexibly constructed, and a much greater mobility of the upper jaw relative to the cranium ('cranial kinesis') is achieved by the development of a number of kinetic joints in the skull, the precise number varying from species to species (Fig. 2.4B). Associated with this "loosening" of the cranium in most squamates is the phenomenon of streptostyly, the freeing of the quadrate bone from its primitive attachments to adjacent bones in the skull so that it becomes more mobile in its mechanical relationship with the pterygoid and the lower jaw (Figs. 2.2E, 2.4A–C). These trends go furthest in the snakes, where kinesis is accentuated by the reduction of most of the bones of the upper jaw to simple, tooth-bearing rods (Fig. 2.4C, D) and highly mobile quadrates are elongated to permit an enormous mandibular gape. The result is a remarkably versatile and efficient prey-handling and ingestive mechanism (Gans, 1961; Boltt and Ewer, 1964; Frazzetta, 1966; Bellairs, 1969; Kardong, 1974). The muscles which control the operation of this mechanism are predictably complex, and have been described in detail (Haas, 1973).

Primitively, reptilian teeth are simple and peg-like, showing little evidence of any significant functional differentiation along tooth rows (Fig. 2.8A). However, differentiation is found in many modern forms associated with dietary or feeding specializations, the most extreme examples being the various kinds of venom fang which have evolved in some snakes and one genus of lizards (Fig. 2.4C) (Edmund, 1969). Many kinds of tooth attachment are found in reptiles, the three most important being (i) the primitive pleurodont condition, common in lizards, in which the tooth is attached to the inner side of the jaw element (Fig. 2.4J); (ii) the acrodont condition, in which the tooth is fused to the summit of the bony element (e.g. *Sphenodon*); and (iii) the thecodont condition, in which the tooth is set in a socket (e.g. crocodilians). Most reptiles shed and replace their teeth throughout life (Edmund, 1969; Bellairs and Attridge, 1975), and do so in orderly and often very complicated sequences (Osborn, 1973), so as to ensure that the jaw always has a full complement of functional teeth. This process of replacement appears to be suppressed in most acrodont reptiles (Edmund, 1969). Turtles lack teeth, and reduce their prey with a horny beak. In certain snakes specialized for egg-eating (e.g.

Dasypeltis, Elachistodon and certain species of *Elaphe*) the eggs are broken in the throat by ventral extensions of the cervical vertebrae (hypapophyses) (Gans, 1974). In the case of *Dasypeltis*, the crumpled shells are then regurgitated.

B. Appendicular Skeleton

The main features of the limbs and girdles of a generalized reptile are shown in Fig. 2.2H and of a chelonian in Fig. 2.3F. In most basic respects, both sets show the standard tetrapod pattern of construction, though adaptive radiation within the reptiles has led to a considerable amount of variation in the detailed morphology as different life-styles and modes of locomotion have been adopted. Typical reptiles are quadrupedal, have pentadactyl limbs extended laterally (rather than under the body), and normally move with their bodies close to the ground. The hind limbs are generally longer than the fore-limbs, except in the sea turtles, where the reverse is true. Limb reduction and loss has occurred independently in many squamate groups, most notably among the ancestors of the snakes. Nearly all modern snakes are totally limbless, though pelvic rudiments are to be found in a number of primitive forms. Limb reduction in lizards, ranging from changes in relative limb size to total loss, is confined to six groups—the Scincidae, Anguidae, Teiidae, Cordylidae, Pygopodidae and Amphisbaenidae—and has usually occurred as an adaptation to burrowing.

C. Muscles and Locomotion

The evolution of morphological and locomotor diversity within the Reptilia has been accompanied by a corresponding diversity of musculo-skeletal arrangements, both in connection with bodily movement and in connection with lung ventilation (see Section IV). The undulating movements of locomotion are brought about by columns of longitudinal muscle which clothe the vertebral column and fill the spaces between neural spines and transverse processes, and between transverse processes and centra. Movements of the fore- and hind-limbs are controlled by a complex series of extensor and flexor muscles connecting limb bones, girdles and body wall. Variations on this theme are numerous, both within and among species, but the basic pattern is essentially the same in all four-legged reptiles, though some groups (e.g. the chelonians) suffer more severe physical limitations than others when they are moving. The limbless reptiles have departed most fundamentally from the reptilian pattern.

Snakes are undulators *par excellence*, so not surprisingly their vertebral musculature has become extremely complicated and specialized (Gasc, 1976) and permits a greater variety of movements and contortions than is found in any other terrestrial vertebrate. The mechanics of the snake's sinuous style of locomotion have been analyzed in great detail by a number of workers (see summaries in Gray, 1968 and Gans, 1974). Four styles of locomotion are commonly differentiated in snakes—undulatory, concertina (moving through a narrow tube), rectilinear (straight creeping) and sidewinding—and most snakes can employ any but rectilinear movement if occasion demands it. Rectilinear movement appears to be an accomplishment only of stout-bodied snakes, in particular boas and pythons and a few of the larger viperids.

IV. Visceral Organization and Homeostasis

The arrangements of the main internal organs of three representative reptiles are shown in Figs. 2.5, 2.6 and 2.7. Reptiles lack a true diaphragm, so that the heart and lungs are never completely separated from the abdominal organs, though in chelonians and some lizards folds of the peritoneal lining of the body cavity separate them to some extent. In crocodilians, an unusual form of diaphragm, not homologous with that of higher vertebrates, separates the heart and lungs from the remaining abdominal organs. The main effects on visceral organization of body elongation in the evolution of the snakes (and, to a lesser extent, in the limbless lizards) have been the displacement of paired, symmetrically located organs into asymmet-

---

Fig. 2.5. Viscera. (A) Contents of body cavity (ventral view) of female lizard (*Lacerta*). The viscera are shown turned over to the right side of the lizard and the cloaca is cut open. The oviduct is shown on one side only. (B) Urinogenital system of male adder (*Vipera berus*), ventral view. (C–F) Lungs of *Sphenodon* (C); *Chamaeleo* (D), showing air sacs; loggerhead turtle, *Caretta* (E); monitor lizard, *Varanus* (F), showing saccular region at caudal extremity of lung. C, E and F are diagrammatic sections of the lung, connective tissue being shown in black. (From Bellairs and Attridge, "Reptiles")

adr, adrenal; bl, bladder; br, bronchus; cae, caecum; cop, coprodaeum; dao, dorsal aorta; duo, duodenum; epd, epididymis; fb, fat body; hp, hemipenis; k, kidney; lin, large intestine; liv, liver; ov, ovary; ovd, oviduct and its opening; ovdf, oviduct funnel; pro, proctodaeum; pvc, posterior vena cava; spl, spleen; sto, stomach; tm, thigh muscles (cut); tr, trachea; ugp, urogenital papilla; ur, ureter and its opening; uro, urodaeum.

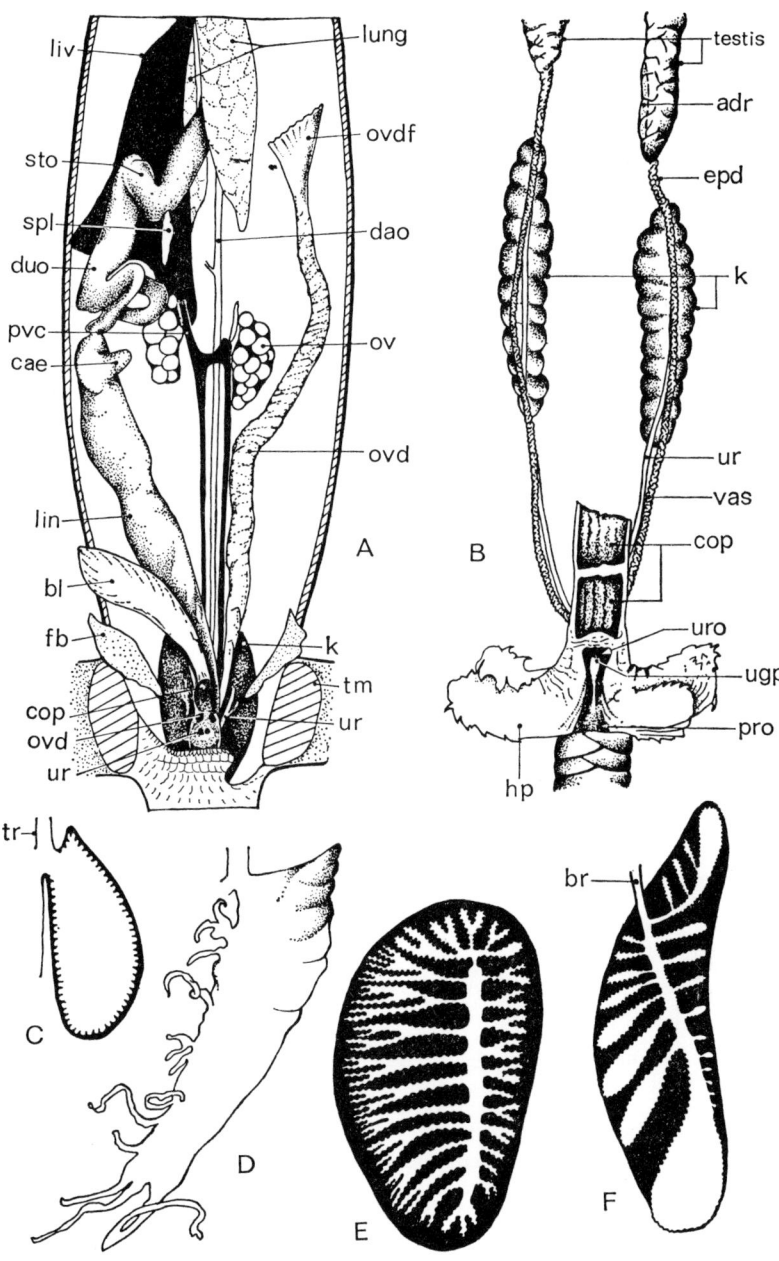

rical arrangements, and the reduction of coiling in the intestine. Both groups of limbless reptiles, with the exception of the amphisbaenians, have suffered a reduction of the left lung, which, in the majority of snakes, has become rudimentary. The right lung, however, tends to be unusually long. The distribution of organs within the body cavity of snakes is remarkably constant in a given species relative to the ventral scales, with the result that the location of particular organs can be predicted quite easily from scale counts (Bragdon, 1953; see also many anatomical studies by Bergman (e.g. 1961)).

A. Gastro-intestinal Tract

Comparatively little is known about the alimentary tract and digestive physiology of reptiles. A number of recent reviews provide a very useful summary of current knowledge of the reptilian digestive system, in particular of the gross interior morphology (Parsons and Cameron, 1977), histology (Luppa, 1977) and physiology (Skoczylas, 1979) of the digestive tract, the biochemistry of digestion (Dandifrosse, 1974), and the pharmacology of reptile venoms (Russell and Brodie, 1974). Anatomically, the reptilian alimentary tract is simple in comparison with that of higher vertebrates (Guibé, 1970).

Buccal cavity Food entering the mouth is subjected to very little mechanical or physiological treatment prior to swallowing, beyond orientation and, in some reptiles, a little preliminary chewing, for which reason salivary gland secretions (with the exception of venoms) are thought to have little if any digestive significance in reptiles, their role being largely lubricatory. Proteolytic activity has been detected in the saliva of the European grass snake, *Natrix natrix* (Skoczylas, 1970a), but only at very low levels, in contrast to that in the venom of

Fig. 2.6. Viscera. Dissection of male *Natrix natrix* (diagrammatic). (From Bellairs, "The Life of Reptiles")

a, right auricle; ao, dorsal aorta; cd, cystic duct; clo, cloacal opening; fb, fat body; gb, gall bladder; hd, hepatic duct; int, intestine; j, junction between alveolar and saccular parts of lung; lcc, left common carotid artery; li, liver; ljv, left jugular vein; lk, left kidney; lsa, left systemic (aortic) arch; lvc, left anterior vena cava; oe, oesophagus; ohp, opening of hemipenis; p, pancreas; pvc, posterior vena cava (cut short); re, rectum; rjv, right jugular vein; rk, right kidney; rl, right lung (alveolar part); rvc, right anterior vena cava; sl, saccular part of lung; sp, spleen; srl, suprarenal or adrenal gland; st, stomach; te, testis; th, thyroid gland; thy, thymus; tr, trachea; tsh, tongue sheath; ugp, urogenital papilla with common opening for ureter and vas on each side; ur, ureter; v, ventricle; vd, vas deferens.

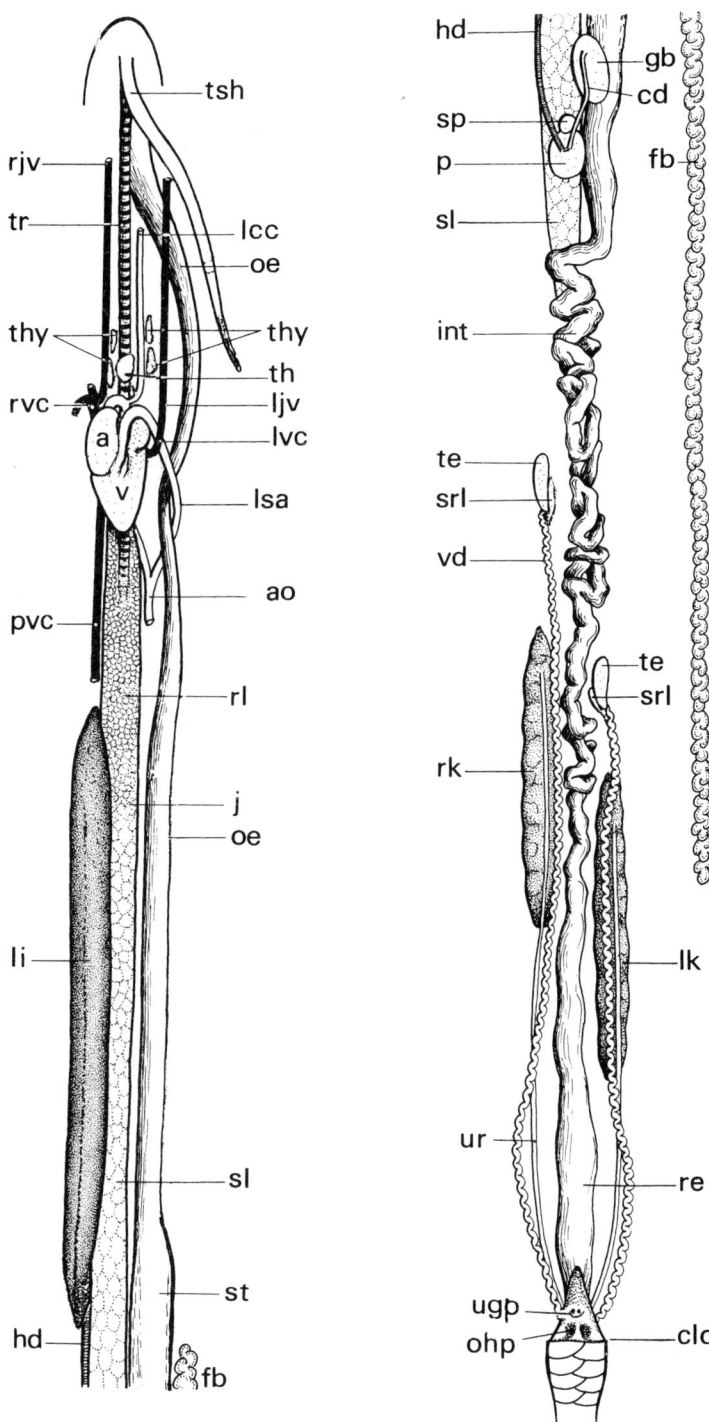

certain snakes—in particular the Crotalidae and (to a lesser extent) Viperidae—the venoms of which are rich in proteolytic enzymes (Russell and Brodie, 1974). Snake venoms in general are chemically very complex, multi-purpose agents, having effects on prey and enemies which can no longer be simply dichotomized as "haemotoxic" or "neurotoxic". They are manufactured in modified salivary glands and delivered through specialized teeth which differ in structure from group to group, some being grooved, as in the "backfanged" or opisthoglyphous snakes, while others are hollow, as in the proteroglyphous (cobras, mambas, sea snakes, etc.) and solenoglyphous snakes (vipers and pit vipers). An ingenious development within the proteroglyphs is the long-range venom delivery apparatus of *Naja nigricollis*, the spitting cobra.

Reptilian tongues are variable both in structure and function, being barely mobile in some cases (crocodilians and chelonians), and highly mobile and protrusible in others (e.g. lizards) where they have become important aids to feeding and drinking. In the snakes and many lizards (e.g. varanids) the mechanical function of the tongue has been lost in the interests of chemosensory specialization. In the chameleons, the reverse appears to have happened, and the sensory function has been lost in the interests of extreme mechanical specialization. In most other squamates both functions are important (see Section VI below).

Alimentary tract A notable feature of the interior morphology of the alimentary tract of reptiles is the presence of extensive longitudinal folding in the gut wall (Parsons and Cameron, 1977), presumably a means of increasing the distensibility of the gut to accommodate bulky food. The stomach is generally divisible into two parts, the corpus and the pars pylorica, though the distinction between the two regions is clearer in some reptiles (e.g. crocodilians) than in others (e.g. squamates). The corpus forms the so-called "gizzard" of crocodiles. As in amphibians and birds, but in contrast to the condition found in mammals, pepsin and hydrochloric acid appear to be secreted by the same (oxynticopeptic) cells in the gastric mucosa. A variety of digestive enzymes is produced by the stomach, pancreas and intestine, but as yet relatively few have been thoroughly investigated in reptiles (Dandifrosse, 1974). The distribution of some of these enzymes is summarized in Table 2.1. Bile salts differ chemically among reptiles as they do among vertebrates generally (Tammar, 1974), but they perform broadly the same role in the digestion and absorption of fats.

Table 2.1. The distribution of some of the digestive enzymes of reptiles (after Dandifrosse, 1974)[a]

Reptile	Organ	Digestive enzyme
Chelonia (Testudines)	Stomach	Amylase; pepsin; trypsin; chitinase; chitobiase
	Pancreas	Amylase; ribonuclease; trypsin; chymotrypsin; carboxypeptidase A; chitinase
	Intestine	Proteinase; invertase; amylase; maltase; chitobiase; trehalase; isomaltase; sucrase
Crocodilia	Pancreas	Chymotrypsin
Sauria (Lacertilia)	Stomach	Chitinase; chitobiase; pepsin
	Pancreas	Chitinase; chymotrypsin; amylase; chitobiase
	Intestine	Chitobiase
Serpentes (Ophidia)	Oesophagus	Amylase; pepsin
	Stomach	Amylase; pepsin
	Pancreas	Amylase; chymotrypsin; trypsin
	Intestine	Amylase; protease

[a] Aggregated data from 14 species of chelonian, 1 species of crocodilian (*Caiman crocodilus*), 11 species of lizards and 5 species of snakes.

The intestine is relatively short in reptiles, although this varies in different groups according to the requirements of body design and diet. The intestines of snakes, most of which are carnivorous, are relatively short, while those of the herbivorous chelonians are relatively long. The lizards are intermediate in this respect. The metabolizable products of digestion and water are absorbed in the intestine, but studies of this phenomenon are very few, and largely confined to chelonians (Dandifrosse, 1974).

The gut terminates in the cloaca, which is often a region of considerable complexity. Typically, it consists of three consecutive chambers (Fig. 2.5A, B): an anterior coprodaeum, into which the faeces are discharged; a middle urodaeum, which receives the urinogenital ducts; and a posterior proctodaeum, which acts as a general collecting area for digestive and excretory wastes before their eventual release into the environment. The male intromittent organ or organs also open into this region and a variety of glands, including scent glands and defensive glands, discharge their products into the cloaca.

A urinary bladder, opening directly into the coprodaeum, is present in some lizards (Fig. 2.5A), in *Sphenodon*, and in chelonians (Fig. 2.7).

Digestion Digestion in reptiles is commonly assumed to be highly efficient, since many ingest their prey whole and appear to egest relatively little. When the progress of such digestive processes is monitored directly with the aid of X-ray photography, the results are certainly impressive (Blain and Campbell, 1942). However, in energetic terms, the efficiency of reptilian digestion (i.e. the ratio of assimilated to consumed energy) appears little different from that of other vertebrates, with values mostly in the range 80–90% (see Section V below). Temperature is known to influence the rate of digestion in reptiles (Benedict, 1932; Skoczylas, 1970b; Windell and Sarokon, 1976) so it would not be unreasonable to expect that it might also affect the efficiency of digestion. However, what little evidence there is suggests that once thermal acclimatisation has taken place, digestive efficiency is relatively insensitive to temperature (Dutton *et al*, 1975; Table 2.4).

B. Excretion and Osmoregulation

Kidneys and salt glands The vital functions of eliminating metabolic waste products from the body, and of regulating water and ionic balance within the body, are performed in reptiles, as in other vertebrates, principally by the kidneys, but with the important support, in the reptilian case, of specialized cephalic salt glands, intestinal mucosa, lungs and skin. The precise extent to which these various components of the excretory and osmoregulatory system contribute to homeostasis in a particular species depends greatly on that species' ecology and life habits.

The kidneys of reptiles lie dorsally in the posterior part of the body cavity (Figs. 2.5A, B, 2.6, 2.7) and differ in shape and relative size from group to group (Fox, 1977). The basic structure of the adult kidney is recognizably similar to that of the more familiar mammal, though there are some notable differences. For example, while there may be as many as a million nephrons in the mammalian kidney, there are only a few thousand in reptiles; the pelvis, pyramids and Henle's loop are absent in most reptiles and glomeruli are poorly developed; and the kidneys of many male snakes and lizards have a unique segment—the so-called "sex segment"—where the tubules undergo seasonal changes of size and secretory activity under the control of testicular androgens (see review by Fox, 1977).

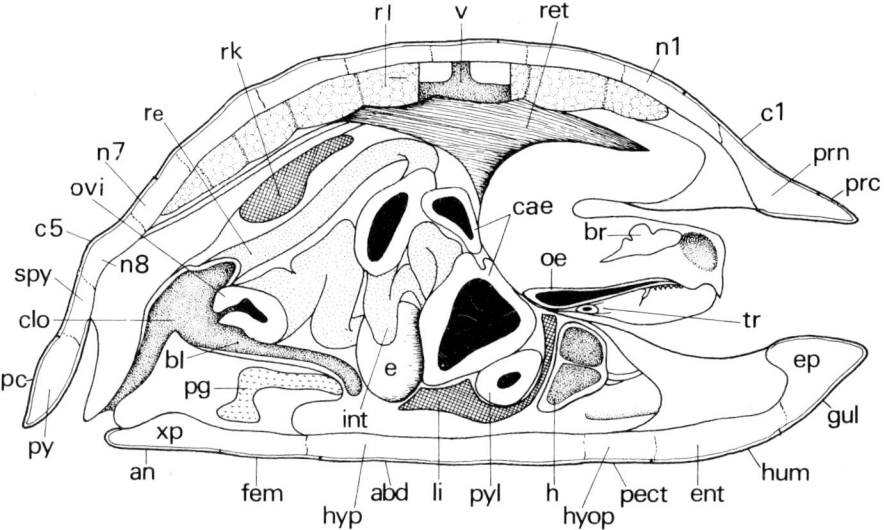

Fig. 2.7. Viscera. Diagrammatic lateral view of female *Testudo graeca* showing viscera in longitudinal section slightly to the right of midline. Part of the right lung has been cut away to show one of the vertebrae attached by its neural spine to the carapace. (From Bellairs, "The Life of Reptiles")

bl, bladder; br, brain; cae, caecum (cut twice with intervening piece left on right half of body); clo, cloaca; e, egg in ovary; h, heart; int, intestine; li, liver (intermediate lobe); oe, oesophagus; ovi, oviduct (left); pg, pelvic girdle; pyl, pyloric part of stomach; re, rectum; rk, right kidney; rl, right lung; ret, retractor muscles of neck; tr, trachea; v, vertebra.

Parts of shell: Horny plates: abd, abdominal; an, anal; cl, c5, centrals 1 and 5; fem, femoral; gul, gular; hum, humeral; pc, postcentral; pect, pectoral; prc, precentral. Bony plates: ent, entoplastron; ep, epiplastron; hyop, hyoplastron; hyp, hypoplastron; n1, n7, n8, neurals 1,7 and 8; prn, proneural or nuchal; py, pygal; spy, suprapygal; xp, xiphiplastron.

Unlike birds and mammals, reptiles are unable to concentrate urine—a deficiency presumably related to the absence of the loop of Henle. Because of this, the reptilian kidney would be unable to eliminate soluble metabolic wastes such as ammonia and urea without a considerable loss of water, a loss which few terrestrial reptiles could in fact afford. Consequently, metabolic wastes are normally excreted in a comparatively insoluble form as uric acid and urate salts. A comparison of the major reptile groups in terms of the composition of their urine reveals a clear correlation with life-style, ammonia and urea being excreted in significant amounts only in aquatic or semi-aquatic forms (Table 2.2). An additional and important means of excreting salts in reptiles is the cephalic salt glands of many (particularly marine) chelonians and squamates (Peaker and Linzell, 1975; Dunson, 1976), which are able to secrete hypertonic solutions of electrolytes (principally sodium, potassium and chloride). These glands are modified lachrymal glands in marine turtles, nasal glands in a wide range of lizards, and sublingual and Harderian glands in sea snakes (Dunson, 1976), and are assumed to be under neuro-endocrine control. No salt glands have been found in either crocodilians or *Sphenodon*.

Water balance Urine flowing into the cloaca from the ureters passes back into the colonic part of the intestine and into the bladder (when present), where both water and salt reabsorption (principally sodium) occurs. Other important sites of water and salt reabsorption in many reptiles are the cloaca itself and the renal tubules. Water reabsorption is clearly related to water conservation in terrestrial reptiles, but salt reabsorption may not necessarily be related to "salt conservation", since salts reabsorbed in the gut may quickly be eliminated via the cephalic salt glands. Schmidt-Nielsen *et al* (1963) suggested that this apparent conservation of urinary salt may in fact be designed to aid water conservation, as salts can be excreted much more economically in terms of "water costs", via the salt glands (which *can* produce a hypertonic solution) than via the kidneys. Reptiles without cephalic salt glands must rely on cloacal avenues of salt excretion, and these can be costly in terms of water. Consequently, where water conservation is at a premium, as for example in desert species, reptiles without salt glands have in many cases acquired the capacity to tolerate considerable salt loads in preference to using valuable water for excretory purposes (Dantzler and Schmidt-Nielsen, 1966; Bradshaw and Shoemaker, 1967).

The partitioning of water exchanges between the various avenues of gain and loss varies considerably between species, and within species depends heavily upon the prevailing ambient conditions of temperature and relative humidity (Cloudsley-Thompson, 1971; Bentley, 1976). For example, the profound influence of temperature on rates of cutaneous and respiratory water loss in the desert lizard *Sauromalus obesus* was shown by Crawford and Kampe (1971). It has long been believed that the major loss of water was via respiration. Bentley (1976) has demonstrated that cutaneous water loss can account for a large proportion of the total water loss, though species vary enormously in the absolute amounts of water lost this way (Table 2.3).

The importance of cutaneous *uptake* is more problematical, since certain lizards once thought to absorb water "like blotting paper" (e.g. *Moloch horridus* and *Uromastix hardwickii*) are now known, at least in the former case, to drink in a special way, by channelling water which falls on the skin through fine capillaries to the corners of the mouth (Bentley and Blumer, 1962). The evidence for cutaneous uptake in crocodilians was, until recently, conflicting (cf. Cloudsley-Thompson, 1968, 1969, with Bentley and Schmidt-Nielsen, 1965). However, Diefenbach (1973) has now confirmed that it occurs in both *Caiman crocodilus* and *Crocodylus niloticus*. Cutaneous uptake also appears to occur in some aquatic chelonians (Bentley, and Schmidt-Nielsen, 1970).

Table 2.2. Approximate percentage of total urinary nitrogen in the form of ammonia, urea and urates (uric acid and urate salts) in reptiles (after Dantzler, 1976)

	% of total urinary nitrogen appearing as:		
	Ammonia	Urea	Urates
CHELONIA			
Wholly aquatic	20–25	20–25	5
Semi-aquatic	6–15	40–60	5
Wholly terrestrial:			
Moist environment	6	30	7
Dry environment	5	10–20	50–60
Gopherus agassizii (Desert tortoise)	3–8	15–50	20–50
Pseudemys scripta (Freshwater turtle)	4–44	45–95	1–24
CROCODILIA	25	0–5	70
SQUAMATA			
Sauria	?	0–8	90
Serpentes	?	0–2	98
RHYNCHOCEPHALIA			
Sphenodon punctatus	3–4	10–28	65–80

The homeostatic control of water exchanges in reptiles is in part physiological (e.g. the regulation of glomerular filtration rate and tubular permeability to water by neurohypophysial hormones—Dantzler, 1976) and in part behavioural (e.g. drinking, or shade seeking), but precisely how overall integration of these control mechanisms is achieved is unknown.

C. Lungs, Ventilation and Gas Exchange

The Respiratory Tract The lungs of reptiles, as of all tetrapods, develop as paired outgrowths of the oesophagus, and differ considerably in form and structure from group to group (Fig. 2.5C–F). Relative to body size, reptilian lungs are larger in total volume than mammalian lungs, but considerably smaller in terms of surface area (Wood and Lenfant, 1976), and contrary to a once widespread belief, are ventilated by both negative (i.e. aspiration) and positive pressure breathing. In terms of structural complexity, most reptilian lungs are intermediate between those of amphibians and those of birds and mammals. Typically, each lung is a sac-like structure with a large central air space into which the bronchus opens directly, and peripherally arranged alveoli (Fig. 2.5C). In the more advanced reptiles, the area of the gas exchange surface is greatly increased by extensive folding of the lung wall and the division of the lung into numerous air chambers lined with alveoli and connected to the bronchus by means of branching secondary bronchi (Fig. 2.5E, F), a development which both reduces the size of the central air space, and gives the lung a sponge-like structure not dissimilar, at least in its extreme form (i.e. in crocodiles), from that of the more familiar mammalian lung. Chameleon lungs are notable for the finger-like air sacs which protrude from the posterior region of each organ (Fig. 2.5D) and function in ventilation and as aids to body inflation when the animal is threatened (Bellairs, 1969). Reptiles breathe mainly through their nostrils, though mouth-breathing is possible and may be important in some cases. Most aquatic and some burrowing reptiles possess a means of closing their nostrils when submerged. Inspired air is drawn through the nostrils into paired nasal sacs which connect with the bucco-pharyngeal cavity via the internal nostrils. These are placed well forward in most reptiles (Fig. 2.8A) and open into the buccal cavity close behind the openings of the organs of Jacobson. The palate is thus short in these cases. In some lizards, particularly those like the monitors, with elongated snout regions (Fig. 2.8B), the internal nostrils are further back and the palate is correspondingly larger. The full development of a bony secondary palate is seen only in the crocodilians (Fig. 2.8C), where the internal nostrils open at the back of the mouth in very close proximity to the glottis. Valve-like flaps of tissue on the roof and floor of the mouth, just in front of the internal nostrils and glottis respectively, enable the throat region to be sealed off from the buccal cavity during submergence, thus permitting the crocodile to grapple with prey underwater without drowning itself, and to breathe via its nostrils even when its mouth is open and full of water.

Table 2.3. Total evaporative and cutaneous water loss in selected reptiles at 23°–27°C (after Bentley, 1976)

	Habitat	Total water loss (mg/cm^2/day)	Cutaneous water loss (mg/cm^2/day)	As % of total
CROCODILIA				
Caiman crocodilus	Aquatic	38	32.9	87
CHELONIA				
Pseudemys scripta	Aquatic	16	12.2	78
Terrapene carolina	Temperate forest	7	5·3	76
Gopherus agassizii	Desert	2	1·5	76
SAURIA				
Iguana iguana	Tropical forest	6·7	4·8	72
Sauromalus obesus	Desert	2	1·3	66
SERPENTES				
Natrix taxispilota	Aquatic	19	16·7	88
Pituophis melanoleucus	Desert	5·6	3·7	64
Spalerosophis cliffordii	Desert	7·4	4·8	65
Cerastes cerastes	Desert	2·3	1·3	57

The trachea is generally long in reptiles, and supported by cartilaginous rings which are complete in chelonians and crocodiles, but mostly incomplete in squamates. It leads into the pharynx through the glottis, which can be opened and closed by muscles attached to the cartilages of the larynx. The glottis of snakes is extremely mobile, and presumably as an adaptation to the ingestion of large mouthfuls, can be extended anteriorly out of the mouth to permit breathing during ingestion.

A respiratory innovation found in some snakes is the so-called "tracheal lung", a development of alveolar tissue on the dorsal side of

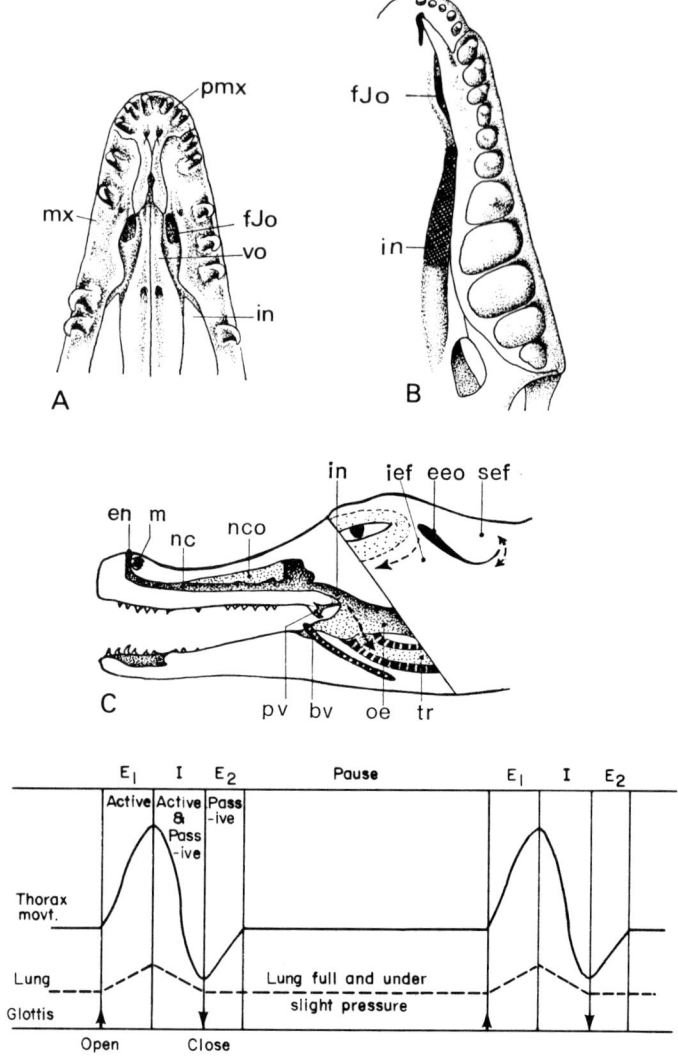

Fig. 2.8. (A) Palate of monitor lizard (*Varanus salvator*) showing pleurodont teeth and separation of openings of Jacobson's organ (fJo) from internal nostrils (in). mx, maxilla; pmx, premaxilla; vo, vomer. (B) Left jaw of the lizard *Dracaena guianaensis*, showing broad, crushing teeth, foramen for the duct of Jacobson's organ (fJo), and internal nostril (in). (From Bellairs, "The Life of Reptiles". (C) Respiratory passages in the head of a crocodile (diagrammatic). Arrows show direction of airway and movements of ear-flaps. (From Bellairs and Attridge, "Reptiles".) bv, basihyal valve; eeo, external ear opening; en, external nostril; ief, inferior ear-flap; in, internal nostril; m, muscles of nostril; nc, nasal cavity; nco, nasal concha; oe, oesophagus; pv, palatal valva; sef, superior ear-flap; tr, trachea. (D) Diagrammatic representation of the breathing movements of a lizard (*Lacerta*), showing the triphasic pattern. An 'up' movement on the thoracic mechanogram is produced by an inward (i.e. expiratory) movement of the thorax. (From Hughes, 1965).

the trachea which enables the snake to breathe even when its lung is wholly compressed by ingested food.

Posteriorly, the trachea divides (except in the majority of snakes) into two bronchi and delivers inspired air, either directly or through numerous secondary bronchi, into the respiratory (alveolar) regions of the lungs. A characteristic of the snake lung and to some extent of the lungs of many lizards, is the functional differentiation of respiratory and non-respiratory regions, the latter being posterior to the former (Fig. 2.6). In the case of snakes, as much as 50% of the lung is relatively avascular and devoid of alveoli, and presumably, therefore, non-respiratory. A number of functions have been suggested for this saccular extension of the lung. McDonald (1959) has suggested that an extension of the lung in snakes is required on mechanical grounds to compensate for the ventilatory consequences of body elongation, in particular for the restrictions imposed by ophidian musculo-skeletal design on the capacity to increase body diameter during breathing. This limitation can be overcome for any required tidal volume by increasing the size of the air sac. Species differences in lung surface area and air sac volume apparently related to the ability to increase oxygen consumption during activity have been reported by Ruben (1976a). Yet another function attributed to the air sac is that of buoyancy control, a suggestion which receives support from the observation that aquatic snakes tend to have longer air sacs than terrestrial snakes.

Breathing The absence of any kind of diaphragm in most reptiles, and the occurrence of rhythmic gular movements in many chelonians and lizards similar to those of amphibians, have together been responsible for a great deal of misunderstanding in the past about the ventilatory mechanisms of reptiles (Wood and Lenfant, 1976), in particular for the belief that air entered the lungs as the result of positive pressure gular pumping, as in amphibians, and not by negative pressure (aspiration) breathing, as in mammals. Recent studies, however, using electromyographic and other techniques have confirmed earlier suspicions that reptiles do employ negative pressure breathing, and that gular pumping is olfactory, not respiratory, in function (Gans, 1970).

The ventilatory movements of the reptilian body are brought about principally by the intercostal muscles, assisted in varying ways and to differing extents by other muscles of trunk and abdomen, and by smooth muscles in the walls of the lungs themselves. In chelonians, where the rigid skeleton prevents the ribs being used in ventilation, other groups of muscles have become important, and intrapulmonary pressure is altered by muscle-induced movements of the viscera, limbs and girdles (Gaunt and Gans, 1969a). Aquatic chelonians are also able to exploit hydrostatic pressure for ventilatory purposes (Jackson, 1971). The only reptiles with a real, if somewhat unusual diaphragm are the crocodilians, which also have an unorthodox ventilatory mechanism (Gans and Clark, 1976), most particularly with respect to the way liver movements are used to change the volume of the pleural cavity.

Ventilation patterns are very varied in reptiles, and no single pattern can be said to be typical of the group as a whole (Wood and Lenfant, 1976). A respiratory cycle fairly typical of lizards is illustrated in Fig. 2.8D. A somewhat different ventilatory pattern—biphasic rather than triphasic—appears to characterize snakes (Clark et al, 1978).

Pulmonary gas exchange is supplemented in many reptiles by exchange across pharyngeal and cloacal epithelia and, to a lesser extent, by exchange across the skin. Aquatic chelonians in particular make use of these extrapulmonary mechanisms, their function being to enable gas exchange to continue (albeit at a reduced level) while the animal is submerged. In the soft-shelled turtles (Trionychidae), pharyngeal exchange is promoted by highly vascularized villiform papillae in the mouth, where about 30% of under water oxygen uptake appears to take place, the remainder occurring across the leathery carapace and plastron (Girgis, 1961). In several chelonian families which have aquatic and semi-aquatic members (though not the Trionychidae), pairs of accessory bladders opening into the cloaca are thought to function as supplementary breathing organs, particularly during periods of prolonged submergence such as hibernation (Bellairs, 1969). Some aquatic turtles, for example *Pseudemys scripta*, appear, in contrast, to have very limited capacities for extrapulmonary gas exchange (Jackson and Schmidt-Nielsen, 1966) and the same appears to be true of crocodilians (Naifeh et al, 1970). Small but significant amounts of cutaneous exchange have been reported for snakes (Standaert and Johansen, 1974).

Control of ventilation Relatively little is known about the control of ventilation in reptiles. Superficial observations which reveal continuously fluctuating blood gas concentrations and blood pH might suggest that control is in fact poor, but such a conclusion is not justified (Wood and Lenfant, 1976; Howell and Rahn, 1976). The misunderstanding arises from a failure to appreciate the importance in many reptiles of the relationship between body temperature and blood pH, which is inverse and almost linear (Howell and Rahn, 1976). This means that the homeostatic "target" at any particular body temperature will be the blood pH appropriate to the temperature, and not one particular "normal" value as in mammals. Hence the apparent variability of blood pH in reptiles, very far from being a sign of the absence of ventilatory control, is an important manifestation of it.

D. Cardiovascular System

The heart The reptilian heart is basically three chambered with a left and right atrium and a single ventricle subdivided to varying extents in different reptile groups by an interventricular septum (Fig. 2.9B, C). Only in crocodilians is the subdivision of the ventricle more or less complete (Fig. 2.9C) (White, 1976). Deoxygenated blood from the systemic circulation empties via the sinus venous into the right atrium. The left atrium receives oxygenated blood from the lungs. In non-crocodilians, both atria open into the same side of the ventricle, which for convenience is shown as the "left" side in Fig. 2.9B, although in life it is more usually the dorsal side since the interventricular septum is horizontal. ("Left" and "right" in this context refer respectively to the left and right hand sides of the animal, not of the diagram.)

As indicated by the arrows in Fig. 2.9B, deoxygenated blood from the right atrium tends to stay on the right side of the ventricle and enter the pulmonary trunk and (to a lesser degree) the left aortic arch, while oxygenated blood from the left atrium tends to remain on the left side of the ventricle and enter both left and right aortic arches. Thus, under normal circumstances, little mixing of oxygenated and deoxygenated blood appears to take place even in reptiles with a minimal interventricular septum, though since the separation is functional rather than anatomical, the degree of mixing will inevitably be influenced by any changes of resistance to blood flow from the ventricle that arise in the pulmonary or aortic circulations. Increased pulmonary resistance, for example, when aquatic reptiles dive, would tend to cause deoxygenated blood destined for the pulmonary circuit to be shunted into the aortic circuit (a 'right-to-left' shunt) along with oxygenated blood from the left atrium, thus increasing mixing. The direction of the shunt is reversed when the animal resurfaces and increases ventilation.

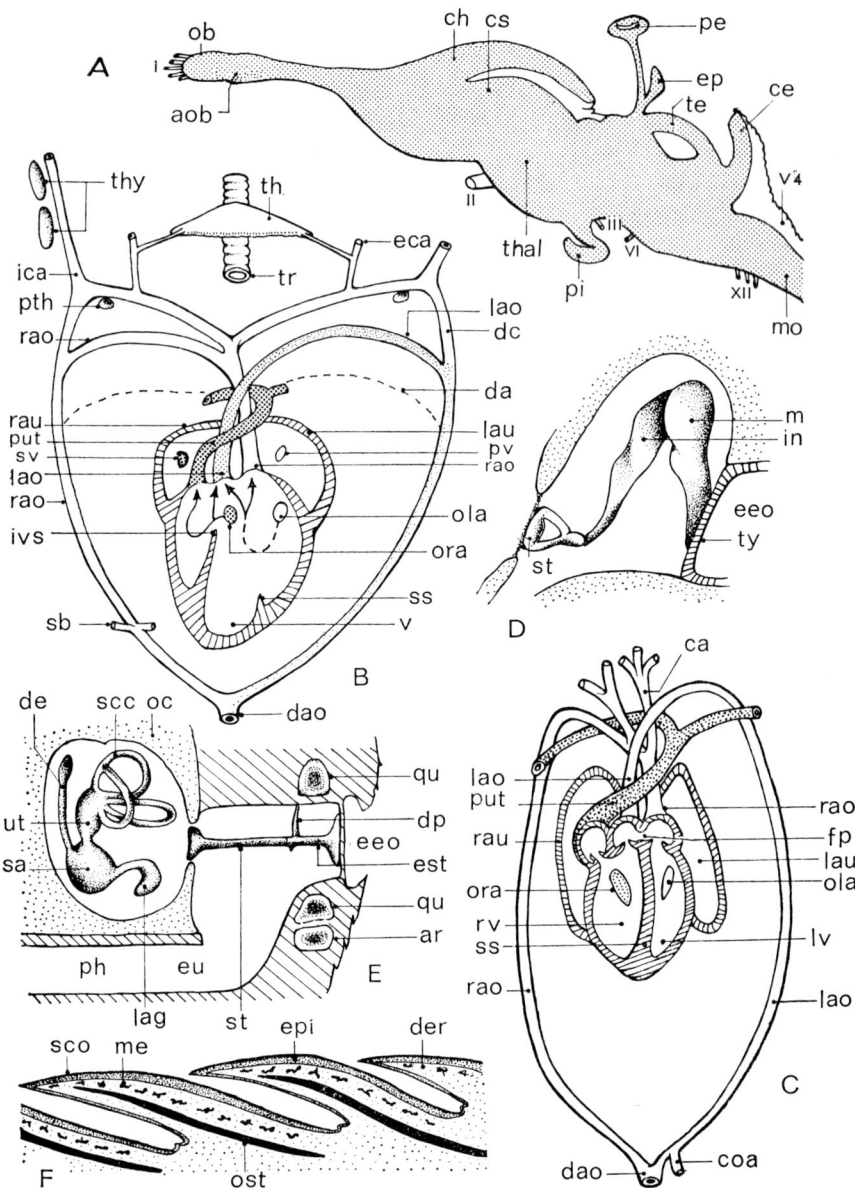

Fig. 2.9. (A) Longitudinal section through brain of lizard. (B,C) Heart, arterial arches etc. of lizard (B) and crocodile (C), with heart structures shown diagrammatically in same plane from ventral side. Vessels carrying venous blood stippled, those carrying mixed blood stippled lightly; arrows in B show direction of blood flow in

In crocodiles, only the retention of the left aortic arch and the presence of a small aperture in the interventricular septum linking left and right ventricles—the foramen of Panizza (Fig. 2.9C)—prevent the circulatory system from being essentially like that of birds and mammals. Nevertheless, these differences are sufficient in principle, to allow some mixing of oxygenated and deoxygenated blood to take place, either through the foramen of Panizza, or in the dorsal aorta if, at systole, deoxygenated blood in the right ventricle were to enter the left aortic arch, as anatomical considerations might lead one to expect (Fig. 2.9C). But in fact, pressure differentials and valve arrangements are such that very little, if any, mixing takes place, for under normal circumstances, deoxygenated blood in the right ventricle passes preferentially into the pulmonary trunk and not into the left aortic arch; and oxygenated blood in the left ventricle enters both the right and (via the foramen of Panizza) the left aortic arches (White, 1976). Only when pulmonary resistance is unusually high (e.g. when diving) or left aortic resistance unusually low, will blood from the right ventricle be shunted into the left aortic arch. Under normal circumstances, therefore, a complete double circulation appears to be the rule in crocodilians.

---

heart. The blood in the left aorta of the crocodile is normally oxygenated (see text). (D) Middle ear and ossicles of mammal. (E) Inner and middle ear of reptile, seen diagrammatically in partial cross-section. (F) Longitudinal section through skin of lizard with osteoderms. (From Bellairs and Attridge, "Reptiles")

aob, accessory olfactory bulb; ar, articular; ca, carotid-subclavian stem (left side); ce, cerebellum; ch, cerebral hemisphere; coa, coeliac artery; cs, corpus striatum; da, ductus arteriosus; dao, dorsal aorta; dc, ductus caroticus; de, ductus endolymphaticus; der, dermis; dp, dorsal process of extra-stapes; eca, external carotid artery; eeo, external ear opening; ep, epiphysial part of pineal complex; epi, epidermis; est, extra-stapes; eu eustachian tube; fp, foramen of Panizza; h, hinge of scale; ica, internal carotid artery; in, incus; ivs, main interventricular septum; lag lagena; lao, left aorta (systemic arch); lau, left atrium; lv, left ventricle; m, malleus; me, melanophore; mo, medulla oblongata; ob, olfactory bulb; oc, otic capsule; ola, opening of left atrium into ventricle; ora, opening of right atrium; ost, osteoderm; pe, parietal eye; ph, pharynx; pi, pituitary; pth, parathyroid; put, pulmonary trunk; pv, opening of pulmonary vein into left atrium; qu, quadrate; rao, right aorta (systemic arch); rau, right auricle; rv, right ventricle; sa, saccule; sb, subclavian artery; scc, semicircular canal; sco, stratum corneum of epidermis; ss, secondary interventricular septum; st, stapes (= columella auris); sv, sinus venosus opening into right atrium; te, tectum of midbrain; th, thyroid; thal, thalamus; thy, thymus bodies (shown on one side only); tr, trachea; ty, tympanic membrane (eardrum); ut, utricle; v, ventricle; v4, 4th ventricle of brain. Cranial nerves: I, olfactory; II, optic; III, oculomotor; VI, abducens; XII hypoglossal.

Blood flow Heart rate is dependent (not always in a simple way—White, 1976) on many variables in reptiles, in particular on body temperature, body size, metabolic rate, respiratory rate and sensory stimulation. The relationship with temperature is a positive one, and the temperature coefficient (Q_{10}) is generally between 2 and 3 (Licht, 1965). Activity causes marked increases in heart rate, and maximal rates at any given temperature can be as much as three times the corresponding resting rate. This heart rate increment (maximal minus resting heart rate) also varies with temperature, becoming maximal just above the mean of the preferred body temperature range (Licht, 1965). By analogy with Fry's (1947) concept of "metabolic scope for activity", this heart rate increment could usefully be described as the "cardiac scope for activity".

The influence of temperature on heart rate in some lizards also appears to be dependent on whether the animal is warming up or cooling down (Bartholomew and Lasiewski, 1965), a relationship most easily interpreted in terms of thermoregulation. In the Galapagos marine iguana, for example, heart rates during cooling are considerably lower at all body temperatures than heart rates during warming (Bartholomew and Lasiewski, 1965). Since heart rates directly determine patterns of heat distribution in the body, the depression of heart rate during cooling would have the effect of reducing heat losses from the body when these lizards plunge into the water to feed. Conversely the relative increase in heart rate during warming would have the effect of facilitating heat gain when the lizards re-emerge from the water and begin basking. Experimental studies reveal that these expectations are in fact fulfilled (Bartholomew and Lasiewski, 1965; Morgareidge and White, 1969; White, 1973, 1976). A similar capacity for cardiovascular adjustment appears to be present in crocodiles (White, 1976).

In addition to their role in thermoregulation and activity, cardiovascular adjustments are known to be important in reptiles, as in higher vertebrates, during diving. In general, submergence is followed by a reduction of heart rate (bradycardia), though the time course and extent of this reduction are very variable (White, 1976), and may, to some degree, depend on other factors. In *Caiman crocodilus*, for example, bradycardia is more intense when diving is "fear-induced" rather than spontaneous (Gaunt and Gans, 1969b), suggesting some kind of physiological "anticipation", in the former case, of a prolonged period of submergence. Vagal inhibition and (in crocodilians at least) intra-pulmonary and/or thoracic pressure appear to be important inducers of bradycardia (White, 1976).

Respiratory properties of the blood Reptilian erythrocytes are oval, biconvex, nucleated, and generally smaller and more numerous than amphibian cells. They vary in size from about 10 × 5 microns to 22 × 12 microns, and number between $0.5–1.5 \times 10^6/mm^3$ of blood (Bellairs, 1969; Saint Girons, 1970; Duguy, 1970). Various kinds of white cell are also found and though considerably less numerous than the erythrocytes, are both absolutely and relatively more abundant in reptilian blood than in the blood of most mammals. The basic structural characteristics of reptile haemoglobin have not yet been described, but there is no reason to suppose that they are any different from those of other vertebrates. The blood chemistry of reptiles, as presently understood, was reviewed by Dessauer (1970) and Sullivan (1974).

Oxygen dissociation curves for a number of reptile species have been described in the literature, which is reviewed by Wood and Lenfant (1976). Eight examples are shown in Fig. 2.10. Attempts to associate the parameters of these curves—in particular their shapes, their P_{50} values and their sensitivities to blood CO_2 tensions and temperature—with life habit have met with varying degrees of success. In chelonians, for example, there appear to be marked differences between the dissociation curve parameters of terrestrial and aquatic species (Fig. 2.10A), which make sense (in terms of life habit) when the physiological significance of these differences is understood. Relative shifts to the right in the position of dissociation curves, whether between species, or within individuals under different conditions, reflect increasing P_{50} values and decreasing oxygen affinity (i.e. a net tendency to unload oxygen). Fig. 2.10A, therefore, reveals that aquatic species (with the exception of the mud turtle) have lower oxygen affinities than terrestrial species, presumably as an adaptation to prolonged submergence, when maximal unloading is desirable. Other parameters of these "aquatic" dissociation curves can be interpreted in the same way, for example their greater "sigmoidicity" (Fig. 2.10A), and their known tendency to shift still further to the right when blood CO_2 tension increases (the so-called "Bohr shift"), as it is bound to do in the tissues of an animal which has ceased to ventilate.

In contrast, the same distinction between aquatic and terrestrial species is not apparent in squamates. Indeed, the reverse is sometimes apparent. For example, the blood of the aquatic snake *Acrochordus javanicus* has a much higher oxygen affinity than that of the fully terrestrial/arboreal boa constrictor (Fig. 2.10B). At the same time, *Acrochordus* has an enormous Bohr shift in comparison with that of the boa (or indeed, with that of most other vertebrates), which seems more in keeping with its highly aquatic habits. This has been interpreted as a system strongly favouring unloading when the snake is submerged, and loading when it is ventilating for brief and irregular periods at the surface (Johansen and Lenfant, 1972; Wood and Lenfant, 1976).

Various blood attributes are known to be dependent on variables such as age, body size, temperature and acclimation. Oxygen affinity, for example, has been found to decline with age in certain snakes (Pough, 1977a), and oxygen capacity (the vol% of O_2 bound by fully saturated blood) to increase (Pough, 1977b). Oxygen affinity is positively related to body size in lizards (Pough, 1977c), negatively related in snakes (Pough, 1977d). Oxygen capacity is temperature sensitive in many reptiles, and, very significantly, tends in some lizards and snakes to become maximal within the normal activity temperature range of the species, where it is also relatively temperature-insensitive (Pough, 1976), a device, presumably, for maintaining maximal oxygen availability when demand is most likely to be high.

The lymphatic system This system is well developed in reptiles, more highly developed, indeed, than the venous system itself, to which the collected lymph is eventually delivered. An extensive review of the subject was provided by Ottaviani and Tazzi (1977).

E. Reproduction and Development

Sexual reproduction is the rule in reptiles, the only known exceptions being a few species of lizards and one snake, which have developed the ability to reproduce parthenogenetically (Maslin, 1971; Porter, 1972; Cole, 1975; Mittwoch, 1978).

The extent to which males and females are different in appearance varies considerably, being marked in some species (especially lizards), moderate in others, and more or less absent in others. On the whole, externally visible sex differences in reptiles are not clear cut, and depend for their usefulness on the availability of several mature specimens for comparison. A number of more objective sexing techniques have been used successfully in certain cases, for example the use of sexing probes in snakes to detect the presence of retracted hemipenes (Laszlo, 1975); manual probing for evidence of the penis in crocodiles (Brazaitis, 1969); the assaying of circulating testosterone levels in lizards (Judd *et al*, 1977).

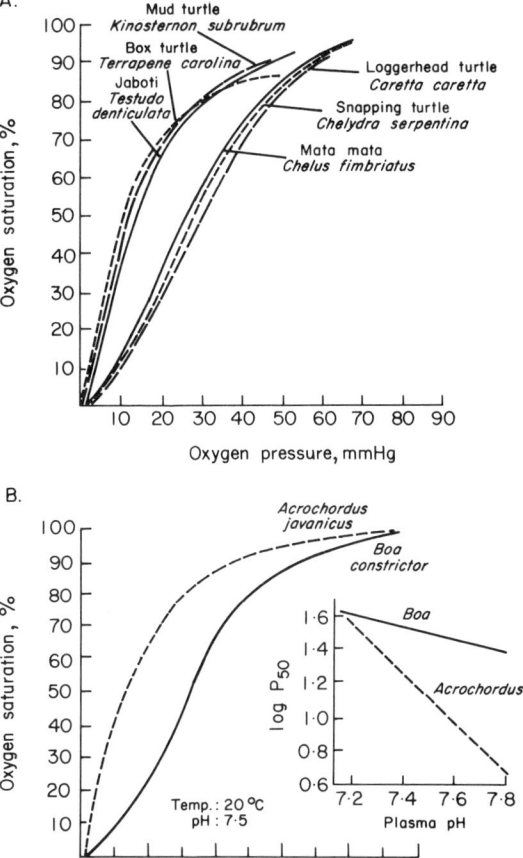

Fig. 2.10. (A) Oxygen dissociation curves for blood of various turtle species. (From Wood and Lenfant, 1976, based on various sources.) (B) Oxygen dissociation curves and Bohr effects in whole blood of the aquatic elephant trunk snake (*Acrochordus javanicus*) and the arboreal boa constrictor (*Constrictor constrictor*)*. (From Johansen and Lenfant, 1972).

Sex organs, ducts and products There is now an extensive literature on the sexual biology of reptiles, much of which has recently been reviewed by Fox (1977). The usually paired gonads lie in the abdominal cavity and discharge their gametic products through ducts which open into the urodaeum of the cloaca (Figs. 2.5A, B; 2.6). Sperm cells produced by the testis collect first in the coiled tubules of

* Throughout the book both *Boa constrictor* and *Constrictor constrictor* are used.

the epididymis, from where they are conveyed to the cloaca via the vas deferens (Figs. 2.5B, 2.6). In the female, ova released into the coelom from the ovaries at ovulation are drawn into the oviducal funnel (Fig. 2.5A), and carried down the oviduct by ciliary and muscular activity. There is no midline fusion of female genital ducts to form a single uterine or vaginal structure, with the result that left and right ducts open separately into the cloaca. Urinary and genital ducts on each side open separately into the cloaca in the great majority of female reptiles, though in some turtles they fuse just before entering the cloaca. Urinogenital fusion is more common in male reptiles.

Fertilization is internal and occurs in the "upper" part of the oviduct, to which region the migration of sperm cells is assisted by ciliary activity. With the single exception of the tuatara, fertilization is effected by male intromittent organs, of which there are essentially two kinds. In chelonians and crocodilians, the penis consists of a fibrous, ventromedial thickening of the cloacal wall, with a pair of spongy longitudinal ridges on the dorsal surface. When engorged with blood these ridges expand to form the walls of the seminal groove along which the semen passes on its way towards the vent. The free end of the penis is also erectile, and by muscular action can be extended through the vent into the cloaca of the female. There is no inversion of the penis during this process.

The squamates have a more elaborate intromittent apparatus. In this group, the male copulatory organs are paired ("hemipenes"), and at rest lie ventrolaterally behind the vent in the anterior region of the tail. During copulation, one hemipenis is extended by the combined action of blood engorgement and muscular contraction, during the course of which the organ is turned inside out (Figs. 2.5B, 2.14E, F). Semen is conveyed from male to female via a seminal groove in the outer wall of the everted hemipenis. The morphology of the hemipenis is extremely variable, particularly in snakes, and this variation is commonly thought to have taxonomic significance.

Reproductive cycles Breeding tends to be seasonal in all reptiles that naturally experience regular cycles of photoperiod, temperature, food availability or rainfall. Clearly it is essential that young are produced only when environmental conditions are likely to be optimal. In the case of most temperate species, the breeding season is relatively short and occurs once during the annual cycle, though it tends to lengthen as latitude decreases. In the tropics, reptiles breed more frequently, and some reproductive activity may be observable at most or all times of the year. Even here, fluctuations in the intensity of reproductive activity occur in association with seasonal cycles of rainfall and food availability.

The physiological basis of reptilian breeding cycles has been investigated to any great extent only in lizards (e.g. Licht, 1972), though other reptiles are now receiving some attention (e.g. Hawley and Alesiuk, 1976). In temperate reptiles, the breeding cycle typically begins when individuals emerge from hibernation in the spring, though the timing of gonadal recrudescence and regression in the annual cycle differs considerably between species (Licht, 1972). In some reptiles, particularly snakes, the annual cycle is complicated by the male's ability to store sperm over winter in the epididymis and vas deferens, thus enabling insemination and fertilization to take place while the testes themselves are still inactive (Licht, 1972).

A number of studies have attempted to identify the principal environmental factors regulating breeding cycles in reptiles and these have been reviewed by Licht (1972). The three most likely factors are temperature, rainfall and photoperiod, especially the first (Licht, 1972). Endogenous, circannual rhythms of physiological activity also appear to be important in the control of breeding cycles, so it is probable that the environmental factors phase the endogenous rhythms, thereby ensuring that breeding and climate are appropriately synchronised. Precisely how these factors exert their physiological influence is uncertain, but it seems highly likely that the interaction is mediated by the same hypothalamic-pituitary-gonadotropin control system that is known to be responsible for controlling the breeding cycle of mammals (Licht, 1972).

Mating, whether seasonal or not, is usually preceded by some form of courtship behaviour, and inter-male rivalry leading to territory formation, often involving complex visual displays and vocalizations, is not uncommon, particularly in lizards. Useful general accounts of reproductive behaviour in reptiles are provided by Bellairs (1969) and Porter (1972), while more specialised studies were reported by various authors at a symposium on reptilian social behaviour (Greenberg, 1977).

Embryonic development Fertilization initiates the process of embryonic development, and normally occurs soon after mating at the beginning of the breeding season. However, the females of some chelonian and squamate species are able to delay fertilization for several months (even years) after mating by storing sperm within their oviducts, a technique quite distinct from storage in the male genital tract during the regression phase of the testicular cycle. Oviducal storage means that sperm obtained from an autumn mating can be used to fertilize eggs the following spring—and to continue fertilizing them, if necessary, during the ensuing summer—without further copulation. Sperm storage of this kind is probably quite common in lizards and snakes (Bellairs, 1969; Porter, 1972; Fox, 1977).

Once fertilization has taken place, the egg passes into the glandular region of the oviduct and becomes enveloped successively in various secretions of the oviducal wall, in particular those producing the albumen layer, the egg membranes, and the shell. In most reptiles, the shell is a tough, flexible material of parchment-like consistency, whereas in many chelonians, crocodilians and some lizards (principally geckos) it is hard and brittle, due to the presence in the shell membranes of crystalline calcium salt deposits. Both types of shell are permeable to water and respiratory gases, and this appears to serve important physiological functions during development (Packard *et al*, 1977).

Embryogenesis is highly temperature-dependent in reptiles, and each species appears to have its own optimum temperature for development. Quite small temperature increases can greatly reduce the period of gestation (Platt, 1969), and substantial departures from the thermal optimum can markedly increase the incidence of developmental abnormalities and embryonic death (Vinegar, 1974). The key to the success of the reptile egg as an instrument of reproduction on land is, as emphasized elsewhere, the development of the amnion, chorion and allantois, extra-embryonic membranes which have essentially the same function in reptiles as they have in higher vertebrates (see Bellairs, 1969). Extensive summaries of the stages of embryonic development in the snapping turtle *Chelydra serpentina*, and the viviparous lizard, *Lacerta vivipara*, will be found, together with excellent illustrations, in Porter (1972).

Yolk, with which reptile eggs are well endowed, provides the main source of nutrients and energy for the developing embryo, and this is true even in those viviparous species which have developed placentation (see below). Though most of the yolk is consumed during embryonic development, the young of some species, instead of discarding what is left at the time of birth or hatching, continue to make use of it by withdrawing the yolk-sac into their bodies and metabolizing its contents during the difficult early days of post-natal life.

An interesting difference exists in the calcium content of the yolk of primitive and advanced reptiles. Chelonian and crocodilian embryos obtain most of the calcium they require for osteogenesis from the inner surfaces of the eggshell. Their yolk is correspondingly poor in calcium. Squamate embryos, on the other hand, obtain most of their calcium from the yolk, and little from the shell. Since the evolution of viviparity requires a progressive reduction of the eggshell, only species whose embryos are not dependent on the eggshell for their calcium will have the evolutionary potential to become viviparous (Packard *et al*, 1977). This may explain why viviparity has evolved several times among the squamates, but never among the chelonians or crocodilians.

Viviparous species are those in which the developing eggs are retained within the oviducts until the young are ready to be born. The shell membranes of such eggs do not contain calcium salts, and they are reduced to varying degrees in different species. Their continuing presence has been sufficient to justify, in the eyes of some writers, the use of the term "ovoviviparity" for this mode of reproduction in reptiles, in order to distinguish it from the "true viviparity" of placental mammals. However, other writers (e.g. Bellairs and Attridge, 1975; Packard *et al*, 1977) have argued that the distinction between ovovivipiarty and viviparity is an artificial one. Viviparity has arisen independently on numerous occasions among the squamates, and is found in some members of most squamate families, though exclusively in only a few (Fitch, 1970; Packard *et al*, 1977). The mode of reproduction is clearly a labile adaptive strategy, for not only do closely related species differ with respect to whether they are viviparous or oviparous, different populations of the same species are known to vary in this respect as well, for example the African skink, *Mabuya quinquetaeniata*. Viviparity in these cases appears to be associated with climates showing greater seasonal temperature fluctuations, where the interior of a thermoregulating reptile would provide a more satisfactory thermal environment for developing eggs than could be obtained by oviposition (Packard *et al*, 1977). This hypothesis is supported by the distribution of many cold-tolerant species, such as *Lacerta vivipara, Anguis fragilis, Vipera berus* and *Thamnophis sirtalis*, all of which are viviparous (Tinkle and Gibbons, 1977; Shine and Bull, 1979).

Associated with the reduction of the eggshell in most viviparous species has been the development of placentation, seen at its most primitive in lizards like *Lacerta vivipara*, where little more than water and respiratory gases are exchanged, and at its most complex in lizards like the European skink, *Chalcides chalcides* and the North American snake genus *Thamnophis*, where the eggs are much less yolky and the exchange of materials, including nutrients (amino acids in particular) and excretory products (urea) is more extensive (Bellairs, 1969; Hoffman, 1970). In *Chalcides* and *Thamnophis*, the placenta is formed by the close application of the extra-embryonic membranes to the uterine wall (the "uterus" in reptiles being that part of the oviduct in which embyronic development takes place). A thinning of the tissues on each side of the placenta makes it possible for the maternal and foetal blood vessels to come into close apposition, thereby facilitating exchange.

The number of eggs or young produced per clutch or brood, and the number of clutches or broods per season, vary considerably between species. Both intra- and inter-specifically, clutch and brood size in lizards depend on body size, larger lizards having larger reproductive outputs. When lizards of the same size and kind are compared, clutches tend on the whole to be larger than broods. Data relating to numbers of eggs per clutch and numbers of clutches per season were tabulated very fully for lizards in Tinkle *et al* (1970) and Porter (1972) and for snakes in Porter (1972). At the end of embryonic development, the young squamate's escape through the eggshell or enclosing membranes is assisted by a special "egg-tooth" attached to the tip of the premaxillary bone and projecting forward (Fig. 2.4I). Young crocodilians and chelonians do not have an egg-tooth, but are equipped instead with a horny thickening at the tip of the snout, the "egg-caruncle", which performs the same function.

V. Metabolism

A. General

The metabolic and thermal physiology of reptiles is of considerable interest to comparative physiologists because of the crucial phylogenetic position of this group in relation to the evolution of birds and mammals. The considerable literature on the subject was reviewed by Templeton (1970), Cloudsley-Thompson (1971) and Bennett and Dawson (1976). Desmond (1977) reviewed the recent upsurge of interest in dinosaur metabolism and thermophysiology initiated by Bakker (1971, 1972).

B. Energy Flow and Utilisation

Metabolism is essentially a complex of physiological and biochemical processes concerned with the production and storage of energy. In recent years, the energetics of reptiles and amphibians has become an area of active research interest, with particular emphasis on (i) chemical energy budgeting and the determination of annual energy budgets for different species (e.g. Fitzpatrick, 1973; Dutton *et al*, 1975; Derickson, 1976a; Andrews and Asato, 1977; Patterson and Davies, 1982b); and (ii) the control of heat exchanges (thermal energy balance) in the interests of body temperature regulation (Templeton, 1970).

In energetics food utilisation is most commonly measured in terms of energy assimilation efficiency (the ratio of energy consumed as food (C), less faeces (F) and urine (U), to energy consumed, multiplied by 100) and production or "conversion" efficiency (the ratio of energy stored as growth, fat deposits, gamete production etc (P) to energy consumed (C) or energy assimilated (A) times 100, depending on whether gross or net conversion efficiencies are being considered). The assimilation efficiencies of reptiles vary with diet, but are generally high in carnivorous species (80–90%). The lower efficiencies (50–55%) of herbivorous species appear to be due to the lack of either cellulase or appropriate gut symbionts. Conversion (growth) efficiency tends to be higher in ectotherms than in endotherms because of the much greater metabolic energy losses in the latter, though this superiority is most evident only under optimal thermal conditions. Conversion efficiency appears to be more temperature-dependent than assimilation efficiency, at least in temperature-acclimatised animals (Table 2.4).

Data of the kind shown in Table 2.4, which are derived from controlled laboratory experiments, can, with the help of a few working assumptions, be used to calculate annual energy budgets for "typical" members of a given species under natural conditions. The budget for *Sceloporus olivaceus*, as calculated by Dutton *et al* (1975), is given in Table 2.5.

An important component of the energy budget not isolated in data of this kind is the allocation of energy to reproduction, perhaps the most important component of "production" (P) from the point of view of the individual's overall energy strategy and adaptive fitness (Tinkle, 1969; Tinkle *et al*, 1970). Evidence now coming to light (e.g. Derickson, 1976a; Patterson and Davies, 1982b) suggests that there are marked and important differences between species with respect to energy allocation for reproduction which correspond in some degree to the expectations of r- and K-selection theory (Gadgil and Bossert, 1970; Pianka, 1970). According to this theory, species designated as "r-selected" are those whose fitness depends primarily on "r", the

Table 2.4a. Energy budgets of the lizard *Sceloporus olivaceus*, under different experimental conditions.

Consumption (C), egestion + excretion (FU), assimilation (A) and production (P) rates in cal/g. day. Metabolic rates (R) were calculated as the mean hourly O_2 consumption rates of each group determined at its acclimation temperature × the oxycalorific coefficient 4.825×10^{-3} cal/μl × 24h (after Dutton et al, 1975).

Acclimation temperature (°C)	N	Mean Wt. (g)	C ($\bar{x} \pm s$)	FU ($\bar{x} \pm s$)	A ($\bar{x} \pm s$)	$\frac{A}{C} \times 100$ (%)	R ($\bar{x}$)	P ($\bar{x} \pm s$)	$\frac{P}{C} \times 100$ (%)	$\frac{P}{A} \times 100$ (%)
15	14	14.41	10.05 ± 8.13	1.09 ± 2.39	8.96 ± 8.05	89	7.45	1.51 ± 9.84	15	17
20	13	15.70	29.45 ±21.26	5.90 ± 4.27	23.55 ±18.60	80	16.91	6.64 ±17.57	22	28
25	9	16.66	113.21 ±85.40	11.44 ± 4.46	101.77 ±86.88	90	15.55	86.22 ±87.14	76	85
30	9	18.17	121.01 ±84.29	22.42 ±16.21	98.59 ±78.63	81	20.60	77.99 ±69.53	64	79

[a] The energy values in this Table and Table 2.5 have been left as originally published and not converted to Joules; in Table 2.6 calories are given for consistency.

Table 2.5. The annual energy budget of *Sceloporus olivaceus* as determined for a typical one year old 16·49 g lizard from the data of Table 2.4 extrapolated to fit known weather conditions and observed body temperatures. All energy entries in Kcal (after Dutton et al, 1975).

C	FU	A	$\frac{A}{C} \times 100$ (%)	R	P	$\frac{P}{C} \times 100$ (%)	$\frac{P}{A} \times 100$ (%)
261·2	43·3	218·0	83·5	98·5	119·5	45·8	54·8
				115·3[a]	102·7	39·3	47·1
				123·7[a]	94·3	36·1	43·3
				131·9[a]	86·0	32·9	39·4

[a] Respiratory losses calculated on the assumption that field rates are 2, 2·5 and 3 × laboratory rates respectively.

intrinsic rate of increase. They are characterised by short life-spans, high reproductive effort (eggs per season) and early sexual maturity. In contrast, species designated as "K-selected" are those whose fitness depends primarily on K, the carrying capacity of the environment. These species are characterised by longer life-spans, low reproductive effort and delayed sexual maturity.

Various reproductive implications of this theory have been tested in reptiles by Tinkle (1969), Tinkle et al (1970), Avery (1975), Derickson (1976a), Patterson and Davies (1982b, c), and in general results have confirmed theoretical expectations. The results of two independent studies are provided in Table 2.6 for the purposes of comparison. Each study itself compares the energy budgets of supposedly r- and K-selected species, and in each case, the ways in which the two types of species differ are strikingly similar. For example, the r-K model predicts that both in weight relative terms and in terms of the percentage of the total annual energy budget allocated to egg production, r-selected species will invest more energy in their annual reproductive effort than K-selected species. This expectation is fully confirmed by the findings of both studies (Table 2.6). Other predictions are also confirmed by the data of Table 2.6—for example, the expectation that assimilation efficiencies will be lower in r-selected than in K-selected species. Studies of this kind can be expected to throw considerable light on the evolution and variability of reptilian reproductive strategies.

Table 2.6. Annual energy allocation to egg production in lizards

Species	Presumed r-K categorization	Mean wet wt. (g)	Mean no. of eggs/♀/year	Total annual energy investment in egg production		Unit annual energy investment in egg production		Assimilation efficiency (%)	Egg production (P_E) efficiency (%)	
				cals/♀	cals/g/yr	cals/egg	cals/g/egg		$\frac{P_E}{C}$	$\frac{P_E}{A}$
Podarcis (Lacerta) hispanica[a] (Spain)	K	2·25	3·75	1999	888·4	533	237	80·6	8·1	10·05
Psammodromus hispanicus[a] (Spain)	r	1·51	6·28	2820	1867·6	449	297·4	75·7	19·2	25·4
Sceloporus g. graciosus[b] (U.S.A.)	K	4·83[c]	10·4	12945	2680·1	1227	254	81·7	*	*
Sceloporus undulatus garmani[b] (U.S.A.)	r	3·70[c]	20·9	15457	4177·6	775	204·1	76·2	*	*

[a] Unpublished data from Patterson and Davies (1982b, c).
[b] Data from Derickson (1976a).
[c] Calculated from lean dry bodyweight data in Derickson (1976a) assuming 70% water content. These estimates exclude viscera.
* Data on annual energy income as food (C) not available.

C. Metabolic Rate

An animal's metabolic rate, which can be measured in terms of several physiological parameters but is usually assessed in terms of oxygen consumption, is commonly assumed to be a measure of that animal's rate of energy expenditure. In the case of oxygen consumption measurements, this assumption is valid providing the energy production is entirely aerobic, which in reptiles it probably is in most normal circumstances, though it is now clear that aerobic energy production can be greatly supplemented during violent activity by anaerobiosis (see later). Metabolic rate is probably the most extensively studied parameter of reptilian physiology, and the topic was reviewed by Bennett and Dawson (1976). By contrast, the cellular and biochemical aspects of metabolism in reptiles are very poorly understood, and have been studied in any detail in only five species (reviewed by Coulson and Hernandez, 1974). Though it is too early yet to be dogmatic, these studies reveal that in most basic respects, reptilian metabolic biochemistry is like that of other vertebrates (Bennett, 1972a).

Rate–Weight relations The relationship between metabolic rate and bodyweight in reptiles is, as in organisms generally, an allometric one of the general form $M = aW^b$, where M is the resting metabolic rate (vols O_2/hr), W is the body weight (g), and "a" and "b" are constants which can be determined empirically by regression analysis of rate-weight data on a double logarithmic plot: "a" is the y-intercept of the regression line and gives the metabolic rate of an hypothetical 1 g animal; "b" is the slope of the regression line. When metabolism is expressed in weight-relative terms (i.e. vols O_2/g/hr), the relationship is then negative and the equation becomes $\frac{M}{W} = aW^{(b-1)}$.

Much discussion and argument has centred around the values of the exponent "b" for reptiles, but the problem now seems to have been resolved by the very extensive re-analysis of rate-weight data and relationships carried out by Bennett and Dawson (1976). Their general equations for reptiles at 20°C and 30°C are as follows:

20°C: M (vols O_2/hr) = $0.102\,W^{0.80}$ or $\frac{M}{W}$ (vols/g/hr) = $0.102\,W^{-0.20}$

30°C: M (vols O_2/hr) = $0.278\,W^{0.77}$ or $\frac{M}{W}$ (vols/g/hr) = $0.278\,W^{-0.23}$

The regression line for the log-transformed rate-specific rate-weight data at 30°C ($\log \frac{M}{W} = \log.\ 0.278 - 0.23 \log W$) is shown in Fig. 2.11. The effect of temperature on rate-weight relationships is evidently to change the elevation of the regression line ("a") but not its slope

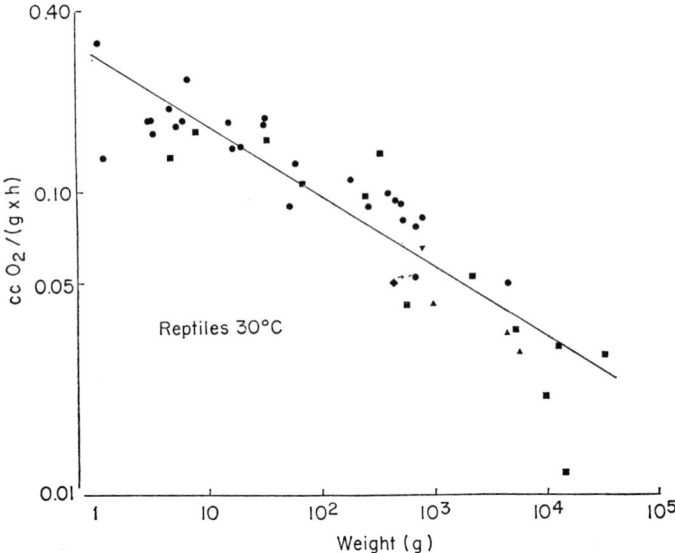

Fig. 2.11. The influence of bodyweight (W) on weight-specific metabolic rate (M/W) in reptiles at 30°C (double logarithmic plot). Circles: lizards; squares: snakes; triangles: turtles; inverted triangles: crocodilians; diamond: tuatara. The equation for the regression line is log M/W = log 0.278 − 0.23 log W. (From Bennett and Dawson, 1976).

("b"), for the regression exponents at 20°C and 30°C do not differ significantly from one another. Furthermore, they are encouragingly close to the exponent of 0·75 (or −0·25) which characterizes the rate-weight regression lines of organisms generally (Hemmingsen, 1960).

When reptiles are compared with birds and mammals, their weight specific resting metabolic rates are considerably lower over the entire weight range, even when comparisons are made at 37°C (Fig. 2.12). These differences appear to be due to certain quantitative differences at the cellular level related to aerobic energy production, in particular to the activity and density of mitochondria (Bennett, 1972a).

Temperature and activity In addition to its consistent (and perhaps primary) dependence on bodyweight, metabolic rate is also profoundly influenced by temperature and activity. This is well illustrated by the R-T curve of the desert lizard *Dipsosaurus dorsalis* (Bennett and Dawson, 1972) shown in Fig. 2.13. In this case, the Q_{10} value is different for each temperature interval in both resting and active

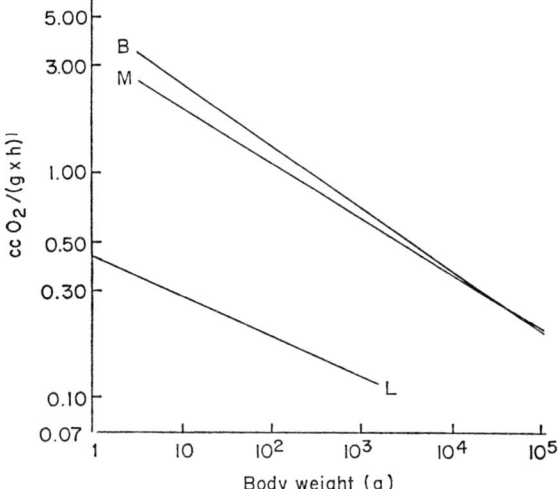

Fig. 2.12. Comparison of the weight-specific metabolic rate-weight lines for lizards (L) resting at 37°C with those of birds (B) and mammals (M) under 'basal' conditions. (From Bennett and Dawson, 1976).

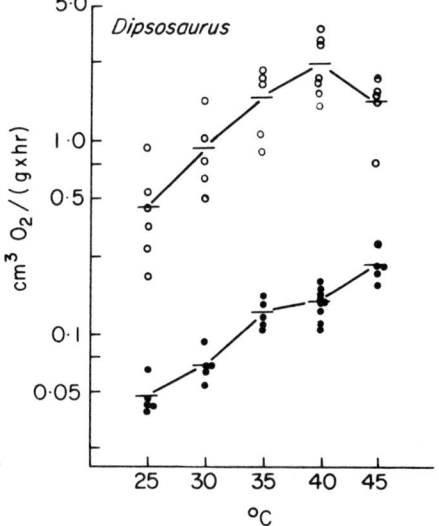

Fig. 2.13. The influence of temperature on resting (shaded circles) and active (open circles) oxygen consumption in the lizard *Dipsosaurus dorsalis* (semi-logarithmic plot). Conditions of maximal activity were produced by electrical stimulation for 2 minutes. Short horizontal lines indicate mean values. (From Bennett and Dawson, 1972).

animals, revealing the complexity of temperature effects in this species. Between 30°–40°C, the resting R-T curve levels off with a Q_{10} not significantly different from 1. This metabolic plateau is interesting, because it coincides with the range of body temperatures most commonly experienced by *Dipsosaurus* in the wild, and points to the existence of some degree of metabolic homeostasis within this range. Such plateaux have been reported in other reptiles (e.g. Aleksiuk, 1976b; Tromp and Avery, 1977; Davies and Bennett, 1981).

The separation between the resting and active curves in Fig. 2.13 represents the "aerobic scope for activity" and this also attains its maximum value at about 40°C, which is near the mean activity temperature of these animals (Bennett and Dawson, 1972). This correlation appears to be typical of reptiles. Being able to maximize energy production at normal body temperatures is clearly of adaptive value from the point of view of both prey capture and predator evasion.

The parameters of R-T lines such as these depend in many cases on thermal history and can be altered by the processes of thermal "acclimation" or "acclimatization", time-dependent compensatory adjustments the function of which is to mitigate in some degree the undesirable biochemical and physiological consequences of imposed body temperature changes (see Chapter 15). It is now quite evident that the ability to acclimate to temperature is widely distributed among reptiles (Bennett and Dawson, 1976; Patterson and Davies, 1978c), though precisely how this ability enhances fitness in the wild is less clear. Some insight is gained by comparing the acute R-T relationships of cold- and warm-adapted individuals and species in the laboratory (Murrish and Vance, 1968; Patterson and Davies, 1978c; Davies and Bennett, 1981). In a typical case, the two R-T curves will be displaced relative to one another, with the cold adapted line substantially above the warm line. Among other things, this means that at high temperatures, warm-adapted animals metabolize less rapidly than animals not adapted to high temperatures; and that at low temperatures, any given level of energy demand (as represented by the metabolic rate) is met by cold-adapted individuals (or species) at lower temperatures than it is by warm-adapted individuals. In both cases, the metabolic compensation observed makes excellent sense in terms of adaptation and survival, as it does in other cases where acclimation occurs over only part of the experienced temperature range (Patterson and Davies, 1978c).

Compensation of a rather different kind appears to be important during hibernation when, in addition to their dependence on reserves of energy in the form of lipids and glycogen (Avery, 1970; Derickson, 1976b; Patterson *et al*, 1978), some species effect physiological adjustments of metabolism which depress energy expenditure during dormancy to the lowest sustainable level, lower indeed than is found at the same temperature in non-dormant animals. In the case of *Lacerta vivipara*, negative compensation of this kind effects an estimated energy saving equivalent to approximately 35% of the total quantity of energy expended during hibernation (Patterson and Davies, 1978b). The occurrence of such metabolic adjustments highlights the importance of the distinction between cold-induced torpor (a passive, non-acclimatory response to low temperature) and true hibernation, or "brumation" as it is sometimes called in reptiles, which involves active physiological adjustments. Very little is currently known about the underlying biochemistry of these adjustments in reptiles (Aleksiuk, 1976a,b).

Anaerobiosis In recent years it has become increasingly apparent that anaerobically derived energy forms a substantial component of the total metabolic power output of reptiles during strenuous activity (Bennett, 1972b; Bennett and Dawson, 1972; Bennett and Licht, 1972; Ruben, 1976b). The low weight-specific metabolic rates of reptiles in comparison with those of birds and mammals and their relatively modest aerobic scopes, place severe limitations on their ability to generate sudden bursts of aerobic power. Reptiles have overcome these limitations to some extent by exploiting glycolytic modes of energy production and acquiring the ability to tolerate high blood lactate concentrations. The result is a remarkably effective, "short-burst" energy producing system.

The expectation that total energy production capacity (aerobic + anaerobic) will correlate with life-style is borne out by studies by Ruben (1976b), who found that agile, active snakes (*Coluber* and *Masticophis*) had markedly greater total energy-producing capabilities of at least ×2 than more heavy-bodied, sluggish species (*Crotalus*). At least 50% of the total metabolic power output in each case was anaerobic. Bennett and Dawson (1972) investigated the influence of temperature on the partitioning of total energy production in the lizard *Dipsosaurus dorsalis*, and found that anaerobiosis contributed 58–83% of the total energy produced during activity, depending on temperature, and that both aerobic scope and lactate production (i.e. total energy production capacity) reached a maximum at 40°C, which is within the normal activity range of this species and very close to the "preferred body temperature" (see below). Considerable oxygen debts are incurred by anaerobiosis in reptiles, and recovery times vary both between species and with temperature (Bennett, 1972b; Bennett and Dawson, 1976).

D. Thermoregulation

Since the pioneering studies of Cowles and Bogert (1944), it has become increasingly clear that reptiles are very far from being the passive, "cold-blooded" conformers to ambient temperature portrayed by earlier physiologists (Bogert, 1959; Avery, 1979). Reptiles are thermoregulators, and given access to adequate environmental sources of heat (usually the sun) are able to maintain body temperatures considerably in excess of ambient for long periods of time. Furthermore, these regulated temperautres tend to cluster about means which are both optimal for certain physiological functions and characteristic of the species (Bogert, 1949; Templeton, 1970; Dawson, 1975).

Preferred body temperature When reptiles are placed in laboratory thermal gradients, they tend to behave in ways which keep their body temperatures within a certain range (e.g. DeWitt, 1967), the extent of which varies from one species to another. Some species—particularly active heliothermic lizards—appear to have relatively narrow preferred body temperature ranges, while others regulate less precisely and have wider ranges. These differences almost certainly have adaptive significance (Patterson and Davies, 1982a). The mean (or sometimes median) of observed body temperatures in thermoregulating reptiles is generally referred to as the "preferred body temperature" (PBT) when the measurements are made in the laboratory, and the "eccritic temperature" when they are made in the field. PBTs vary between species, and are listed for many species in Licht *et al* (1966), Cloudsley-Thompson (1971) and Dawson (1975). Though commonly supposed to be genetically "set", PBT is known to vary seasonally and between the sexes in at least one reptile (*Lacerta vivipara*— Patterson and Davies, 1978a). There is also evidence that significant head–body temperature differences exist in some thermoregulating reptiles, and that head temperature is more precisely regulated than body temperature (Hammerson, 1977).

Since rate processes in biological systems are highly temperature dependent, it has long been assumed that the PBT represents an optimum for certain key physiological processes and capacities, though precisely which is only now beginning to become apparent.

Dawson (1975) lists the following processes as ones which have been shown to proceed optimally near the PBT in many species: metabolic capacities for activity, elimination of lactate levels incurred during activity, auditory sensitivity, digestion and egestion, immunological response, secretion and action of certain hormones, aspects of renal function, and certain reproductive processes.

Control mechanisms Body temperature regulation is achieved largely by behavioural means in reptiles, through the exploitation of the physical principles governing heat exchange (radiation, conduction, convection and evaporation). The behaviour patterns and postural orientations employed can often be quite complex (Heath, 1965; Smith, 1975) and in some species are assisted by morphological and physiological specializations (such as colouration, colour changes, vascular shunts and heat exchangers and even cardiovascular adjustments—see Section IV) which function as modulators of the rate of heat flow between the animal and its environment (Templeton, 1970; Cloudsley-Thompson, 1971). Unlike the birds and mammals, reptiles—with the single exception of the brooding Indian python (Hutchison *et al*, 1966)—have no capacity for endogenous thermogenesis in response to cold, and no insulative body covering to restrict the loss of what little metabolic heat is produced by the body.

The evident temperature dependence of many reptilian activities and processes, and the demonstrable phenomenon of thermoregulation, have prompted a number of workers to search for sites of thermo-regulatory control in the central nervous system. Several thermo-sensitive areas have been identified in various reptilian brains (Hammel *et al*, 1967; Cabanac *et al*, 1967; Heath *et al*, 1972), those located in the hypothalamus being the most intriguing because of the known importance of this structure in the body temperature regulating mechanism of mammals. However, the evidence for functional equivalence is suggestive rather than confirmed at present. Various neurosensory-control models have been proposed for reptilian thermoregulation, with considerable disagreement centering around the nature of the "thermostat" which controls thermo-regulatory behaviour. No general agreement has yet been reached (Templeton, 1970; Berk and Heath, 1975).

VI. Neuro-endocrine control

The integration of physiological and behavioural activities depends on the co-ordinated functioning of the nervous and hormonal systems. In general organization and functioning, these systems are essentially like those of other vertebrates, though in detail each vertebrate and reptilian group has its own peculiarities of structural and functional design, representing distinct adaptive responses to particular life-styles. Only an outline of reptilian neuro-endocrinology can be provided here.

A. Nervous system

Brain and spinal cord The gross anatomy of a typical reptilian brain is shown in Fig. 2.9A. The perceptual and behavioural advances of the reptiles over the amphibians are reflected in the increased complexity of most parts of the brain, but most notably in the enlargement of the cerebral hemispheres, optic lobes and cerebellum. In addition, the size of the brain relative to the size of the body has increased, cephalic flexure (the bending of the brain with respect to the line of the spinal cord, so pronounced in mammals) is apparent for the first time in the vertebrate evolutionary series, and two additional cranial nerves (the XIth and XIIth) have been added to the traditional ten. The reptilian spinal cord, unlike that of mammals, extends the whole length of the body to the tip of the tail, and possesses locomotor control centres which still retain a considerable amount of functional autonomy with respect to the controlling operations of the brain.

Sense organs The major senses of chemoreception, sight and hearing are well developed in most reptiles, though to differing extents in the different groups (Bellairs, 1969; Gans and Parsons, 1970a; Porter, 1972). One additional and quite remarkable sensory system is well developed only in certain snakes—thermoreception (Gamow and Harris, 1973).

Olfaction is a dual chemosensory system in most reptiles, mediated in part by sensory cells within the nasal chambers, and in part by the organs of Jacobson (Fig. 2.14D), ontogenetic derivatives of the embryonic nasal sac which, in lepidosaurians, develop into more or less separate olfactory structures with their own ducts into the mouth (Figs 2.4D, 2.14D) (Parsons, in Gans and Parsons, 1970a). This "vomeronasal" system reaches the highest level of development in the tongue–Jacobson organ complex of snakes, but precisely how its function differs, if at all, from that of the nasal olfactory system is not clear. A chemosensory system analogous to taste is also present in reptiles, in the form of taste buds (and occasionally sensory papillae—Burns, 1969) scattered liberally thoughout the oral epithelium (Luppa, 1977).

Reptilian eyes (Fig. 2.14A, B) differ from mammalian eyes in a number of interesting respects, many of them connected with the process of accommodation (Walls, 1942; Bellairs, 1969; Underwood, in Gans and Parsons, 1970a). However, the most aberrant reptilian eyes of all, apart from the degenerate eyes of certain burrowing species, are the eyes of snakes (Fig. 2.14B) which appear to have been reduced and then re-designed anew during the evolution of this group (Walls, 1942). The novel nature of the snake eye is nowhere more apparent than in the method of accommodation: instead of changing shape, as in other reptiles, the lens of the snake eye moves bodily forwards and backwards in response to pressure changes within the internal fluids of the eyeball. Varying degrees of colour vision (present in lizards and chelonians, largely absent in snakes and crocodiles) and binocular vision are present in reptiles, the latter being most highly developed in certain arboreal lizards (e.g. chameleons—Harkness, 1977) and snakes (e.g. *Ahaetulla*). Nocturnal habits are typically associated with a predominance of retinal rods and vertically elliptical pupils. Nocturnal geckos have serrated pupils (Fig. 2.14C), which help to increase visual acuity in poor light. The eyes are protected by a variety of accessory structures, in particular the eyelids and nictitating membrane. In snakes and geckos, the eyelids have become transparent and fused together to form an immobile spectacle, and the nictitating membrane has disappeared.

Many lizards and the tuatara possess a well developed "third", "pineal" or "parietal" eye on the top of the head, just below a hole in the parietal bone (Fig. 2.9A). Though the existence of this organ has been known for a long time, its function remains a mystery. Some experimental evidence suggests that it may be concerned with thermoregulation (Stebbins and Cohen, 1973; Ralph *et al*, 1979).

Though hearing is the most familiar function of the vertebrate ear, bodily equilibrium is its primitive role, and may well still be its most important function in reptiles. The basic structure of a typical reptilian ear is shown in Fig. 2.9E. It is less complex than the mammalian ear, most notably with respect to the absence of the coiled cochlea in the inner ear, and of the malleus and incus in the middle ear (Fig. 2.9D) (Baird, in Gans and Parsons, 1970a). Hearing is well developed in many reptiles, particularly those with an externally visible eardrum. In snakes and some lizards, the eardrum and cavity of the middle ear have disappeared, and the stapes articulates instead

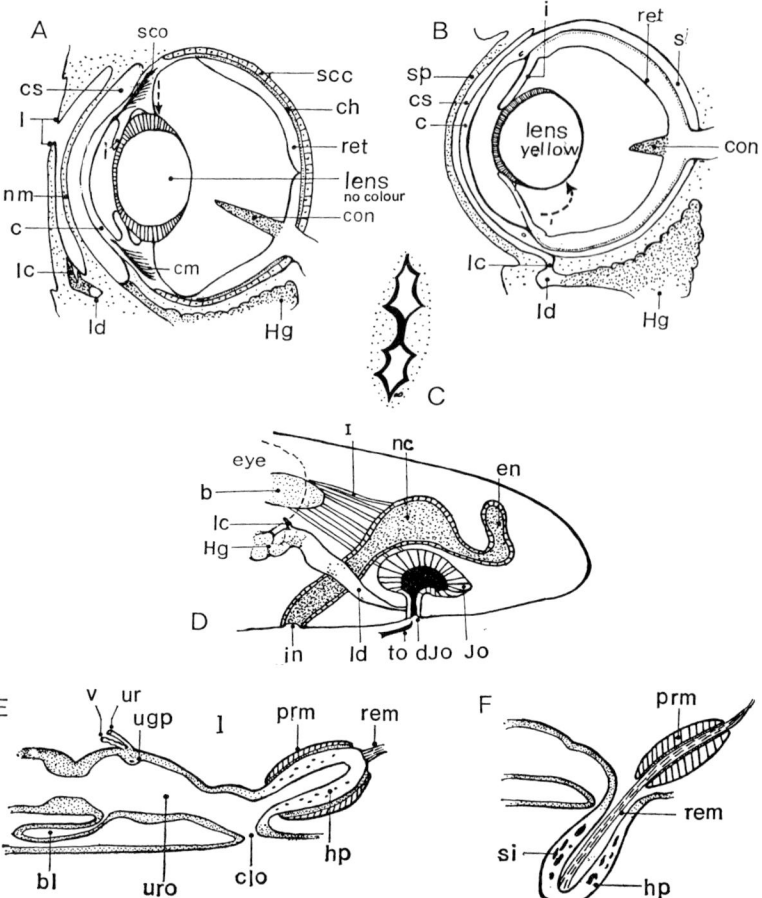

Fig. 2.14. (A,B) Cross-sectional diagrams of the eye in lizards (A) and snakes (B). The lachrymal duct and nictitating membrane actually lie near the front of the eye, not the middle as shown. Arrows show direction of force applied in accommodation. (C) Serrated pupil of gecko eye. (D) Diagram showing nose and organ of Jacobson in the snake, as seen in partly reconstructed longitudinal section. (E,F) Diagrams showing hemipenis of a squamate reptile in longitudinal section. E, retracted. F, everted. Left of figure is anterior. (From Bellairs and Attridge, "Reptiles")

b, brain (olfactory bulb); bl, bladder; c, cornea; ch, choroid; clo, cloacal opening; cm, ciliary muscle; con, conus papillaris; cs, conjunctival space; djo, duct of Jo; en, part of nasal cavity leading to external nostril; hg, Harderian gland; hp, hemipenis; i, iris; in, internal nostril; Jo, Jacobson's organ; lc, lachrymal canaliculus; ld, lachrymal duct; nc, nasal cavity; nm, nictitating membrane; prm, propulsor muscle of hemipenis; rem, retractor muscle of hemipenis; ret, retina; s, sclera; scc, scleral cartilage; sco, scleral ossicle; si, blood sinus; sp, spectacle; to, tongue tip; ugp, urogenital papilla; ur, ureter; uro, urodaeum; v, vas deferens; I, olfactory and vomeronasal nerves to Jo.

with the quadrate bone (Fig. 2.4C). This arrangement has lent support to the popular view that snakes cannot hear airborne sounds, and are sensitive instead only to vibrations carried through the substrate and bones of the body. However, electrophysiological studies by Wever and Vernon (1960) and Hartline (1971) have shown conclusively that in addition to being very sensitive to vibrations, snakes have an auditory system capable of hearing airborne sounds as well, over a limited and relatively low frequency range (150–600Hz), though what significance this ability has in their lives is not known. Hartline (1971) also produced evidence that the lung may be involved in this auditory system as a sound transmitter. The whole subject of hearing in reptiles has recently been reviewed at length by Wever (1978).

Thermoreception is most highly developed among crotaline vipers ("pit vipers"), but thermosensitive pits (or areas) of a less specialized nature occur around the lip margins of certain pythons and boas (Barret *et al*, in Gans and Parsons, 1970a; Gamov and Harris, 1973). The pit vipers have a richly innervated, thermosensitive pit between each eye and nostril which faces forwards, and together they act as a "stereoscopic" heat receptor, enabling these largely nocturnal animals to strike very accurately in the dark. The thermoreceptors are highly sensitive to infra-red radiation, and will respond to a temperature change within the pit of as little as 0·002°C (Bullock and Diecke, 1956). Other kinds of skin receptor probably exist but little is known about them. Nerve endings of the same basic kind that occur in the skin of mammals have been found in reptilian skin, and presumably serve the same range of sensory functions (Miller and Kasahara, 1967). Many lizards have hair-like epidermal structures which are thought to have a sensory function.

B. Endocrine system

The major components of the endocrine system were described in Gans and Parsons (1970b). The functional aspects of this system are perhaps less well understood in reptiles than in any other vertebrate class, but the available evidence suggests that in most basic respects, the system has not departed markedly from that of the amphibians (Porter, 1972).

Thyroid gland The thyroid is of variable size and shape and lies beneath the trachea just anterior to the heart (Figs 2.6, 2.9B). Thyroidectomy affects the sloughing cycle, growth rates, development and metabolism in various reptiles, confirming expectations that the gland produces a thyroxine-like hormone. The thyroid responds in a conventional way to the administration of thyroid stimulating hormone (TSH), suggesting that it is under pituitary control (Lynn, in Gans and Parsons, 1970b).

Parathyroid glands Not far from the thyroid, and close to the carotid and systemic arteries, are usually two pairs of parathyroid glands. In those few reptiles that have been studied, the evidence of experimental parathyroidectomy suggests that the hormone produced by this gland is involved in the regulation of blood calcium and phosphate levels, as it is in other vertebrates (Clark, in Gans and Parsons, 1970b).

Islets of Langerhans Pancreatic islets appear to contain both α and β cells in reptiles, though their relative abundance and pattern of distribution within the islets differ from group to group. α cells secrete glucagon, β cells secrete insulin, and experimental pancreatectomy causes diabetes, a clear indication that pancreatic hormones have the same blood sugar-regulating role in reptiles as they have in mammals (Miller and Lagios, in Gans and Parsons, 1970b).

Adrenal glands A pair of adrenal glands is present in all reptiles, closely associated with the gonads and urinogenital ducts in most cases (Figs 2.5B, 2.6), but with the kidneys in chelonians (Gabé, in Gans and Parsons, 1970b). Additional adrenal tissue may be found elsewhere, as for example in the kidneys of chelonians and crocodilians. Medullary and cortical tissues are distinguishable, but the former is usually scattered within the latter and does not form a separate layer as in mammals. Each of these tissues is assumed to produce the standard array of hormones—adrenaline and noradrenaline in the case of medullary tissue, and various corticosteroids in the case of cortical tissue. Adrenalectomy, in addition to interfering with the stress response mechanism (see Chapter 15), interferes with the regulation of salt and water balance.

Gonads When acting as endocrine glands, the gonads are responsible for secreting the sex hormones, androgens (e.g. testosterone) in the case of the testes, oestrogens in the case of the ovaries. Androgens are known to influence the development of secondary sexual characteristics in male reptiles, and will masculinize the development of female reproductive ducts and renal sex segments if administered experimentally to females. Sex hormone secretion is controlled by the pituitary, and the sex hormones themselves exert a feedback controlling influence on the pituitary. The corpora lutea of lizards and snakes produce progesterone, but since this hormone does not appear to be essential for the maintenance of pregnancy in these animals, its precise function is unclear.

Pituitary gland   As in other vertebrates, the pituitary appears to be the 'master gland' of the endocrine system, sitting as it does at one of the major crossroads of the neuroendocrine system (Fig. 2.9A) in intimate association with the hypothalamus, exercising a controlling influence over the secretory activities of all the other endocrine glands, and yet itself responsive to their secretions (Saint Girons 1970; Licht, 1974). Experiments involving hypophysectomy and the administration of mammalian hormones have revealed that reptilian pituitary hormones, like those of mammals, are profoundly implicated in the regulation of growth, reproduction, reproductive cycles, thyroid and adrenal activity. In addition, secretions of the pituitary similar in function to vasopressin (influencing kidney function and water resorption) and intermedin (influencing colour change) have been identified. However, the details of pituitary function and control have yet to be worked out in reptiles, and it may be premature to assume that they are identical in all important respects to those of other vertebrates.

References

Aleksiuk, M. (1976a). *Copeia* 1976, 170–178.
Aleksiuk, M. (1976b). *J. thermal Biol.* **1**, 153–156.
Andrews, R. M. and Asato, T. (1977). *Comp Biochem. Physiol.* **58A**, 57–62.
Avery, R. A. (1970). *Comp. Biochem. Physiol.* **37**, 119–121.
Avery, R. A. (1975). *Oecologia* **19**, 165–170.
Avery, R. A. (1979). "Lizards—a Study in Thermoregulation". Arnold, London.
Baer, J. G. (1964). "Comparative Anatomy of Vertebrates". Butterworth, London.
Bakker, R. T. (1971). *Evolution* **28**, 636–658.
Bakker, R. T. (1972). *Nature, Lond.* **238**, 81–85.
Bartholomew, G. A. and Lasiewski, R. C. (1965). *Comp. Biochem. Physiol.* **16**, 573–582.
Bellairs, A. d'A. (1969). "The Life of Reptiles". Weidenfeld and Nicholson, London.
Bellairs, A. d'A. and Attridge, J. (1975). "Reptiles". 4th edition. Hutchinson, London.

Benedict, F. G. (1932). "The Physiology of Large Reptiles". Carnegie Institution, Washington.
Bennett, A. F. (1972a) *Comp. Biochem. Physiol.* **42B,** 637–647.
Bennett, A. F. (1972b). *J. comp. Physiol.* **79,** 259–280.
Bennett, A. F. and Dawson, W. R. (1972). *J. comp. Physiol.* **81,** 289–299.
Bennett, A. F. and Dawson, W. R. (1976). *In* "Biology of the Reptilia". (C. Gans and W. R. Dawson, eds.), Vol 5, pp. 127–223. Academic Press, London and New York.
Bennett, A. F. and Licht, P. (1972). *J. comp. Physiol.* **B1,** 277–288.
Bentley, P. J. (1976). *In* "Biology of the Reptilia". (C. Gans and W. R. Dawson, eds.), Vol 5, pp. 365–412. Academic Press, London and New York.
Bentley, P. J. and Blumer W. F. C. (1962). *Nature, Lond.* **194,** 699–700.
Bentley, P. J. and Schmidt-Nielsen, K. (1965). *J. cell. comp. Physiol.* **66,** 303–309.
Bentley, P. J. and Schmidt-Nielsen, K. (1966). *Science* **151,** 1547–1549.
Bentley, P. J. and Schmidt-Nielsen, K. (1970). *Comp. Biochem. Physiol.* **32,** 363–364.
Bergman, R. A. M. (1961). *Acta. morph. neerl.-scand.* **4,** 195.
Berk, M. L. and Heath, J. E. (1975). *J. thermal Biol.* **1,** 15–22.
Blain, A. W. and Campbell, K. N. (1942). *Am. J. Roentg.* **48,** 229–239.
Bogert, C. M. (1949). *Evolution* **3,** 195–211.
Bogert, C. M. (1959). *Sci. Am.* **200,** 105–120.
Boltt, R. E. and Ewer, R. F. (1964). *J. Morph.* **114,** 83–106.
Bradshaw, S. D. and Shoemaker, V. H. (1967). *Comp. Biochem. Physiol.* **20,** 855–865.
Bragdon, D. E. (1953). *Anat. Rec.* **117,** 145–161.
Brazaitis, P. J. (1969). *Br. J. Herpet.* **4,** 54–58.
Bullock, T. H. and Diecke, F. P. J. (1956). *J. Physiol. Lond.*, **134,** 47–87.
Burns, B. (1969). *Copeia* 1969, 617–619.
Cabanac, M., Hammel, H. T. and Hardy J. D. (1967). *Science* **158,** 1050–1051.
Clark, B. D., Gans, C. and Rosenberg, H. I. (1978). *Respir. Physiol.* **32,** 207–212.
Cloudsley-Thompson, J. L. (1968). *Nature, Lond.* **220,** 708.
Cloudsley-Thompson, J. L. (1969). *Br. J. Herpet.* **4,** 107–112.
Cloudsley-Thompson, J. L. (1971). "The Temperature and Water Relations of Reptiles". Merrow, Watford, Herts.
Cole, C. J. (1975). *In* "Intersexuality in the Animal Kingdom". (R. Reinboth, ed.), pp. 340–355. Springer-Verlag, Heidelberg.
Coulson, R. A. and Hernandez, T. (1974). *In* "Chemical Zoology, IX, Amphibia and Reptilia". (M. Florkin and B. T. Scheer, eds.), pp. 217–247. Academic Press, New York and London.
Cowles, R. B. and Bogert, C. M. (1944). *Bull. Am. Mus. Nat. Hist.* **83,** 261–296.
Crawford, E. C. and Kampe G. (1971). *Am. J. Physiol.* **220,** 1256–1260.

Dandifrosse, G. (1974). *In* "Chemical Zoology, IX, Amphibia and Reptilia". (M. Florkin and B. T. Scheer, eds.), pp. 249–275. Academic Press, New York and London.
Dantzler, W. H. (1976). *In* "Biology of the Reptilia". (C. Gans and W. R. Dawson, eds.), Vol 5, pp. 447–503. Academic Press, London and New York.
Dantzler, W. H. and Schmidt-Nielsen, K. (1966). *Am. J. Physiol.* **210**, 198–210.
Davies, P. M. C. and Bennett, E. L. (1981). *J. comp. Physiol.* **142**, 489–494.
Dawson, W. R. (1975). *In* "Perspectives in Biophysical Ecology". (D. M. Gates and R. B. Schmerl, eds.), Ecological Studies 12, pp. 443–473, Springer-Verlag, Heidelberg.
Derickson, W. K. (1976a). *Ecology* **57**, 445–458.
Derickson, W. K. (1976b). *Am. Zool.* **16**, 711–723.
Desmond, A. J. (1977). "The Hot-Blooded Dinosaurs". Futura, London.
Dessauer, H. C. (1970). *In* "Biology of the Reptilia". (C. Gans and T. S. Parsons, eds.), Vol 3, pp. 1–72. Academic Press, London and New York.
DeWitt, C. B. (1967). *Physiol. Zool.* **40**, 49–66.
Diefenbach, C. O. Da C. (1973). *Physiol. Zool.* **46**, 72–78.
Duguy, R. (1970). *In* "Biology of the Reptilia". (C. Gans and T. S. Parsons, eds.), Vol 3, pp. 93–109. Academic Press, London and New York.
Dunson, W. A. (1976). *In* "Biology of the Reptilia". (C. Gans and W. R. Dawson, eds.), Vol 5, pp. 413–445. Academic Press, London and New York.
Dutton, R. H., Fitzpatrick, L. C. and Hughes, J. L. (1975). *Ecology* **56**, 1378–1387.
Edmund, E. G. (1969). *In* "Biology of the Reptilia" (C. Gans, A. d'A. Bellairs and T. S. Parsons, eds.) Vol I, pp. 117–200. Academic Press, London and New York.
Enlow, D. H. (1969). *In* "Biology of the Reptilia". (C. Gans, A. d'A Bellairs and T. S. Parsons, eds.), Vol 1, pp. 45–80. Academic Press, London and New York.
Fitch, H. S. (1970). *Univ. Kansas Mus. Nat. Hist. Misc. Pub.* **52**, 1–247.
Fitzpatrick, L. C. (1973). *Ecol. Monogr.* **43**, 43–58.
Flaxman, B. A. (1972). *Am. Zool.* **12**, 13–25.
Fox, H. (1977). *In* "Biology of the Reptilia". (C. Gans and T. S. Parsons, eds.), Vol 6, pp. 1–157. Academic Press, London and New York.
Frazzetta, T. H. (1966). *J. Morph.* **118**, 217–296.
Fry, F. E. J. (1947). *Publs. Ontario Fish. Res. Lab.* **68**, 1–62.
Gadgil, M. and Bossert, W. H. (1970). *Am. Nat.* **104**, 1–25.
Gamow, R. I. and Harris J. F. (1973). *Sci. Am.* **228**, 94–100.
Gans, C. (1961). *Am. Zool.* **1**, 217–227.
Gans, C. (1970). *Forma et Functio* **3**, 61–104.
Gans, C. (1974). "Biomechanics". Lippincott, Philadelphia.
Gans, C. and Clark, B. (1976). *Respir. Physiol.* **26**, 285–301.
Gans, C. and Parsons, T. S. (eds.) (1970a). "Biology of the Reptilia". Vol 2. Academic Press, London and New York.

Gans, C. and Parsons, T. S. (eds.) (1970b). "Biology of the Reptilia". Vol 3. Academic Press, London and New York.
Gasc, J. P. (1976). *In* "Morphology and Biology of Reptiles". (A. d'A. Bellairs and C. B. Cox, eds.), pp. 177–190, Linn. Soc. Symp. Series, No. 3, London.
Gaunt, A. S. and Gans, C. (1969a). *J. Morph.* **128,** 195–218.
Gaunt, A. S. and Gans, C. (1969b). *Nature, Lond.* **223,** 207–208.
Girgis, S. (1961). *Comp. Biochem. Physiol.* **3,** 206–217.
Gray, J. (1968). "Animal Locomotion". Weidenfeld and Nicolson, London.
Greenberg, N. (1977). *Am. Zool.* **17,** 153–286.
Guibé, J. (1970). *In* "Traité de Zoologie". (P. P. Grasse, ed.), Vol. 14(2), pp. 521–548. Masson, Paris.
Haas, G. (1973). *In* "Biology of the Reptilia". (C. Gans and A. S. Parsons, eds.), Vol 4, pp. 285–490. Academic Press, London and New York.
Halstead, L. B. (1969). "The Pattern of Vertebrate Evolution". Oliver and Boyd, Edinburgh.
Hammel, H. T., Caldwell, F. T. and Abrams, R. M. (1967). *Science* **156,** 1260–1262.
Hammerson, G. A. (1977). *Comp. Biochem. Physiol.* **57A,** 399–402.
Harkness, L. (1977). *Nature, Lond.* **267,** 346–349.
Hartline, P. H. (1971). *J. exp. Biol.* **54,** 349–371.
Hawley, A. W. L. and Aleksiuk, M. (1976). *Comp. Biochem. Physiol.* **53A,** 215–221.
Heath, J. E. (1965). *Univ. Calif. Publ. Zool.* **64,** 97–136.
Heath, J. E., Williams, B. A., Mills, S. H. and Kluger, M. J. (1972). *In* "Hibernation and Hypothermia: Perspectives and Challenges". (F. E. South, J. P. Hannon, J. R. Willis, E. T. Pengelley and N. R. Alpert, eds.), pp. 605–627. Elsevier, Amsterdam.
Hemmingsen, A. M. (1960). *Rep. Steno Mem. Hosp. Nord. Insulinlab.* **9,** 1–110.
Hoffman, L. H. (1970). *J. Morph.* **131,** 57–87.
Hoffstetter, R. and Gasc, J-P. (1969). *In* "Biology of the Reptilia". (C. Gans, A.d'A. Bellairs and T. S. Parson, eds.), Vol 1, pp. 201–310. Academic Press, London and New York.
Howell, B. J. and Rahn, H. (1976). *In* "Biology of the Reptilia". (C. Gans and W. R. Dawson, eds.), Vol 5, pp. 335–363. Academic Press, London and New York.
Hughes, G. M. (1965). "Comparative Physiology of Vertebrate Respiration". Heinemann, London.
Hutchison, V. H., Dowling, H. G. and Vinegar, A. (1966). *Science* **151,** 694–696.
Jackson, D. C. (1971). *Am. J. Physiol.* **220,** 754–758.
Jackson, D. C. and Schmidt-Nielsen, K. (1966). *J. cell Physiol.* **67,** 225–232.
Johansen, K. and Lenfant, C. (1972). *In* "Oxygen Affinity of Hemoglobin and Red Cell Acid Base Status". (M. Rorth and P. Astrup, eds.), pp. 750–783. Munksgaard, Copenhagen.

Judd, H. L., Bacon, J. P., Ruëdi, D., Girard, J. and Benirschke, K. (1977). *Int. Zoo Yb.* **17,** 208–209.
Kardong, K. (1974). *Forma et Functio* **7,** 327–354.
Laszlo, J. (1975). *Int. Zoo. Yb.* **15,** 178–179.
Licht, P. (1965). *Physiol. Zool.* **38,** 129–137.
Licht, P. (1972). *Gen. comp. Endocr.* Suppl. **3,** 477–488.
Licht, P. (1974). *In* "Chemical Zoology IX, Amphibia and Reptilia". (M. Florkin and B. T. Scheer, eds.), pp. 399–448. Academic Press, New York and London.
Licht, P., Dawson, W. R., Shoemaker, V. H. and Main A. R. (1966). *Copeia* 1966, 97–110.
Luppa, H. (1977). *In* "Biology of the Reptilia". (C. Gans and T. S. Parsons, eds.), Vol 6, pp. 225–313. Academic Press, London and New York.
Maderson, P. F. A. (1964). *Br. J. Herpet.* **3,** 151–154.
Maderson, P. F. A. (1965). *J. Zool. Lond.* **146,** 98–113.
Maderson, P. F. A. (1972). *Am. Zool.* **12,** 12–171.
Maderson, P. F. A. and Chiu, K. W. (1970). *Herpetologica* **26,** 233–238.
Maslin, T. P. (1971). *Am. Zool.* **11,** 761–780.
McDonald, H. S. (1959). *Herpetologica* **15,** 193–198.
Miller, M. R. and Kasahara, M. (1967). *Proc. Calif. Acad. Sci.* **34,** 549–568.
Mittwoch, U. (1978). *New Scientist* **78,** 750–752.
Morgareidge, K. R. and White, F. N. (1969). *Nature, Lond.* **223,** 587–591.
Murrish, D. E. and Vance, V. J. (1968). *Comp. Biochem. Physiol.* **27,** 329–337.
Naifeh, K. H., Huggins, S. E. and Hoff, H. E. (1970). *Respir. Physiol.* **10,** 338–348.
Osborn, J. W. (1973). *Am. Sci.* **61,** 548–559.
Ottaviani, G. and Tazzi, A. (1977). *In* "Biology of the Reptilia". (C. Gans and T. S. Parsons, eds.), Vol 6, pp. 315–462. Academic Press, London and New York.
Packard, G. C., Tracy, C. R. and Roth, J. J. (1977). *Biol Rev.* **52,** 71–105.
Parsons, T. S. and Cameron, J. E. (1977). *In* "Biology of the Reptilia". (C. Gans and T. S. Parsons, eds.), Vol 6, pp. 159–223. Academic Press, London and New York.
Patterson, J. W. and Davies, P. M. C. (1978a). *J. thermal. Biol.* **3,** 39–41.
Patterson, J. W. and Davies, P. M. C. (1978b). *J. thermal Biol.* **3,** 183–186.
Patterson, J. W. and Davies P. M. C. (1978c). *Nature* **275,** 646–647.
Patterson, J. W. and Davies, P. M. C. (1982a, b, c). (in preparation).
Patterson, J. W., Davies, P. M. C., Veasey, D. A. and Griffiths, J. R. (1978). *Comp. Biochem. Physiol.* **60B,** 491–493.
Peaker, M. Linzell, J. L. (1975). "Salt Glands in Birds and Reptiles". Cambridge University Press.
Pianka, E. R. (1970). *Am. Nat.* **104,** 592–597.
Platt, D. R. (1969). *Univ. Kansas Pub. Mus. Nat. Hist.* **18,** 253–420.
Porter, K. R. (1972). "Herpetology". W. B. Saunders, Philadelphia.

Pough, F. H. (1976). *Physiol. Zool.* **49**, 141–151.
Pough, F. H. (1977a). *J. exp. Zool.* **201**, 47–56.
Pough, F. H. (1977b). *J. comp. Physiol.* **116**, 337–345.
Pough, F. H. (1977c). *Comp. Biochem. Physiol.* **57A**, 435–441.
Pough, F. H. (1977d). *Physiol. Zool.*, **50**, 77–87.
Ralph, C. L., Firth, B. T., Gern, W. A. and Owens, D. W. (1979). *Biol. Rev.* **54**, 41–72.
Romer, A. S. (1956). "Osteology of Reptiles". University of Chicago Press, Chicago.
Romer, A. S. (1966). "Vertebrate Paleontology". University of Chicago Press, Chicago.
Romer, A. S. and Parsons, T. S. (1977). "The Vertebrate Body". 5th edition. W. B. Saunders, Philadelphia.
Ruben, J. A. (1976a). *J. Exp. Zool.* **197**, 313–320.
Ruben, J. A. (1976b). *J. comp. Physiol.* **109**, 147–157.
Rudall, K. M. (1947). *Biochem. biophys. Acta* **1**, 549.
Russell, F. E. and Brodie, A. F. (1974). *In* "Chemical Zoology, IX, Amphibia and Reptilia". (M. Florkin and B. T. Scheer, eds.), pp. 449–478. Academic Press, New York and London.
Saint Girons, M-C. (1970). *In* "Biology of the Reptilia". (C. Gans and T. S. Parsons, eds.), Vol 3, pp. 73–91. Academic Press, London and New York.
Schmidt-Nielsen, K., Borut, A., Lee, P. and Crawford, E. (1963). *Science* **142**, 1300–1301.
Shine R. and Bull J. J. (1979) *Am. Nat.* **113**, 905–923.
Skoczylas, R. (1970a). *Comp. Biochem. Physiol.* **35**, 885–903.
Skoczylas, R. (1970b). *Comp. Biochem. Physiol.* **33**, 793–804.
Skoczylas, R. (1979). *In* "Biology of the Reptilia". (C. Gans and K. A. Gans eds.). Vol 8. pp. 589–719. Academic Press, London and New York.
Smith, E. N. (1975). *Physiol. Zool.* **48**, 177–194.
Standaert, T. and Johansen, K. (1974). *J. comp. Physiol.* **89**, 313–320.
Stebbins, R. C. and Cohen, N. W. (1973). *Copeia* 1973, 662–668.
Sullivan, B. (1974). *In* "Chemical Zoology, IX, Amphibia and Reptilia". (M. Florkin and B. T. Scheer, eds.), pp. 377–398. Academic Press, New York and London.
Tammar, A. R. (1974). *In* "Chemical Zoology, IX, Amphibia and Reptilia". (M. Florkin and B. T. Scheer, eds.), pp. 337–351. Academic Press, New York and London.
Templeton, J. R. (1970). *In* "Comparative Physiology of Thermoregulation". (G. C. Whittow, ed.), Vol 1, pp. 167–221. Academic Press, New York and London.
Tinkle, D. W. (1969). *Am. Nat.* **103**, 501–516.
Tinkle, D. W. and Gibbons, J. W. (1977). *Misc. Publ. Mus. Zool. Univ. Mich.* **154**, 1–55.
Tinkle, D. W., Wilbur, H. M., and Tilley, S. G. (1970). *Evolution* **24**, 55–74.
Tromp, W. I. and Avery, R. A. (1977). *J. thermal Biol.* **2**, 53–54.
Vinegar, A. (1974). *Herpetologica* **30**, 72–74.

Walls, G. L. (1942). "The Vertebrate Eye and Its Adaptive Radiation". Cranbrook Institute of Science, Michigan, Bull. No. 19.
Webb, J. E., Wallwork, J. A. and Elgood, J. H. (1978). "Guide to Living Reptiles". Macmillan, London.
Wever, E. G. (1978). "The Reptile Ear: Its Structure and Function". Princeton University Press, Princeton, USA.
Wever, E. G. and Vernon, J. A. (1960). *J. Aud. Res.* **1,** 77–83.
White, F. N. (1973). *Comp. Biochem. Physiol.* **45A,** 503–513.
White, F. N. (1976). *In* "Biology of the Reptilia". (C. Gans and W. R. Dawson, eds.), Vol 5, pp. 275–334. Academic Press, London and New York.
Wilson, L. D. (1968). *J. Herpetol.* **1,** 93–94.
Windell, J. T. and Sarokon, J. A. (1976). *Herpetologica* **32,** 18–23.
Wood, S. C. and Lenfant, C. J. M. (1976). *In* "Biology of the Reptilia". (C. Gans and W. R. Dawson, eds.), Vol 5, pp. 225–274. Academic Press, London and New York.

Note added in proof:

Since this chapter was written, two further volumes of the "Biology of the Reptilia" have been published which provide a very extensive review of reptilian neurobiology: Gans, C., Northcutt, R. G. and Ulinski, P. (eds.) (1979) Biology of the Reptilia, Vols 9 and 10, Academic Press, New York and London. Included among the contributions to Vol 9 is a paper by W. B. Quay on the parietal eye-pineal complex.

3 Pathology and Histopathological Techniques

E. ELKAN

Department of Histopathology, Mount Vernon Hospital, Northwood, Middlesex, England

> Accuse not nature, she hath done her part
> Milton, *Paradise Lost*

I. Introduction

The pathologist who deals with reptiles is at a considerable disadvantage compared with his counterparts in human and veterinary medicine. There are over 6000 species of reptile (Goin and Goin, 1962) and many of these differ considerably in appearance and structure; in some cases little is known of their normal biology. Reptiles are not of great economic importance and therefore financial support, which can so often be obtained for research on mammals, birds and fish, is rarely forthcoming.

Although there are important scientific arguments for more work on pathology in reptiles, the need for a text on the subject arises mainly from the ever repeated requests by amateur herpetologists, zoos and laboratories for assistance over the causes of death of specimens in their care. However, the pathologist who is presented with this kind of material soon realizes that his task is very different from that facing human or veterinary pathologists. In particular, the latter have at their disposal text books dealing with the basic normal histology of the species to be investigated. There are but a few publications on reptiles—for example, on the tuatara (*Sphenodon punctatus*) (Gabe and Saint Girons, 1964)—although some more general texts include these animals in their remit (Leake, 1975). Data on the normal biology of the Reptilia may also be found in the series of volumes edited by Gans (1966 and continuing); this monumental work covers both morphology and physiology of the Class. Relevant scientific publications on the pathology of reptiles are dispersed within journals of many countries and the few existing text books are not detailed enough to cover the enormous field. For some guidance, readers are referred to "Krankheiten der Reptilien" (Reichenbach-Klinke, 1977) which reviews publications up to 1976 and "The Principal Diseases of Lower Vertebrates" (Reichenbach-Klinke and Elkan, 1965). Examples of pathological lesions are also depicted in the "Color Atlas of the Diseases of Fishes, Amphibians and Reptiles" (Elkan and Reichenbach-Klinke, 1974). The paucity of published data on reptilian pathology is, perhaps, due partly to a tendency for lower vertebrates to be excluded in comparative texts; for example, in a fairly recent book on comparative pathology (Gresham and Jennings, 1962) the word "reptile" does not even appear in the index. A large comparative histopathology of the lower vertebrates would be invaluable.

In the investigation of diseases of reptiles it is not, unfortunately, sufficient for the pathologist to extrapolate from human or veterinary pathology. The cellular responses are often different and some of the conditions encountered are unusual. Many factors may contribute towards disease, amongst them parasites, trauma, inadequate housing, poor hygiene, malnutrition, metabolic disturbances, a multiplicity of infections and infestations and—less commonly—congenital malformations and tumours. Many reptilian specimens submitted for pathological examination come from establishments where the animals have been kept for varying periods under unsatisfactory conditions. As a result much of the material is of poor quality and the pathological lesions observed are frequently a manifestation of poor husbandry rather than indicative of underlying disease.

There is, as was implied earlier, an urgent need for more experimental research on reptile disease. There are many topics that warrant investigation, for example, cardiovascular disease in the iguana (*Iguana iguana*) (see Chapters 12 and 15). However, acquisition of material poses many problems and often the pathologist, domiciled thousands of miles away from his subject's country of origin, can only keep his doors open, hoping that the mail will bring him specimens in an investigable condition.

This last prerequisite is, unfortunately, unlikely to be fulfilled. On

April 30th 1977 the British Medical Journal, under the heading "Materia non Medica" published the lament of a retired dentist and his melancholic reminiscences on surveying the part of his garden set aside as a cemetery for the cats, hamsters, guinea-pigs, fish and other animals which he and his family had nursed over the years to the bitter, though inevitable, end. Not one of these specimens, some of which may have died from unusual or otherwise interesting conditions, was offered to a laboratory where their sad demise might have contributed to veterinary pathology. As it happens, this dentist was no herpetologist, but if he had been, he would certainly, instead of rodents, cats and fish, have interred snakes, lizards and tortoises with the same sentiment and the same disregard for animal pathology. Nor would he have been alone in this negative attitude towards science. Innumerable small vertebrates are maintained as "pets" in Europe and North America. Few of them survive for very long. Most end up like the dentist's hamsters. In spite of repeated appeals for material, the author's experience is that only the smallest trickle finds its way to a pathological laboratory. It is therefore necessary to repeat what has often been said before. Every specimen which has died is worthy of examination; the results may appear trivial, but frequently they are of great interest.

II. Pathological Examination

Reptiles for pathological examination should be examined as soon as possible after death. A detailed *post mortem* examination should be carried out and note taken of the appearance and position of the organs. Details of *post mortem* technique will not be given here. The reader is referred to the section on the removal of tissues later in this chapter and to the descriptions given in Reichenbach-Klinke and Elkan (1965).

Gross *post mortem* examination of reptiles should be coupled with laboratory techniques. Although histopathological examination is of great importance and will be discussed later, other disciplines must not be ignored, amongst them parasitology, haematology and microbiology. In addition, it should not be forgotten that radiography may help in the evaluation of some cases, even *post mortem*.

Whenever possible, blood smears should be made while the animal is still alive because *post mortem* samples often show artefacts. The techniques for blood sampling are discussed in Chapter 16 and for haematological investigation in Chapter 4.

Microbiological techniques are discussed in detail in Chapter 4. The detailed identification of pathogenic bacteria is rarely possible outside a suitably equipped laboratory. It is important to take swabs from the affected organs and to plate these out on culture media without delay; if this is not done, commensal bacteria, which multiply speedily after death, will invade the internal organs, making the identification of the original causal organism very difficult.

It might be concluded that these difficulties could be overcome by freezing the specimen and sending it to the nearest laboratory when thoroughly refrigerated. But this method too has its limitations. If a specimen is frozen, ice crystals form inside the cells and will rupture them; as a result the histological picture becomes completely distorted, particularly so in the parenchymatous organs like the liver, the spleen, the kidney or the brain. If, therefore, a specimen cannot be immediately examined it may be cooled but it should not be frozen. If histopathological examination alone is intended, the best method of fixing the entire specimen is immersion in either 5–10% formaldehyde or 70% alcohol.

It is quite useless, however, to have a general "stock pot" filled with either solution, into which the specimens are deposited and forgotten. The skin of all reptiles is far too tough and impermeable for such a technique to be successful; while the solution may fix the skin, putrefaction continues apace within. Again and again specimens are submitted which look normal enough from the outside, while the internal organs are transformed into a indefinable mass.

In the case of small specimens, the body cavity should be well filled by injection with fixing solution immediately after death. Large specimens must be dissected and the relevant parts of organs fixed separately. These pieces must be small—preferably only 1 cm cube—and fixed in ten times their own volume of fixative. If the brain is to be fixed adequately, the skull can be split or a small hole drilled into the brain case so that fixative can penetrate.

An important consideration is how specimens should be packed if they are to be sent by post. Small lizards, tortoises or terrapins should be pinned down on cork mats, allowed to harden overnight and then packed in plastic bags. Snakes should not be wound up like a ball of wool. Once they harden in that position they are extremely awkward to dissect. They should either be wound up in the form of a spiral or in the shape of a sidewinder before they are allowed to harden. Either way they are easy to pack. In any case, their length should be recorded before they are hardened. Care must be taken to follow the appropriate postal regulations when despatching such material; in

Britain, for example, suitable containers must be used and these should be sent by First Class Post, marked "Pathological Specimen" (see Chapter 4).

Although the whole carcass is best for examination, specific tissues can be submitted. A person accustomed to work with a scalpel, scissors and forceps can remove the internal organs, fix and pack them. For this purpose a midline incision should be made, circumventing the anus on either side and continuing to the tip of the tail; anteriorly it should extend to the mandibular symphysis (see Fig. 3.1). It is then possible to remove all the viscera including the tongue

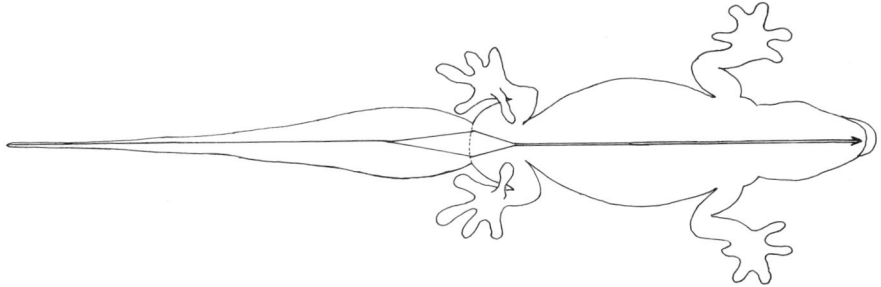

Fig. 3.1. Diagram showing the ventral incision of a lizard or snake for the *en bloc* removal of the viscera. The incision is made with scissors and a scalpel. Note the circumvention of the cloaca; the latter should be kept in continuity with the large intestine and the penes. Stronger scissors are needed for the cutting of the pectoral and pelvic girdles.

and the penes—if present—in one block. In the case of chelonians heavier scissors or a wire saw may be needed to cut the bridges between the plastron and the carapace. Altogether the dissection of chelonians needs more care than that of other reptiles and a working knowledge of their anatomy is important (see Chapter 2).

III. The Preparation of Sections

A. General

Histopathological examination depends upon the production of sections of high quality. The techniques used differ little from those used in human and veterinary work and reference should be made to a standard text such as that by Cook (1974). The microtomist may prefer to make frozen sections which, in addition to being available rapidly, are necessary for demonstrating certain substances such as fat. Plastic media have been little used in work with reptiles but are likely to become more popular in future.

Usually, however, tissues are thoroughly fixed in formaldehyde, dehydrated through alcohols and xylene and eventually embedded in paraffin blocks. The blocks are used for sectioning with the conventional wax microtome. Electron-microscopy will not be discussed here but where available has an important part to play. However, it is not the extreme resolution and the highest magnification which are usually required for routine work on herpetological material. The more instructive pictures are very frequently obtained by the use of low power objectives with a wide flat field. Regrettably, routine laboratory microscopes are rarely equipped with such lenses, nor do they have condensers suitable for wide-field photography.

Specimens which contain bone must be decalcified prior to embedding. Several methods are available and were reviewed in a recent paper by Eggert and Germain (1979). Decalcification is indispensable for all sections through the head, vertebral column or other specimens that include bone. When small specialized organs such as the parietal eye are to be examined, the whole head must be decalcified before the surplus tissue is removed and the central portion embedded. It is then necessary to prepare "serial" (consecutive) sections because only a few of them are likely to produce the optimal result. This is time-consuming but, in the end, a rewarding procedure.

B. Staining

The staining of tissues is of the utmost importance. There is no great difference between the methods employed by human and veterinary histologists and similar techniques are usually satisfactory for reptiles. As a routine procedure the time honoured haematoxylin–eosin method, invented by Ehrlich and subsequently modified in a number of ways, is still completely satisfactory. Where the staining quality of the material is poor, mordanting with celestin-blue sometimes improves the result. Many methods are suitable for bacteria, but the author's choice is that of Gram-Weigert. Gram-negative organisms, which are often a cause of disease in reptiles (see Chapter 6), are not easy to demonstrate in tissues, but two stains that have proved useful for reptilian material are Brown and Brenn (Holt et al, 1979) and Gram-MGPLG (Cooper et al, 1978). The Ziehl–Neelsen stain is used for acid-fast organisms while Giemsa and periodic acid Schiff (PAS) methods are useful for protozoal parasites. Some of these stains are described in Chapter 4; details of others may be obtained from standard histological texts (see, for example, Cook, 1974).

Some of the chemical qualities of tissues or their components can be demonstrated by staining procedures. This applies particularly to mucous substances, calcium and fat. Muco-polysaccharides may be demonstrated by prestaining the haematoxylin–eosin sections with Alcian Blue or by using the periodic acid Schiff method; the results depend upon the type of muco-polysaccharide involved. Calcium and its salts are demonstrable by von Kossa's method and fat is stained, in frozen sections only, by osmic acid, oil red o or one of the Sudan dyes.

Canada balsam which was formerly used world-wide for the final mounting of the sections under glass, has now been superseded by many variants of plastic material which have the advantage that they do not turn yellow with age. A popular example is DPX (Distrene 80 and dibutyl phthalate in xylene).

C. Whole Mounts

It is sometimes desirable to make whole mounts of small worms or even tissues. These must be flattened between glass slides while fresh and then fixed in that position for several days. They are subsequently dehydrated, positioned on the glass slide and covered with successive layers of mountant. When they are completely covered, a final layer of mountant is applied and the whole covered by a cover slip. With a little patience and experience it is possible, by this method, to make satisfactory whole mounts without the ever-intrusive air bubbles. Very small worms or flukes can, before dehydration, be stained with alum carmine solution. Helminthology is by no means a closed chapter and new species, particularly those affecting reptiles, may yet be discovered by anyone with sufficient patience to look for them. Parasites should, therefore, either be submitted for identification whole or preserved as described above. It is also possible to prepare histological sections of parasites but a specific identification of the offending species is rarely possible.

D. Biopsies

Tissues from living animals can also be examined and should be dealt with in the same way as *post-mortem* material. The taking of biopsy specimens is discussed in Chapter 17.

IV. Photography of Pathological Material

Those involved in dissections of reptiles should be equipped with a good photographic outfit so that pictures, both in colour and in black and white, can be taken as soon as anything unusual is discovered and while the specimen or lesion is still *in situ*. This prerequisite is of great importance, since few pathological conditions make good and instructive pictures once the respective organs have been separated from the carcass and from the remaining viscera. Such pictures need an adaptable lighting system and a reliable exposure meter. Dishes of various size and depth are useful because some specimens may need to be photographed under water to avoid disturbing reflections. Background sheets of various colours and shades of grey should be used to provide the necessary contrast.

V. Pathological Responses in Reptiles

Interpretation of pathological lesions in reptiles is not easy, as examples later in this chapter will demonstrate. There is a paucity of information available on the responses of these animals to such insults as trauma, infection and parasites and the need for experimental work must again be emphasized.

Nevertheless, there is increasing evidence from routine histopathological examination of reptiles that these species can react in a variety of ways to injury and infection. Many of the changes seen are similar to those in mammals: for example, cells may show degeneration and death or, in other cases, may proliferate or demonstrate metaplasia. Both acute and chronic inflammation are recognized in reptiles but they are less distinct than in mammals. "Chronic" inflammatory cells, usually lymphocytes and histiocytes, are often a feature of inflammatory processes while the more "acute" type of cells such as eosinophils and heterophils are more frequently associated with parasitic infestations and bacterial infection. Fibrosis can occur and is very often seen in healed wounds, as a response to parasites and around abscesses or "pseudotumours" (see later).

Further examples of the pathological responses of reptiles may be found in the succeeding portion of this chapter. In addition, a useful paper is that by Cowan (1968) who described a number of conditions and pathological lesions in reptiles including amyloidosis, hepatitis, pancreatic and skin lesions.

An important point is that pathological processes in reptiles are temperature-dependent; this has been demonstrated in experimental work—for example on renal disease (Zwart, 1963).

VI. Some Pathological Conditions of Reptiles

In order to demonstrate the role of pathology in the investigation and diagnosis of reptile disease a selection of cases will be discussed and attention drawn to particularly interesting features.

A. Accidents

Traumatic injuries are discussed in detail in Chapter 11.

Predation occurs both in captivity and in the wild and in some cases the circumstances are bizarre. For example, a small green lizard (*Lacerta viridis*) was placed in a cage with a female slow-worm (*Anguis fragilis*). The slow-worm gave birth to several young. The lizard swallowed one of them but this resulted in impaction of the stomach and death of both predator and victim.

A surprising cause of death was diagnosed in a Gaboon viper (*Bitis gabonica*) which, having thrived during four years of captivity, died for no obvious reason. *Post mortem* examination revealed the presence of two of its own fangs which had pierced the duodenum, causing a large pancreatic abscess, septicaemia and death. It is probably normal for vipers to swallow their own fangs when they are replaced but one would expect them either to be decalcified or to pass through the intestinal tract uneventfully. This case demonstrates the value of a *post mortem* examination in elucidating the cause of death.

Accidents can, in certain circumstances, be "iatrogenic", i.e. they can be due to the efforts of the owner to cure the animal of diseases it may—or may not—have. A fully grown specimen of an African sand snake (*Psammophis punctulatus*) died three days after an attempt to treat it with an anthelmintic. The snake was long and agile and had, not surprisingly, objected to the introduction of a catheter into its mouth. The combined efforts of the owner and an assistant were insufficient to steady the snake.

At *post mortem* examination gross inspection revealed what appeared to be perforation of the stomach. Microscopy, however, revealed that the mucosa of the stomach was detached over a large area; this had induced the formation of multiple abscesses and the largest of these had perforated the muscular coat of the stomach, thereby causing peritonitis, septicaemia and death. It should be mentioned, as a postscript to this case, that no intestinal parasites were found in the specimen.

Finally there are accidents which do not lend themselves to an immediate explanation. A captive boa constrictor (*Constrictor constrictor*) died suddenly, having refused food for several months. The only abnormality which could be found on dissection was an intussusception of the small intestine. That this was not an agonal condition was shown by the fact that the affected part of the gut was firmly embedded in adhesions. The intussusception had produced an obstruction so that food could not pass down the intestinal tract and the snake had died without showing any significant clinical signs.

B. Infectious and Parasitic Diseases

Diseases due to infectious agents and parasites are of great importance in reptiles and are discussed in detail in other chapters of this book. Relatively little is known about the natural viral and bacterial ecology of reptiles, but it is probable that the latter, coming into captivity, find themselves assailed by a number of infectious agents against which they have little or no resistance. Their susceptibility to such infections is often enhanced by other factors such as poor nutrition or adverse environmental factors. Examples abound of cases where human communities have been decimated because of exposure to new pathogens, and a similar situation may apply to reptiles. An overwhelming challenge of organisms may have a similar effect. The moral may be to leave reptiles where they occur naturally and not to expose them to the trauma and challenges of captivity.

Details of bacteria responsible for infections in reptiles will be found in Chapter 6 and information on the microbiological examination of samples in Chapter 4. Here it should only be re-emphasized that all bacterial investigations must be carried out immediately after death or, preferably, *ante mortem*. Even a delay of a few hours can produce false results. Histopathology plays an important role in confirming the diagnosis—for example, in demonstrating organisms and lesions (such as micro-abscesses or pneumonia) in the tissues.

Viruses and fungi are discussed in Chapters 5 and 7 respectively. The isolation of such agents needs specialized techniques but histopathology can again aid diagnosis.

Protozoal infections (see Chapter 8) can sometimes be diagnosed clinically, especially if the causal organisms are excreted in the faeces. The difficulty is that many produce few or no clinical signs and are therefore often not suspected. Diagnosis is often made *post mortem* when the parasites are seen in blood smears or histological sections.

Helminths are of great importance in reptiles and are discussed in Chapter 9. Some of these parasites may manifest themselves quite openly if they are seen in the buccal cavity or excreted in the faeces. Others may remain undetected for a long time and are often only found at *post mortem* examination. For example, an Australian water lizard (*Physignathus lesueuri*) lived in captivity in England for nine years and showed no clinical signs. When it died, nematodes of the genus *Capillaria* were found throughout the body, including the cerebral capillaries. This and other cases emphasize that it is always important to open the alimentary tract of reptiles *post mortem* in order to search for parasites and to take samples for histopathological examination.

It is not only the intestinal tract that may yield helminths at *post mortem* examination. Trematodes are frequently found in the ureters, the renal pelvis and the kidney where they can cause hydronephrosis. In one case examined by the author, nearly every Bowman's capsule was distended and filled with nematode larvae. Other helminths may be found encysted, for example in the body wall or on the peritoneum, while the nematode *Capillaria recurva* distributes her eggs under the stratum corneum of the ventral skin of crocodiles (see Chapter 9).

Ectoparasites are discussed in detail in Chapter 10. Ticks and mites are common ectoparasites of reptiles and can cause disease or death due to blood loss or transmission of blood-borne infections. Such parasites should be detected during clinical investigation but are often only found when the reptile is examined *post mortem*.

C. Effects of Captivity

Knowledge of disease in free-living reptiles is limited and most information is based upon investigation of animals in captivity. As was implied earlier, captivity itself plays an important part in the cause or exacerbation of disease. When assessing the effect of captivity on a reptile, the pathologist dissecting the specimen will pay particular attention to (1) the fat body, (2) the liver, and (3) the cardiovascular system, especially the large arteries.

Only prolonged starvation or an extreme burden of parasites will reduce the fat body visibly. If, therefore, the fat body is reduced or absent it can be assumed that the specimen has been exposed to severe hardship. This can be the case in reptiles which fail to feed in captivity. Such animals may take several months to die and at *post mortem* examination are found to be emaciated; often there are secondary infections such as stomatitis.

Occasionally one finds large amounts of fat still stored in the fat bodies of reptiles known to have died of starvation or following a long, debilitating disease. This syndrome has been recognized since 1934 when Rollinat divided these deposits into two parts: the élément constant and the élément variable. The élément variable is relatively labile and can be readily mobilized. The élément constant, however, is part of the anatomical structure of the reptile and is not available for metabolic needs, apparently even *in extremis*.

Death due to inanition is probably not caused by lack of disposable fat alone but by equally severe disturbances in the carbohydrate, nitrogen and protein metabolism; reviews of this subject were published by Butler (1889), Baldwin (1970) and Elkan (1980).

In a freshly caught or recently imported reptile the liver is a deep brown-red colour and firm to the touch. In reptiles which have been kept in captivity for a long period the liver is often enlarged, grey to yellow, friable and, when examined histologically, contains large quantities of fat. There can be little doubt that this state of affairs is due to two factors associated with captivity, (a) overfeeding, and (b) lack of exercise. In its normal habitat a reptile spends much of its waking hours hunting for food. In this pursuit it is by no means always successful and most reptiles are able to survive without food for considerable periods. The herpetologist who keeps these animals in captivity is inclined to overfeed them and to feel that to deny them a constant supply of food is an act of cruelty. Yet one dissection after another shows that more cruelty lies in confining normally active animals in small cages and in overfeeding them. An easy solution to this problem cannot be offered, because captivity means new, changed and uncongenial surroundings and, as is pointed out in Chapter 15, the reptile often cannot adequately adapt or "acclimatize" itself to these.

In the case of the reptile's arteries the situation is less clear. The author has frequently seen cases of atheromatosis and calcification of the media in reptiles, especially the common iguana (*Iguana iguana*). The cause of these conditions is uncertain and there is a need for research on the subject (see Chapter 12). It is very difficult to obtain exact data on these cases and usually impossible to examine control animals. Ideally the latter should be freshly caught and not subjected to any artificial diet. In such an experimental role the iguana might prove a suitable model for unravelling some of the controversies regarding cardiovascular disease.

Age has a bearing on the losses in herpetological collections. In its natural habitat an old, debilitated reptile will soon be killed by predators or succumb to intercurrent disease. Aged specimens are therefore not likely to be caught by collectors. In captivity, however, reptiles may live for a considerable length of time and under such circumstances certain pathological processes may show an apparent increased incidence, such as neoplasia and cardiovascular disease (see Chapter 15).

While neoplasia and medial calcification are probably diseases of old age, other conditions tend to affect young reptiles. In the case of avitaminosis A, the patients most severely affected are very young terrapins, many of which die at the hands of ignorant owners (see Chapter 12). The clinical features of avitaminosis A are typical (Elkan and Zwart, 1967). The eyelids swell until they meet, causing blindness. A chelonian which cannot see refuses to feed and ultimately dies of starvation. The diagnosis is confirmed *post mortem*. Histological sections reveal severe metaplasia of the Harderian gland and identical changes in the renal pelvis and the ureters. The epithelium in these latter sites becomes stratified and desquamates profusely; as a result it blocks the passage of urine, resulting in renal damage as well as starvation. Many young terrapins also suffer from a calcium/phosphorus imbalance due to an inadequate supply of calcium. As a result the "shell" fails to harden properly and later becomes deformed. This condition is usually diagnosed clinically but may also be detected at *post mortem* examination. Any dead chelonian which appears to have a soft shell should be radiographed and tissues taken for histopathological examination.

Metabolic disorders are frequently a feature of captivity and are discussed elsewhere in this book. Gout is probably the most important. If one knew more about such diseases and had better means of investigating them one might well find that they play a much larger role in reptiles than is commonly assumed. The pathologist, in particular, is limited to a few histochemical procedures in order to make a diagnosis. A case examined by the author serves to demonstrate the difficulties which may arise.

A Russell's viper (*Vipera russelli*), died three weeks after being imported from Thailand. Its previous history was unknown. The specimen was well preserved in formaldehyde when it arrived at the laboratory. The only obvious abnormality noted was the presence of innumerable brilliant white foci throughout the parenchyma of the liver.

Histological sections showed that most of the liver had been destroyed and replaced by small granulomata and that between these were deposits, sometimes fan-shaped, sometimes clumped, of highly birefringent material. It required the collaboration of histochemists to demonstrate that the crystals were, in fact, urates in a particularly insoluble form, since they remained unaffected by all the various solvents used in processing the sections.

Urates are the normal end product of protein metabolism. They are usually produced by the liver but eliminated by the kidneys. However, in the event of renal damage or certain other circumstances they accumulate in the blood and are deposited in visceral organs, especially the liver and pericardium (see Chapter 12).

Search for urate deposits in other organs of the viper proved unsuccessful. It appeared, therefore, that this snake died of an unusual kind of gout which has not previously been recorded.

D. Tumours and Pseudotumours

The dictionary definition of the word "tumour" is a "swelling". In everyday medical language the term usually means a malignant growth or, in the case of the "benign" tumour, a growth which displaces but does not invade adjacent tissues. In reptiles, however, one encounters well-defined swellings which are of bacterial origin. If they appear under the skin they can be removed surgically without difficulty. If they affect the liver or other internal organs, they usually cannot be treated. The author refers to these growths as "psuedotumours" because their structure is totally different from the "true" tumours, whether benign or malignant. Some pseudotumours show features of chronic abscesses, with a central core of caseous debris surrounded by a fibrous capsule and inflammatory cell reaction, but others are predominantly cellular and resemble granulomata. They can only be investigated in detail in histological sections. A series of such cases was described by Elkan and Cooper (1976). *Enterobacter*, *Escherichia coli* and *Staphylococcus epidermidis* were isolated but it was not possible to determine whether any of these was the aetiological agent. This condition is also commonly seen in other reptile species. A striking case was a pigmy rattlesnake (*Sistrurus catenatus*) which presented with a severely distorted head, suggesting a tumour of the skull. However, dissection and histopathological examination revealed a large subcutaneous granuloma covering the whole dorsal aspect of the head. Other smaller lesions were subsequently found disseminated among the intestinal tract.

True tumours (neoplasms) occur in reptiles and are discussed in detail in Chapter 13. They can only be diagnosed accurately if examined histopathologically. Of the relatively benign tumours only the dermal papilloma occurs with any frequency. Like the mammalian wart, it is a response to a viral invasion through a minute breach of the skin—made, perhaps, by the stylus of a tick. Once started, the cauliflower-like growth can spread to other sites. The mouth and cloaca are most frequently involved. An enormous acanthosis develops and bacteria and fungi may multiply between the layers of desquamating skin. The worst cases occur in lizards, where the whole head may become involved, including the nares which become totally blocked by desquamating keratin. In chameleons cloacal papillomata have been found accompanied by a profuse infestation with the protozoan parasite *Entamoeba invadens*. Whether the parasite appeared on the scene as an opportunist or as the prime cause of the disease remains uncertain.

Malignant tumours have been recorded from reptiles on a number of occasions and may involve a variety of tissues. For example, Elkan and Cooper (1976), cited earlier, described a mesenteric adenocarcinoma in a boa constrictor which produced a metastatic deposit close to the thyroid and a fatal mesenchymosarcoma in the left forelimb of a *Lacerta sicula*. The latter invaded the body cavity and spread to the lung and the mesentery. Tumours may be detected incidentally during *post mortem* examination, as instanced by the finding in a boa constrictor of a cardiac rhabdomyosarcoma too small to be the cause of death.

The pathologist investigating neoplastic diseases in reptiles must be prepared to carry out a detailed and systematic search of the body organs. For example, a melanoma in a snake was characterized by deposits of malignant cells in nearly every organ (Elkan, 1974). No secondary deposits were found in the brain though one was found in the ventricle, another in the pulp of a tooth and a third on the surface of the penis.

E. Developmental Abnormalities

Developmental abnormalities are relatively uncommon in reptiles and warrant careful scrutiny by the pathologist. In addition to those described in Chapter 14, hamartomata are worthy of mention. An example diagnosed by the author was a splenic hamartoma in a Russell's viper (*Vipera russelli*). The lobular tumour contained splenic cells in a reticulum totally different from that of the spleen. Such lesions are not usually pathogenic.

F. Conditions of Uncertain Aetiology

Despite increased knowledge of reptile pathology, lesions are regularly encountered which cannot be explained or interpreted (see also Chapter 15). It is important that such conditions are investigated and documented and here the pathologist has an important part to play. Three cases recently reported by the author (Elkan, 1979) will be used as examples.

The first was a Sinai cobra (*Walterinnesia aegyptia*) which died of a disease of the kidneys indistinguishable from sarcoidosis: no organisms could be detected. The second concerned two specimens of the Columbian terrapin (*Pseudemys ornatus callirostris*) which died from a type of granuloma, one splenic, one renal, which has not been seen elsewhere. The granulomata occurred in the form of sterile microabscesses lined with giant cells in palisade formation. A detailed description of this interesting condition is given elsewhere (Reichenbach-Klinke, 1977). The third case was a Florida king snake (*Lampropeltis getulus floridana*); this regularly developed subcutaneous multilobular cysts which gradually filled with calcified debris. The cysts were not adherent to the surrounding tissue and could be "shelled out" without difficulty. Several of them were removed surgically from the live snake but new ones appeared at different sites. Early in 1979 the snake had to be killed on account of a fibrosarcoma which, however, appeared to be unconnected with the dermal condition. Examination of a portion of skin *post mortem* revealed cysts of 2–6 mm diameter in the dermis. All the cysts were lined with typical epithelium and enclosed in a connective tissue capsule. They contained keratinous debris and many rectangular prisms of calcium phosphate. Gram staining showed a profusion of intracystic bacteria but no bacteria were seen outside the cysts. Bacteriological culture yielded *Staphylococcus aureus*, *Escherichia coli* and a *Pseudomonas* sp. No definitive diagnosis has yet been made on this case. Originally it was felt that the most appropriate diagnosis was one of tumoral calcinosis, a condition described in humans by Slavin *et al* (1973). However, it remains to be seen whether this is correct.

These and many other cases indicate the importance of pathological examination of tissues removed surgically from live reptiles and emphasize that any specimen which dies or has to be killed should be submitted for a full macroscopical and microscopical examination.

In this chapter the pathological investigation of reptiles has been outlined. It plays an important role in disease diagnosis and research and every effort should be made to ensure that it is used to the full.

References

Baldwin, E. (1970). "An Introduction to Comparative Biochemistry". 4th edition. Cambridge University Press.
Butler, G. W. (1889). *Proc. zool. Soc. Lond.* 602–631.
Cooper, J. E., Needham, J. R. and Griffin, J. (1978). *Lab. Animals* **12**, 91–93.
Cowan, D. F. (1968). *J. Am. vet. med. Ass.* **153**, 848–859.
Cook, H. C. (1974). "Manual of Histological Demonstration Techniques". Butterworth, London.
Eggert, F. M. and Germain, J. P. (1979). *Histochemistry* **5a**, 215–224.
Elkan, E. (1974). *J. comp. Path.* **84**, 51–57.
Elkan, E. (1979). *Br. J. Herpet.* **6**, 15–17.
Elkan, E. (1980). *Br. J. Herpet.* **6**, 75–77.
Elkan, E. and Cooper, J. E. (1976). *J. comp. Path.* **86**, 337–348.
Elkan, E. and Reichenbach-Klinke, H. (1974). "Color Atlas of the Diseases of Fishes, Amphibians and Reptiles." T.F.H. Publications, Reigate, England.
Elkan, E. and Zwart, P. (1967). *Path. Vet.* **4**, 201.
Gabe, M. and Saint Girons, H. (1964). "Histologie de *Sphenodon punctatus* Gray." Centre National de la Recherche Scientifique, Paris.
Gans, C. (1966 and continuing). "Biology of the Reptilia." Academic Press, New York and London.
Goin, C. J. and Goin, O. B. (1962). "Herpetology." W. H. Freeman and Co., San Francisco and London.
Gresham, G. A. and Jennings, A. R. (1962). "Introduction to Comparative Pathology." Academic Press, New York and London.
Holt, P. E., Cooper, J. E. and Needham, J. R. (1979). *J. small Anim. Pract.* **20**, 269–286.
Leake, L. D. (1975). "Comparative Histology." Academic Press, New York and London.
Reichenbach-Klinke, H. (1977). "Krankheiten der Reptilien." 2nd Edition. G. Fischer, Stuttgart and New York.
Reichenbach-Klinke, H. and Elkan, E. (1965). "The Principal Diseases of Lower Vertebrates." Academic Press, New York and London.
Rollinat, E. (1934). "La Vie des Reptiles de la France Centrale". Librairie Delagrave, Paris.
Slavin, G., Klenerman, L., Darby, A. and Bansal, S. (1973). *Brit. med. J.* **1**, 147–150.
Zwart, P. (1963). "Studies on Renal Pathology in Reptiles". Thesis, University of Utrecht.

4 Microbiology and Laboratory Techniques

J. R. NEEDHAM

Division of Comparative Medicine, Clinical Research Centre, Watford Road, Harrow, Middlesex, England

I. Introduction

Before treatment of an infectious disease can be carried out it is advisable to diagnose the infection and, where possible, to isolate the causative agent. In this chapter methods will be described that will assist a successful diagnosis. As many reptile collections are in the care of persons without formal scientific background it is the author's intention to detail several basic tests as well as the more complex diagnostic investigations. Particular emphasis will be laid upon bacteriology with brief mention of parasitology, haematology and clinical chemistry; other techniques are discussed in more detail elsewhere in the book.

II. Equipment and Techniques for Bacteriology

A. Equipment

If only basic procedures are envisaged, with referral of specimens to reference laboratories, it will only be necessary to set aside a small area for the work and this can be equipped on a small budget. If, however, a wide spectrum of investigations is to be undertaken, a laboratory will be required and the financial outlay will necessarily be much greater.

Essentials include a variable temperature incubator, two refrigerators (4°C), a waterbath, microscope and a portable autoclave or pressure cooker. In addition to these, a cabinet or hood should be constructed to enable *post mortem* examinations to be undertaken (see later). When choosing these items there are several points that should be considered. As will be shown later, it is advantageous to carry out the incubation of microbiological cultures at several temperatures with an adjustable incubator. Two refrigerators are essential, one for infected materials, including carcasses, and the other for uncontaminated items such as culture media and reagents. In a large laboratory one refrigerator may be replaced by a cold room, in which culture material can be stored. Freezer space should be available for the storage of sera and cadavers not required for microbiological or histopathological examination. A waterbath is desirable for several tests, particularly when a steady temperature is required. This can easily be achieved if the bath is fitted with an impeller which mixes the water. A binocular microscope has many advantages over a monocular model, particularly because it induces less eye strain when used for a long period. It is essential that it is equipped with several objective lenses, including an oil immersion lens, a sub-stage condenser with diaphragm and, for ease of operation, an integral light source. A portable autoclave has been included in the list because of its many functions such as the decontamination of waste materials and the sterilization of instruments and culture media.

If specimens suitable for microbiological investigation are to be collected from cadavers at autopsy, it is desirable to carry out *post mortem* examination in a protective hood or cabinet. The primary object is to protect the worker from possible infection by organisms present in the carcass and liberated as an aerosol. The cabinet may be totally enclosed and fitted with high efficiency filters on both the air inlets and extracts. This arrangement will also ensure that the specimen is protected from contamination by the environment. More simply the worker can be protected by an open fronted structure with a perspex lid through which the worker can see the carcass (Fig. 4.1). In most cases it is not necessary to use an enclosed cabinet. Working in these cabinets is restrictive because of the limited space available and the difficulties do not justify their routine use, except when it is suspected that the carcass may be infected with a zoonotic organism. However, if *post mortem* examinations are carried out regularly, their use is desirable and staff soon become accustomed to them.

Numerous other small items that will be required include microscope slides, cover slips, staining racks and instruments. These will be covered in subsequent sections.

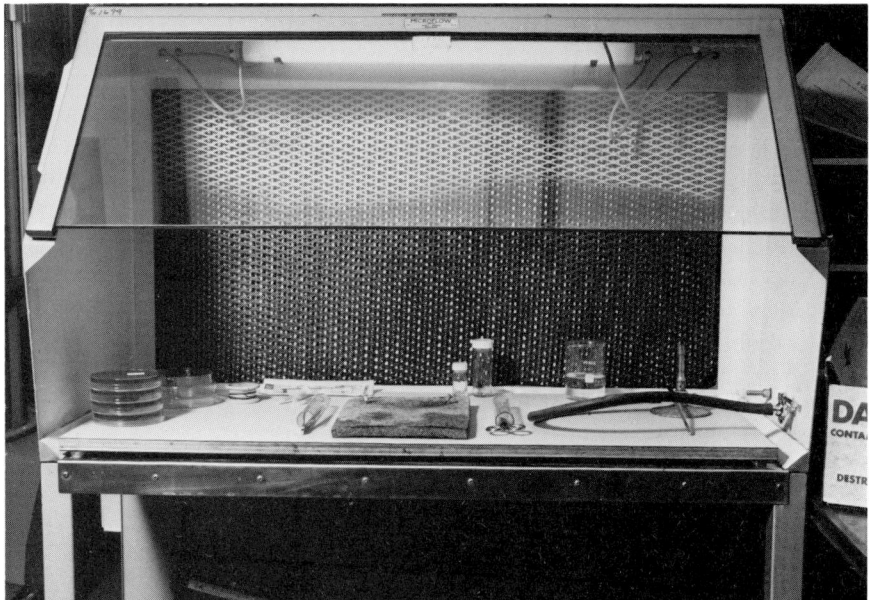

Fig. 4.1. Simple open fronted cabinet for *post mortem* examinations, complete with Bunsen burner, bacteriological agar plates, cork board and instruments.

B. Disinfection, Disposal and Hygiene

There are several categories of waste. Contaminated waste includes all carcasses, body fluids and exudates, cultures of micro-organisms and the various types of containers that have been in contact with them. Disposal of these items must be accomplished so as not to endanger workers and other animals in the collection. Carcasses should be incinerated; if this is not practical they may be sterilized in the autoclave before disposal. All plastic items, such as petri dishes containing agar cultures, should be rendered sterile by autoclaving and not by incineration, as many will not burn. Contaminated glassware may be autoclaved but pipettes should be placed immediately in a solution of sodium hypochlorite containing 10 000 parts/million of chlorine and left for at least 24 hours before rinsing and washing.

The inside of the *post mortem* cabinet deserves special mention. When an enclosed version is used, the air inlets and extracts may be sealed and the cabinet fumigated with formalin, a particularly efficient method (Newsom and Walsingham, 1974). The extract filters can also be evaluated microbiologically (Needham, 1981) after fumigation. Non-enclosed models may be disinfected by wiping with sodium hypochlorite solution.

The second category consists of items that may be described as contaminated and combustible. These include all paper waste from the laboratory, as well as material from the cage or vivarium, and these items should be treated as described for infected carcasses. A third category comprises non-contaminated glassware, which is best dealt with by adequate washing, but it should be remembered that corrosive waste products must be adequately labelled to avoid accidents.

It is essential that disinfectants employed in the laboratory are used correctly. Details are given by Maurer (1974). Disinfectants should be applied at suitable concentrations to achieve quick effective disinfection of articles (Needham, 1978).

C. Stains and Reagents

Many microbiological identification procedures rely on various staining techniques and specialized reagents. Some of the reagents required need to be used freshly prepared and hence cannot be purchased in their final form.

Simple stains may be used to show the morphology of bacterial cells, the easiest method being that using Löeffler's methylene blue (Baker, 1967).

However, a preferable technique utilizes Gram's stain. This is probably the most important stain used in bacteriology and enables bacteria to be divided into two groups—Gram-positive or Gram-negative. The original method was described by Gram in 1884. Since then various modifications have been suggested, including those by Kopeloff and Beerman (1922) and Preston and Morrell (1962). The latter is of value to those workers who wish to simplify the differentiation stage of the technique, as it incorporates iodine–acetone in place of 100% acetone. The author has found the following method to give a very reliable result when dealing with smears of bacteria and swabs taken from reptiles.

1. Flood smear after fixing with 0·5% aqueous crystal violet for 30 seconds and then wash off with water.
2. Flood smear with Lugol's iodine (Baker, 1967) for 1 minute and then wash off.
3. Differentiate with acetone. The acetone should be poured on the smear and washed off after 5 seconds. (If the smear is very thick this stage should be repeated.)

4. Counterstain the smear with 0·5% aqueous safranin for 30 seconds and then wash off with water.

After blotting dry the smear should be viewed using oil immersion.

This method has always given clear results. Gram-positive organisms stain blue-black, whereas Gram-negative organisms are red. It must be remembered that it is not uncommon for non-viable Gram-positive rods to stain Gram-negative.

It is sometimes of value to demonstrate the presence of spores. This is desirable because small spores inside a bacillary body may be missed and the position of the spore acts as a diagnostic aid. A simple staining method can be used and is described below:

1. Prepare, dry and fix a thin smear of the organism.
2. Flood the smear with 5% aqueous malachite green, gently warm and leave for 5 minutes before washing with water.
3. Counterstain with 0·5% aqueous safranin for 30 seconds and wash off.

Blot dry and view the slide under oil immersion, when the spores will be seen stained green and vegetative bacteria red.

The third commonly used stain is the Ziehl–Neelsen method for the staining of acid-fast bacilli. Originally Ehrlich (1882) reported a method which was modified by Ziehl and Neelsen and described by Johne (1885). The method uses basic fuchsin in alcoholic phenol which, when heated, penetrates the bacillus.

A smear is made.

1. Flood the smear with filtered carbol fuchsin and warm until steam rises. The time required is 10 minutes and at intervals the slide must be reheated. It is essential that no part of the slide becomes dry.
2. Wash with distilled water.
3. Decolourize with 20% sulphuric acid. The end of this process is taken when the smear is a very faint pink in colour.
4. Counterstain with Löeffler's methylene blue for 30 seconds. Wash and blot dry.

When viewed with an oil immersion objective the small bacilli are bright red and the background a pale blue.

Other less common stains can also be used, such as capsule stains and flagellar stains, and details can be found in standard bacteriological reference books.

In addition to the staining techniques described above, the identification of micro-organisms also relies on reagents that cannot be readily purchased. Some will be described later, together with details of the technique in which they are applied.

D. Collection of Specimens

A variety of specimens may be useful in disease diagnosis.

Swabs

Probably the greatest number of samples arrive at a microbiological laboratory on a swab. There are many different types available. The use of cotton wool swabs is not a recent innovation but dates back to the turn of the century (Hewlett and Nolan, 1896). Since that time the use of swabs has been studied with particular reference to the survival of organisms and their subsequent recovery in the laboratory.

Swabs may now be purchased readily from laboratory equipment suppliers and it is only necessary to stock three different types. Plain cotton wool swabs are probably most satisfactory when there is to be a short time interval between collection of the specimen and its examination. Serum coated swabs, however, are beneficial when a long delay is likely, as occurs when specimens are posted to the laboratory, or when fastidious organisms are involved. Both these types of swab have fairly large plegets of wool measuring some 15 mm in length by 7 mm in width, wound round a wooden stick. This, however, means that they may be too large to sample small sites accurately, and in these cases the use of nasopharyngeal swabs is advocated. These consist of a fine wire handle with a small pleget of alginate wool at one end (Fig. 4.2). Because of their thin wire support these swabs may also be considered safer to use when taking, for example, cloacal samples.

Sites

Often the living animal has a surface lesion that is easily sampled—for example, the skin, shell, mouth or throat.

Skin lesions are frequently encountered in reptiles and often involve ulcers. It is easy to obtain material from these using a small swab (Fig. 4.3). The swab should be rubbed against the lesion, if possible towards the periphery as this is where active multiplication of

4 MICROBIOLOGY AND LABORATORY TECHNIQUES

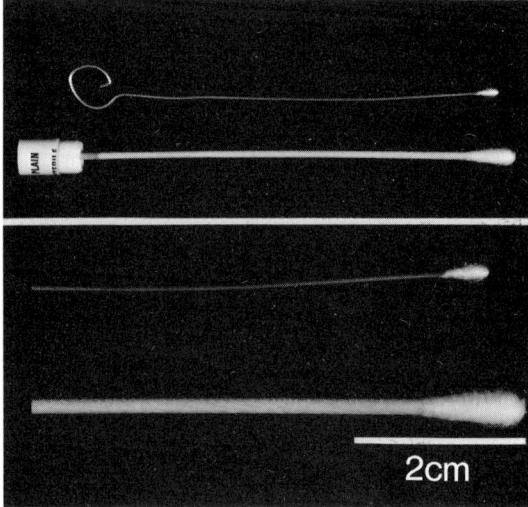

Fig. 4.2. Bacteriological swabs. Top photograph shows a nasopharyngeal swab and plain cotton wool swab. Bottom photograph shows comparison of the size of the wool pleget.

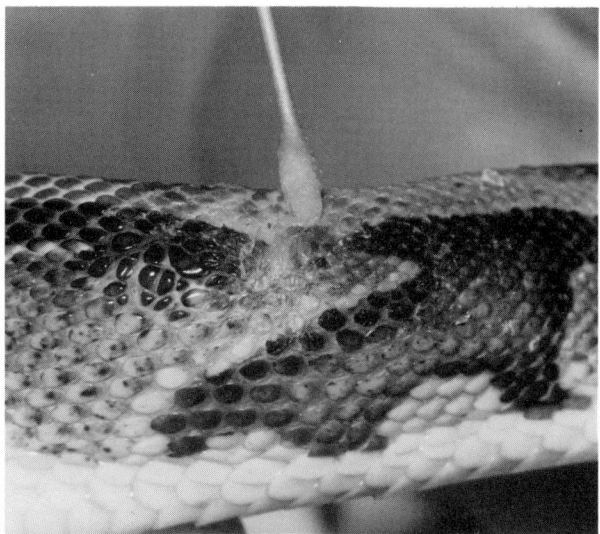

Fig. 4.3. Swab being taken from the outside of a skin lesion on a young boa constrictor.

organisms occurs. Care should be taken to avoid contact between the swab and any other part of the animal, including intact skin.

Shell lesions of tortoises, terrapins and turtles can present problems. The lesions may penetrate deeply into the shell (Holt *et al*, 1979) and it is necessary to examine and expose them carefully. Wallach (1977) described a method for the examination of lesions in turtles where the shell plates had sloughed off and the lesions were covered by a pseudomembrane. The author has examined terrapins with "shell-rot" and found the following method suitable for use during a *post mortem* examination. The shell is examined and a small lesion selected as it is reasoned that this is a likely site of active infection. Using a sterile scalpel the plate is lifted to expose the soft lesion underneath. A sample is then taken with a nasopharyngeal swab which is used to inoculate various media, including Sabouraud's dextrose agar for fungi.

When using this method it is advisable to use a small swab as this reduces the risk of contamination of the specimen.

Mouth lesions are common in reptiles and occur in chelonians (Holt and Cooper, 1976) as well as in snakes. Specimens may easily be obtained (Figs. 4.4 and 4.5) using an appropriate swab. Once again, care must be exercised to ensure that the lesion alone is

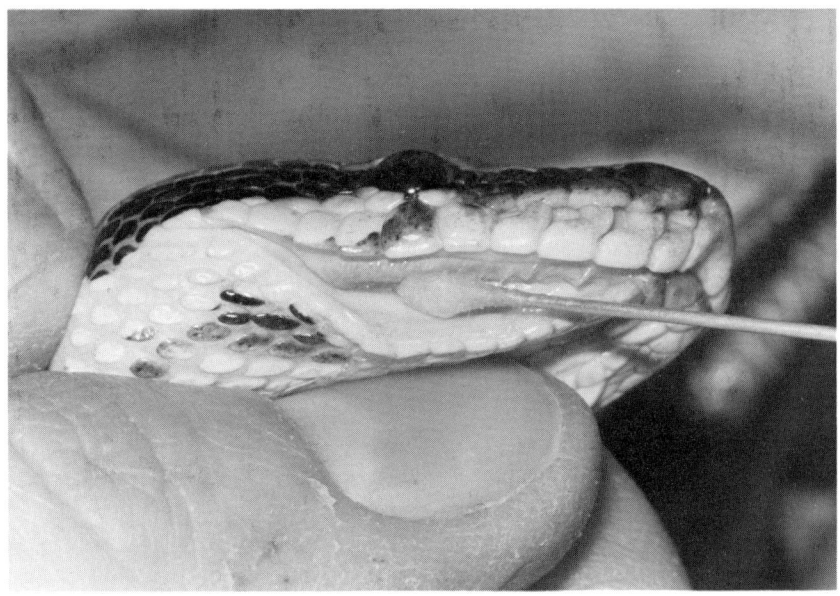

Fig. 4.4 Collection of specimen from the side of the mouth.

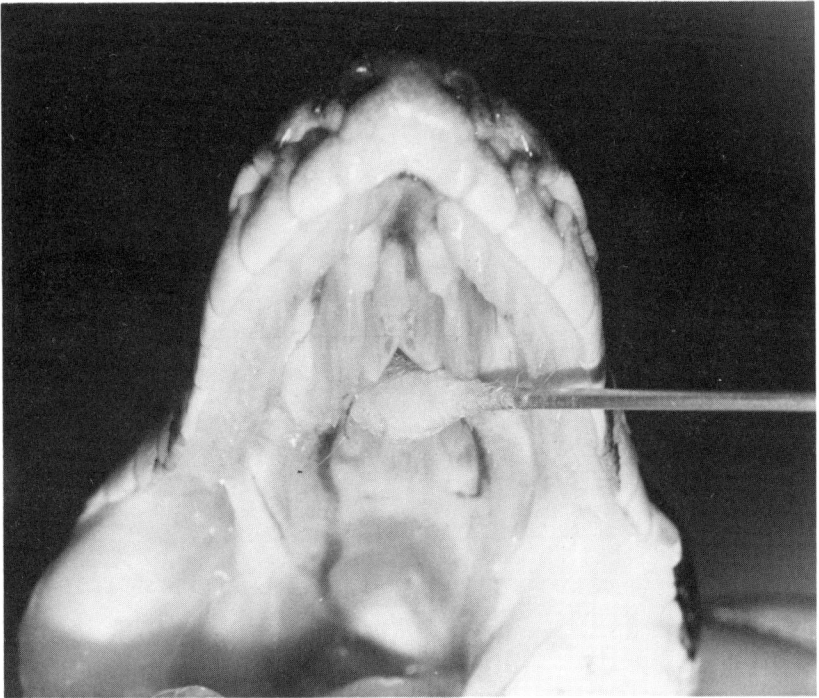

Fig. 4.5. Deep mouth swab. Care must be taken to avoid touching the teeth and tongue.

swabbed. It may be necessary to place a gag in the jaws, and this must not touch the affected area.

Abscesses have been frequently investigated by the author and appear to fall into two groups. The first group present as very hard swellings and can be excised easily as a discrete lump. They should be placed immediately in a sterile bottle and stored at 4°C until they can be examined. In the laboratory it is simple to tip such lesions into a petri dish and to bisect them with a sterile scalpel blade. Once cut the interior will be found to be hard and caseous (Fig. 4.6) and a specimen can be collected from this area using a small swab. The second, rarer group of abscesses are those which are not found as clearly defined lumps, but are soft and filled with pus. The lesion may be incised and a sample of pus collected on a swab, but it is important to obtain an adequate quantity.

The faeces of reptiles are regularly examined for pathogens, particularly bacteria and parasites. The collection of faeces must not

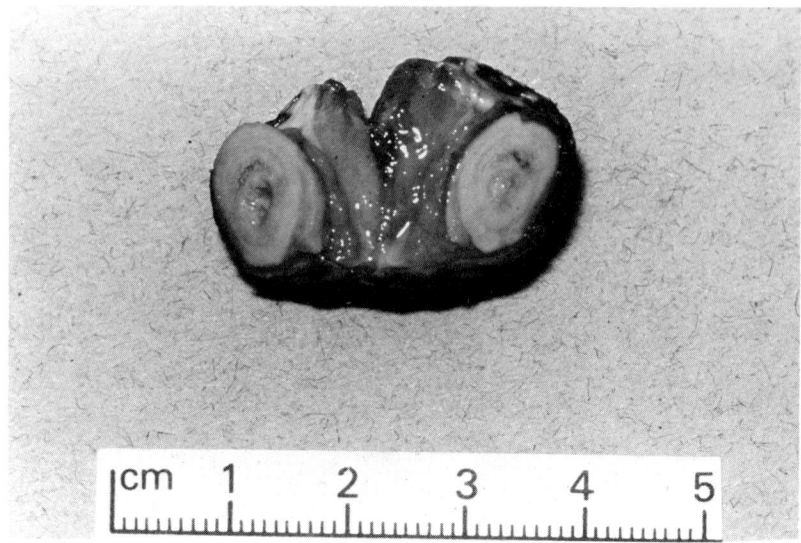

Fig. 4.6. Lesion excised from the flank of an iguana. It has been cut to expose the interior which is hard and caseous.

be undertaken lightly, as there are many errors which can seriously interfere with laboratory tests (Needham, 1977). Fresh faeces are desirable if accurate results are to be obtained. This may be difficult to achieve with reptiles and it is sometimes easier to take a swab from the cloaca (Fig. 4.7). The presence of urates in the cloaca may complicate such sampling but is unlikely to influence the microbiological findings.

Post Mortem Examinations

When an animal is found dead, or has to be killed, the carcass should be sent for autopsy or, if facilities allow, examined immediately. This permits the prompt collection of samples for microbiological and histological tests. In some cases autolysis may render the specimen unsuitable for microbiology as the natural flora may have overgrown the causative organism.

Adequate preparation for a *post mortem* examination is essential. Two sets of dissecting instruments should be available, one for opening the skin or shell of the animal and the other for working with the internal organs. Facilities should be available to sterilize the latter

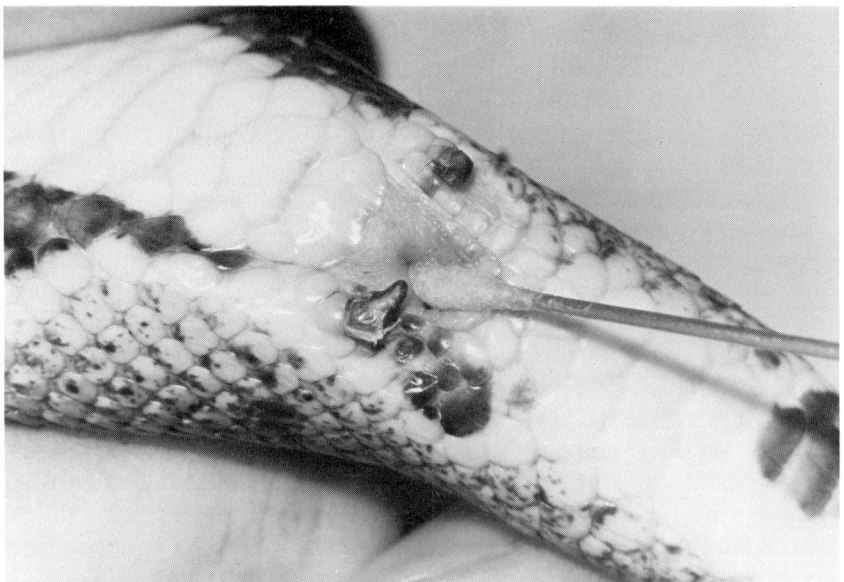

Fig. 4.7. Collection of faecal material directly from the cloaca.

set between organs and it is usually sufficient to soak them in alcohol which is burnt off immediately before use.

If the cause of the illness or death is not known, the *post mortem* examination and collection of material for microbiological investigation must be conducted in a logical manner. The head should be examined first and a throat swab taken. This is followed by examination of the thorax and respiratory system. If lung lesions are suspected specimens may be examined in one of two ways. Verstraete (1973) described one method. He took small pieces of tissue, incubated them in a nutrient broth and identified the bacteria from agar plate subcultures. Another method (Needham, 1979) is somewhat simpler and involves cutting through the affected organ and rubbing the freshly cut surface on to a culture medium. This technique gives reliable results and is time saving. The liver, kidneys and other internal organs must be inspected and specimens collected as described above. Finally the alimentary tract should be examined. Samples of ingesta and faeces can easily be obtained from the different portions of the intestine and provide the most satisfactory specimens for laboratory examination.

From time to time the microbiologist may be asked to examine eggs or embryos, especially from captive breeding programmes or during the course of studies on low fertility or embryonic mortality in wild populations. Little is known of the role of bacteria in such circumstances (see Chapter 6) and the protocol to be followed must be formulated by the individual microbiologist.

The author's approach is exemplified by the following incident. A breeder of pythons (*Python molurus*) with a collection of 50 snakes, contacted the author when he found that fertilized eggs were dying during incubation. In the laboratory three eggs were carefully examined and it was noticed that on each there were damp patches. The outside of the shell of each egg was wiped with 70% alcohol prior to opening the shell with scissors. Inside, the developing snake could be seen surrounded by dark foetid fluid. A sample of fluid was collected by puncturing the membranes with a needle. The fluid withdrawn into a syringe was then examined by several methods and a pure culture of a *Pseudomonas* sp. was obtained. This result, combined with the damp patches seen on the shell, prompted investigation of the incubator; it was finally concluded that the eggs were being kept in too moist conditions, in which the *Pseudomonas* was able to multiply.

Environmental Samples

Bacteriological investigation of the environment of reptiles is not regularly carried out. However, samples may be collected with relative ease in the event of an epizootic.

Swabs moistened with sterile saline can be used to take samples from the walls of vivaria; this can be particularly useful if fungal infections are suspected. Settle plates can also be used and provide an indication of airborne contamination. Settle plates are blood agar plates which are placed in suitable sites, uncovered and left exposed for at least 6 hours. After this time the plates are incubated, the micro-organisms counted and, where appropriate, identified. Plates placed in different localities will usually yield different numbers of colonies.

Other items that may require sampling include water containers and, of particular importance, the water in terrapin tanks. In such cases bacteriological examination is best carried out on a volume of water withdrawn from below the surface with a sterile syringe. In the case of terrapin water, where *Salmonella* spp. are sought, a large volume (at least 20 ml) may be required since only a small number of bacteria may be present in each ml of water. Another method of testing water was suggested by Shotts *et al* (1972) who used gauze sponges to collect samples from lakes.

Carriage of Specimens

A specimen may need to be sent to a laboratory by post. In such cases it is important to comply with relevant requirements of the postal authorities, since many countries have regulations governing the transport of pathological specimens by post. These have two objects in mind; protecting other mail from soiling as a result of badly packed specimens and speeding the passage of samples to their destination. In order to illustrate the requirements, reference will be made to the Post Office Regulations in Great Britain.

The Post Office has no objection to handling pathological specimens but has made the stipulation that they must be sent by First Class Post. The specimen should be enclosed in a sealed container which must itself be placed in an approved box. It must be packed so that it cannot move about in the box and the packing should be of sufficient absorbency that if a leak occurs no material will contaminate the outside of the package. Once the packet has been wrapped the outside must be marked "Fragile with Care" and also "Pathological Specimen". The Authorities reserve the right to stop any package that infringes the regulations and may destroy it. Further, there are legal provisions for the prosecution of any person who does not comply with the regulations.

Many types of container marketed by commercial companies are acceptable for postal transit. If, however, a container has not been approved, it must be sent to the Post Office for examination before it is used. Although the regulations stipulate wooden or metal packing boxes, there are several strong cardboard containers that have received approval and in each case the maximum contents to be sent are printed on it. It is essential to ensure that the package is addressed clearly and it is also advisable to include the address of the sender so that, in the event of an accident, he can be notified.

Pathological specimens may also be sent overseas between recognized laboratories. They must be sent by letter packets and are classified as "Perishable Biological Substances". Speedy delivery is made possible by the use of air mail. The packing and labelling of the letters require special attention and it is necessary to refer to the postal authorities for guidance. In some cases it is necessary to arrange for Customs clearance at the country of receipt and some countries will not accept specimens without a clearance certificate from their agricultural authorities.

Another method of transport overseas is to use air freight. This is very much more expensive than using the post, but does have the advantage of speed of carriage. The specimen will be delivered directly to the airport closest to its final destination, where it can be collected. This is the method of choice for very delicate or urgent specimens but the airline concerned must be consulted beforehand.

Many specimens posted to a laboratory consist of swabs or body fluids. Since there is likely to be a delay of at least 24 hours between despatch of the specimen and its collection it is important to ensure that the specimen does not deteriorate appreciably. Organisms can die during transport or those such as *Pseudomonas aeruginosa* may overgrow others, thus giving a false picture. This can be prevented by the use of transport media for swabs and by keeping other specimens cool, preferably packed in ice.

Stuart (1946a) described a transport medium for swabs. The medium is a semi-solid non-nutritional substrate and effectively preserves fastidious organisms; it prevents them from drying and also protects them against overgrowth by other organisms. It is also satisfactory for the long-term storage of specimens. Stuart *et al* (1954) recorded successful cultivation of organisms after 5 days and Cooper (1957) reported the isolation of enteric pathogens after 8–12 weeks' storage. The author has found that organisms from reptiles can easily be recovered up to 3 weeks after the specimens have been collected. It is advisable to allow the transport medium to warm to room temperature before the swab is placed in it so that the organisms are not killed by a sudden change in temperature. However, once in the medium, specimens are best kept at 4°C until they can be processed. Recently several manufacturers have introduced a pack which contains a swab and a tube of transport medium. The swab is removed from the package, the specimen collected and the swab pushed into the transport medium tube which can be sealed and labelled. This pack is of great value to any worker who does not wish to keep large supplies of transport media and is particularly recommended for collecting field specimens from reptiles.

Whilst considering the collection of specimens it is worth detailing the information that must accompany them to the laboratory. Correct data must be supplied with the sample if the necessary diagnostic tests are to be performed and should include:

The name of the sender

The date of collection of the specimen
The sender's reference number
The animal species, age and sex
A description of the specimen
The type of examination requested
Clinical information

All these items may be easily embodied into a request form issued by the laboratory. This may include a section for the laboratory to fill in the results before a copy is sent back to the clinician.

It is particularly important that, whenever possible, specimens should be collected before starting antimicrobial therapy. If treatment has commenced full details must be given on the form.

E. Bacterial Cultivation

In order to identify bacteria, it is necessary to grow them on, or in, a suitable medium. A wide variety of media will be needed if the many different requirements of the various bacteria are to be satisfied. The media must provide different chemical substrates at the correct hydrogen ion concentration. The temperature, moisture and atmospheric conditions must be controlled. Some bacteria are relatively hardy and can grow on a wide range of media, including basic forms such as nutrient agar, whereas others are more fastidious and supplements must be added to the medium.

The materials used in culture media have been selected for their ability to provide nutrients in a form easily assimilated by the organisms. Peptone provides nitrogen; it is a product of the peptic digestion of protein and is present in most media. Carbon is derived from carbohydrates following breakdown by enzymes. All organisms are dependent on mineral salts particularly for metabolism involving enzymic reactions. Certain bacteria may need the addition of other substances, such as serum, to the medium.

Culture media were originally prepared from their separate constituents. Nowadays, however, there are many commercial companies producing media ready for use. They may be purchased as dehydrated powder, or, at a slightly higher cost, already made up and sterilized. If the latter are used it is wise to place standing orders for weekly delivery so as to ensure fresh supplies of media.

Media used in the bacteriological laboratory may be divided into two groups; liquids and solids. Liquid media of many different types exist and may contain one or more nutrients.

Solid media have the advantage of promoting growth of bacteria as individual colonies which can be picked off for pure culture, whereas liquid media may have mixed growth undetected by the eye. The experienced worker is often able to recognize the colonial morphology of the various species and from this information, together with a Gram stain result, set up confirmatory tests. Solid media are made by adding a gelling agent to liquid medium. The agent used is agar-agar, known normally as agar, and 1% is usually sufficient to produce a satisfactory solid medium when added to a nutrient base.

Before considering incubation it is worth mentioning the groups of media that are used. The first group is made up of simple media and comprises the various nutrient broths and agars. The second group are termed enriched media. Essentially these are simple media with an additive such as blood, serum or hydrocoele fluid. These promote a better growth of most organisms and hence give rise to bigger, more recognizable, colonies. The third group comprises the differential media which are very useful in the diagnosis of disease. An example is MacConkey medium which will differentiate between lactose fermenting and non-lactose fermenting enteric bacteria. The fourth group is the selective media. These, as their name suggests, are used when specific organisms are being studied. They include very specialized constituents which are able to eliminate many of the species of organism not required. This group is of particular importance when screening animals for infection. The final group consists of enrichment media. These are used particularly when a specimen contains only small numbers of the organism in question. The medium promotes the growth of the required organism and sub-cultures yield sufficient colonies to permit studies to be made.

Having inoculated the specimen on to a suitable medium, the latter must be incubated at the optimum temperature and in an atmosphere likely to promote maximum growth of the test organism. The different atmospheres available for cultivation may be broken down into three groups; normal air or aerobic, no free oxygen or anaerobic and a modified atmosphere such as 10% carbon dioxide.

Cultures incubated by the aerobic method do not require any special attention and may be placed inside an incubator in petri dishes, bottles or tubes. Organisms which grow in this way are termed facultative aerobes and this is useful information in identification.

Some bacteria require minimal amounts of oxygen in the atmosphere and are called micro-aerophilic. Incubation of these may be carried out by making tube cultures. Test tubes or universal bottles are filled to three-quarters of their capacity with a suitable agar medium. This is then stab-inoculated with the culture in question. Micro-aerophilic organisms will grow at some point below the surface of the agar.

A very large number of bacteria, including such pathogens as *Clostridium* spp., are known as anaerobic organisms since they must be grown in media free of oxygen. Because of this requirement specialized techniques must be used. Anaerobic culture was formerly a very neglected method of bacterial isolation because of the difficulties in setting up the necessary methods. This frequently resulted in a failure to diagnose correctly. However, in recent years, a much easier method of achieving an anaerobic atmosphere has been devised and this has put anaerobic incubation within the scope of the smallest laboratory.

The easiest method of anaerobic culture is similar to that used for micro-aerophilic organisms. A stab culture is set up, making sure that the straight wire used to inoculate the medium is pushed to the bottom of the container. The anaerobic organisms will multiply at the bottom of the stab. The addition of 0·5% glucose to the medium assists the production of anaerobic conditions.

Another medium which gives excellent results is Robertson's cooked meat medium. This was first recorded in 1916 by Robertson and is now produced by commercial companies. The author has used this medium very successfully when isolating organisms from swabs from reptiles—particularly *Clostridium* spp. but also, on occasion, such bacteria as staphylococci which have failed to grow on blood agar under aerobic conditions.

As mentioned above, agar plates may be incubated anaerobically. The original method used a jar known as the McIntosh and Fildes' Jar. This has valves to admit the hydrogen gas necessary for incubation. Inside the jar, fixed to the lid, is a catalyst to ensure complete removal of the oxygen within the jar. Recently a much simpler method of creating an anaerobic atmosphere has been introduced. This is the Gas-Pak system (Becton-Dickinson, Wembley, Middlesex, England). The system consists of a transparent perspex jar, with a lid containing a pelleted catalyst. After placing the medium within the jar, a generator envelope is charged with 10 ml of water and this will produce hydrogen mixed with a little (10%) carbon dioxide. Finally an indicator strip is placed in the jar so that the maintenance of anaerobic conditions can be monitored. This simple apparatus enables any laboratory to carry out anaerobic culture with ease.

Many bacteria require a modified atmosphere before growth is satisfactory; for example *Haemophilus* spp. require additional carbon dioxide. The agar plates can be placed in a metal container and a lighted candle put inside. The candle will burn until there is approximately 10% carbon dioxide, which is sufficient to allow the growth of organisms.

A very important consideration when setting up cultures of organisms is the temperature of incubation. It is generally assumed that pathogenic organisms can be readily isolated following incubation at 37°C. This is true for many of the organisms normally encountered in veterinary science. However, in the case of the Reptilia, this is not necessarily the correct temperature of incubation, as the animal's natural body temperature may be considerably lower. The author has conducted a large series of investigations comparing incubation at 25°C and 37°C. In many cases more species of organism have been isolated from the cultures at 25°C than those at 37°C and it is believed that this occurs because at the lower temperature, fast growing organisms do not overgrow other, slower growing, bacteria. One case (Fig. 4.8) illustrates a typical series of results. Swabs were taken from a royal python (*Python regius*) with stomatitis. Duplicate agar plates were set up at 37°C and 25°C. After incubation, *Proteus* spp. and *Aeromonas* spp. were isolated at both temperatures, but in addition *Escherichia coli* was grown at 25°C. As well as favouring the growth of certain bacteria, the lower temperature is advisable whenever cultures have been set up for the isolation of fungi (see later).

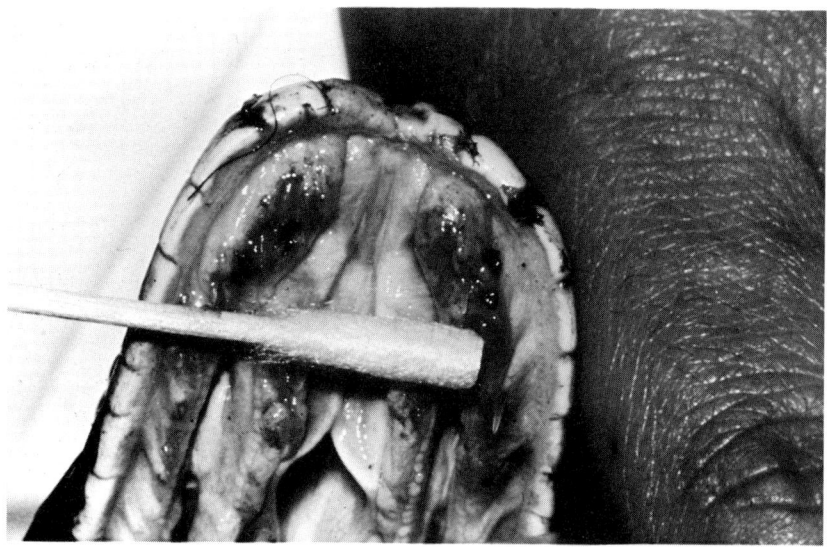

Fig. 4.8. Python with stomatitis showing the use of a large cotton wool swab for the collection of a specimen.

Laboratory Examination

After collection of samples the next stage is to select the appropriate methods of incubation and the necessary media. In this section guidelines are provided for the treatment of specimens so that the worker will have the best chance of recovering and isolating microorganisms.

When dealing with specimens from reptiles it is important to remember that the organisms may not be as specific or significant as those isolated from non-reptilian species. For example, the buccal cavity may yield intestinal bacteria acquired from the prey. Isolation methods must, therefore, be less selective than is advocated in many microbiology reference works.

When dealing with the respiratory system (including the buccal cavity and pharynx), it is wise to include cultures in an atmosphere of increased carbon dioxide, which simulates the elevated levels in expired air. A blood agar plate, chocolate agar plate and MacConkey agar plate should be incubated at 37°C and 25°C, the chocolate agar being placed in a carbon dioxide atmosphere. In addition, a sample of the specimen should be incubated in cooked meat medium as described earlier. Sub-cultures can be made from the various primary cultures and identification attempted.

Internal organs may be treated in a similar manner. Using the cut surface technique a blood agar plate and MacConkey plate should be inoculated; one set is incubated at 37°C and the other at 25°C. In addition, a further blood agar plate must be incubated at 37°C in an anaerobic atmosphere. If a swab is taken in preference to a cut surface technique this also should be placed in cooked-meat medium after plating on to agar.

Samples of gastro-intestinal contents are treated in a different manner. Often it is important to screen the material for the presence of *Salmonella* spp. A portion of the sample should be inoculated on to deoxycholate citrate agar (DCA) (Hynes, 1942), which is incubated at 37°C, and a portion into selenite F. (Leifson, 1936). After incubation for 24 hours sub-culture on DCA should be made. Recently it has been suggested that prolonged incubation of selenite yields a higher rate of isolation of *Salmonella* (Chattopadhyay and Pilford, 1976), and hence a further sub-culture should be made after 72 hours. If it is necessary to examine faeces for a wider spectrum of organisms than the above specific pathogen, MacConkey agar may be used in combination with or instead of DCA.

Parasitological examination may also be carried out on faeces and this will be dealt with in a subsequent section.

The author's experience of abscesses in reptiles is that they rarely yield organisms encountered in mammalian abscesses, for instance *Staphylococcus aureus*, but correspond more to the picture seen in chronic skin ulcers. For example, an abscess from a crocodile (*Crocodylus niloticus*) yielded two strains of *Escherichia coli*, Providence group A, *Proteus mirabilis* and *Proteus rettgeri* and *Bacillus alvei*. Because many abscesses have been found to contain gut flora, it is recommended that material from abscesses is plated on to a blood agar plate, MacConkey agar plate at 37°C and 25°C and into cooked meat medium. In addition a smear should be made and stained by Gram's technique. It must always be borne in mind that abscesses may contain *Mycobacterium* spp. and it is a wise precaution to stain a smear by the Ziehl–Neelsen technique; culture may also be attempted on Löwenstein-Jensen medium (Jensen, 1955).

Another large group of specimens comprises body exudates such as peritoneal fluid. If presented to the laboratory as fluid, a portion should be inoculated into cooked meat medium and nutrient broth. If a swab is sent the material should be inoculated on to blood agar and MacConkey agar as already described.

Blood taken from the heart is very suitable for the isolation of organisms from cases of septicaemia (see Chapter 6). Unfortunately, it is often only practicable to consider this after death of the reptile, when the heart may be removed at *post mortem* examination. (Holt *et al*, 1979; Holt, 1979.) The wall of a heart chamber is cut with a sterile scalpel and forceps used to make the cut gape. A sample of heart blood is easily obtained by introducing a swab through the hole. The blood should be incubated on blood agar and in cooked meat medium.

There are many other possible sites that may provide specimens and, in most cases, there will be little indication as to which organisms are likely to be encountered. In view of this the author suggests the following general culture regime which will usually ensure the maximum chance of successful isolation of organisms. The material should be cultured on blood agar and MacConkey agar at 37°C and 25°C. A blood agar plate should also be incubated anaerobically and a portion of the specimen inoculated into cooked meat medium which should be incubated at 37°C for at least 48 hours before sub-culture on blood agar.

The scheme above employs blood agar because of its value as a general purpose enriched medium. MacConkey agar will help to differentiate the gut flora so often encountered in reptile specimens. One of these, *Proteus* species, can swarm over blood agar and a specimen may be rendered unidentifiable (Wallach, 1977) but MacConkey medium, particularly if prepared without salt, will inhibit such swarming. The usefulness of cooked meat medium and the essential nature of anaerobic incubation has already been discussed.

F. Bacterial Identification

Specimens collected from both living and dead reptiles will often contain many different species of organisms; before a diagnosis can be successfully made it is necessary to identify them. This is achieved by obtaining pure cultures of the organisms, by one or more of the methods already described, and then performing identification tests.

In this section attention will be paid to the laboratory tests which must be carried out once the specimen has been incubated on culture medium and its morphology has been ascertained by staining. The tests are mostly of a biochemical nature, but also include serological (immunological) methods. The entire process of identification is the gradual build-up of information gathered from the results of many separate investigations.

At the start, the growth characteristics of the organism should be noted. It is important to record at what temperature growth occurs and which media support the organism. The shape, size and colour of the colony must be described. Next staining must be carried out. Other than in the case of a suspected acid-fast organism, the Gram stain is essential, perhaps combined with a spore stain. The majority of the biochemical tests are selected depending on the shape and Gram-staining reaction of the culture. For example, different tests are conducted to confirm *Staphylococcus aureus* from those for *Aeromonas liquefaciens*.

Biochemical tests are fairly simple and in many cases are designed to assess the ability of the organism to utilize a certain substrate. Often an indicator is incorporated into the medium so that the reading of the test is simplified. There are several ways in which the biochemical reagents can be employed and each has its own advantages and disadvantages. The most common method is to perform each test in a separate vessel such as a small test tube or bijou bottle. When required for use the appropriate bottles may be assembled and inoculated individually. After incubation the tests are read; reference books may be consulted to obtain the identification. Another method, particularly for the Enterobacteriaceae, is to purchase a card containing a series of test systems, each of which is inoculated with a suspension of the culture. After reading the result is obtained from a code which forms part of the kit. This method has the advantage that the necessity to consult reference books is largely eliminated and, also, the tests are confined to one card. There are other methods available but the author, having tried several different systems, is of the opinion that the best method is the first—that of individual bottles for each test. This has the advantage that the tests used can be varied according to the suspected organism and therefore there is greater scope. With the regular use of this system the worker can familiarize himself with the significance of each individual test and hence speed his diagnoses.

There are some important points to remember relating to the setting up of biochemical tests. By far the most significant is to ensure that the tests are inoculated with a pure culture. It is therefore essential to check the purity of the inoculating suspension by setting up a purity plate. This must be checked before the biochemical tests and, if found to be supporting the growth of more than one species of organism, the tests must be discarded and set up again. Each worker should become familiar with the correct way of inoculating the tests. Some require longer times of incubation than others. It has also been shown that the result of the test may depend upon the volume of the inoculum and the quality of the medium used (Stevens, 1977). It is therefore suggested that, as far as is possible, one supplier is chosen and all biochemical tests are performed using media from that supplier. Further, control organisms should always be inoculated into several bottles of each batch of medium so that the latter may be checked for both positive and negative reactions. The author has found that reliable results are obtained by making a suspension of the organism under test in the following manner. Peptone water (4·5 ml) is placed in a bijou bottle and sufficient of the organism is emulsified so that the peptone water becomes slightly cloudy. This suspension is then used to inoculate the bottles of biochemical test reagents.

There are many biochemical tests common to a number of bacteria. They include the production of hydrogen sulphide gas, the production of urease and the incorporation of different carbohydrates into peptone water, for example, lactose, glucose, sucrose and mannitol. It must be the decision of the individual worker as to whether it is necessary to identify fully every bacterium or whether it is sufficient to determine the genus only. Fewer tests are needed for the latter.

In order to simplify the biochemical tests necessary for identification the tests required for the main groups of bacteria encountered by the author in material from reptiles will be described.

Members of the Enterobacteriaceae are frequently isolated including *Proteus* spp. *Enterobacter* spp., *Escherichia coli* and, less commonly, *Salmonella* spp. These can be identified using sucrose, lactose, glucose, mannitol, dulcitol peptone waters, citrate utilization, hydrogen sulphide production, lysine and ornithine decarboxylases and arginine dihydrolase, production of urease, indole production and gelatine hydrolysis. This same set of tests may also be used for *Klebsiella* spp., *Pasteurella* spp. and *Aeromonas* spp. A modified series of tests may be utilized for *Pseudomonas* spp. The isolate should be examined for its ability to hydrolyse gelatine, utilize citrate and mannitol and to produce urease and indole. In addition a culture should be incubated at 5°C and 42°C.

Bacteroides spp. are obligate anaerobes and tests must be conducted in an anaerobic atmosphere. The tests used are the same as those for the Enterobacteriaceae with the exclusion of urease production, citrate utilization and enzyme reactions.

For other Gram-negative organisms, such as *Acinetobacter*, *Haemophilus* and *Neisseria* spp., the tests required are described in standard laboratory books.

Gram-positive organisms are isolated infrequently from reptiles and are usually *Clostridium* and *Staphylococcus* spp. Clostridial species may be identified using a similar set of tests to those used for the Enterobacteriaceae with the addition of tests to demonstrate whether the organism can digest serum or meat; anaerobic culture is necessary. The identification of *Staphylococcus* spp. and the differentiation between *S. aureus* and *S. epidermidis* are relatively straightforward. The organism is identified by its characteristic colonial morphology, haemolytic reaction on blood agar and positive catalase test. Further tests are the coagulase test (Fisk, 1940) and the production of deoxyribonuclease. The latter two tests are in wide use in medical microbiology and Needham (1974) demonstrated their ability to differentiate staphylococci from animal sources.

There are many other biochemical tests applicable to different species of organisms and details of these can be found in Cowan and Steel (1966).

It is not possible to discuss the isolation and identification of all the organisms that are associated with disease in reptiles. However, two genera deserve special mention as the techniques for their diagnosis are very different from the other bacteria described earlier. The organisms concerned are *Mycobacterium* spp. and *Leptospira* spp.

The acid-fast bacilli, *Mycobacterium* spp., are well recognized pathogens of reptiles (Aronson, 1929; Vogel, 1958). They produce characteristic lesions in organs and material from these can be stained by the Ziehl–Neelsen technique described earlier in this chapter. If the bacterium is present typical short thick acid-fast bacilli will be seen. Culture of the lesion can be attempted using specialized medium. The material should be treated with sodium hydroxide (Aronson, 1929) and after neutralization the sediment may be placed on to Dorset's egg medium and Löwenstein-Jensen medium. Duplicate cultures should be set up for incubation at 25°C and 37°C. The species are slow growing and several weeks may be needed before colonies are seen. For this reason a rapid diagnosis will be best achieved if specimens are also examined histopathologically.

The bacteria comprising the genus *Leptospira* have been isolated from many animals including reptiles (Ferris *et al*, 1961). The organisms may be found in the organs and body fluids of reptiles, including the urine. A special medium is required for their growth (Stuart, 1946b) and, if organs are suspected of being infected, it is necessary to make a suspension of them before the medium is inoculated (Ferris *et al*, 1959). Blood can be tested for the presence of agglutinins by the method of Gochenour *et al* (1953) although it appears that positive titres can be obtained from reptiles that do not yield the organism on culture (Andrews *et al*, 1965). The bacteria can be demonstrated by dark ground microscopy. Because of the difficulties involved in the diagnosis of leptospiral infections it is advisable that specimens should be sent to a reference laboratory where appropriate facilities are available.

It is often possible to obtain a presumptive diagnosis. If a *Pseudomonas* or *Neisseria* sp. is suspected an oxidase test may be performed. A 1% solution of tetramethyl-p-phenylenediamine is made up and a little is placed on filter paper with a pipette. Using a piece of glass, a colony is streaked over the solution. An immediate purple colour indicates a positive oxidase result and therefore the colony could be one of the two bacteria.

Finally, mention must be made of two further investigations that are carried out before confirming the identity of the organism. The first is a check on motility. The most satisfactory method is that utilizing a hanging drop (Cruickshank, 1969) which eliminates errors caused by air currents. The second test is for the production of catalase. A saline suspension of the organism is made on a glass slide and one drop of 20 volumes hydrogen peroxide is added. Immediate effervescence is taken as positive. Alternatively, the hydrogen peroxide may be applied directly to a nutrient agar culture of the organism; again effervescence indicates catalase production.

Having gathered all the various test results it is necessary to refer to a book of tables, such as that by Cowan (1974). In addition, help with the identification of morphological characteristics and interpretation of biochemical and other tests can be obtained from colour atlases, such as that of Gillies and Dodds (1968). Research is now in progress using information stored in computers to identify organisms (Curtis *et al*, 1972). When making reference to tables or any other sources of information, it must be remembered that organisms may be present in atypical forms. For example, Cooper *et al* (1978), working with frogs, reported the isolation of the atypical coccal form of *Acinetobacter*; this is normally isolated as a Gram-negative rod.

In certain cases the identification of an organism can be confirmed using serological methods. This is very relevant to *Salmonella* spp. and *Escherichia coli*. The former in particular can present a threat to the health of personnel working with reptiles. Many different strains of *Salmonella* have been identified serologically and a number have been isolated from reptiles, particularly terrapins and tortoises (Anğ *et al*, 1973; Clegg and Heath, 1975; Borland, 1975). Serological methods are the only way in which the identification of individual strains within the species may be accomplished easily. Similarly, entero-pathogenic *Escherichia coli*, which may pose a health threat to young children, can be identified serologically. These strains of the organism have been demonstrated in laboratory animals (Schiff *et al*, 1972) and, since these are often fed to captive reptiles, it is possible that the latter may harbour the strains in question. The tests utilize specific antisera to cause agglutination. Each test is simple to carry out. A thick suspension of the organism is made in a loopful of saline on a glass slide, and to this, one loopful of specific antiserum is added and mixed well. The slide must be gently rocked and viewed for clumping, which indicates a positive reaction. It is helpful to hold the slide against a black background when checking for agglutination. In the case of some organisms it may only be necessary to check for agglutination against one antiserum, but for a correct serological identification of *Salmonella* and *Escherichia coli* several will be required. Whenever a test is carried out it is essential that a saline suspension is examined for auto-agglutination.

It is sometimes not possible to identify fully an organism in the laboratory and on these occasions help must be sought from a reference laboratory. In the United Kingdom the Central Public Health Laboratory at Colindale, London is the reference laboratory for *Salmonella* spp. and will assist in determining strains. At the same locality are reference laboratories for *Streptococcus* and *Staphylococcus* spp.—and, incidentally, disinfectants!

The ultimate object of all the methods listed in this chapter is the quick and correct identification of organisms. Normally this requires at least 24 hours and more often 48. On occasions it is highly desirable to achieve a presumptive diagnosis before 48 hours and this can be accomplished by utilizing quick micro-methods. The necessary reagents and test methods were listed by Breach (1972). They do not include those for the utilization of carbohydrates but are those which detect the production of enzymes. It must be stressed, however, that these techniques do not replace the standard biochemical tests, which should always be performed so that the presumptive diagnosis can be confirmed.

The author has found one micro-method to be of great practical value. This involves the differentiation between *Salmonella* and *Proteus* spp. When these two organisms are grown in primary culture on deoxycholate citrate agar both appear as non-lactose fermenters i.e. yellow colonies. Because the swarming of *Proteus* is inhibited on this medium differentiation between it and *Salmonella* must be based on biochemical methods. Colonies of the suspect organism are inoculated on to commercially produced urea agar slopes. The slopes are incubated in a 37°C waterbath and the development of a purple colour after 1 hour is indicative of urease production—a feature of *Proteus*. If no colour is present after 4 hours it is highly probable that the organism is not a *Proteus* spp. and hence further biochemical and serological tests must be performed. This test enables time to be saved by eliminating *Proteus* from samples of faecal material cultured on agar.

G. Sensitivity Tests

Probably the second most frequent investigation undertaken in the microbiology laboratory is the determination of the sensitivity of an organism to antimicrobial agents. This plays an important role in work with reptiles. Some of the agents involved have been used in veterinary medicine for many years, while new ones are regularly being added. The selection of chemotherapeutic agents must be left to the person responsible for the treatment of the reptile, as there are many factors to be considered (Sanford, 1976). The prime object of the tests carried out in the laboratory is to provide information so that a reasoned judgement may be made.

There is a variety of possible tests available to the worker and each has been designed to give a speedy and accurate result. The method used in an individual laboratory must depend to a large extent upon

4   MICROBIOLOGY AND LABORATORY TECHNIQUES   119

the facilities and manpower available. In this section three methods will be described and one suggested for general use. All three methods are based upon diffusion of the agent through agar: the former is contained in a paper disc placed on the surface of the agar. This procedure was recommended by the Expert Committee on Antibiotics of the World Health Organisation (W.H.O., 1961) and is in widespread use.

The simplest test utilizes several discs of paper, each impregnated with a different agent. These may be purchased as single discs or made up into sets fixed to a central core (Fig. 4.9). A suspension of the test organism is made in saline. Agar plates are then inoculated with

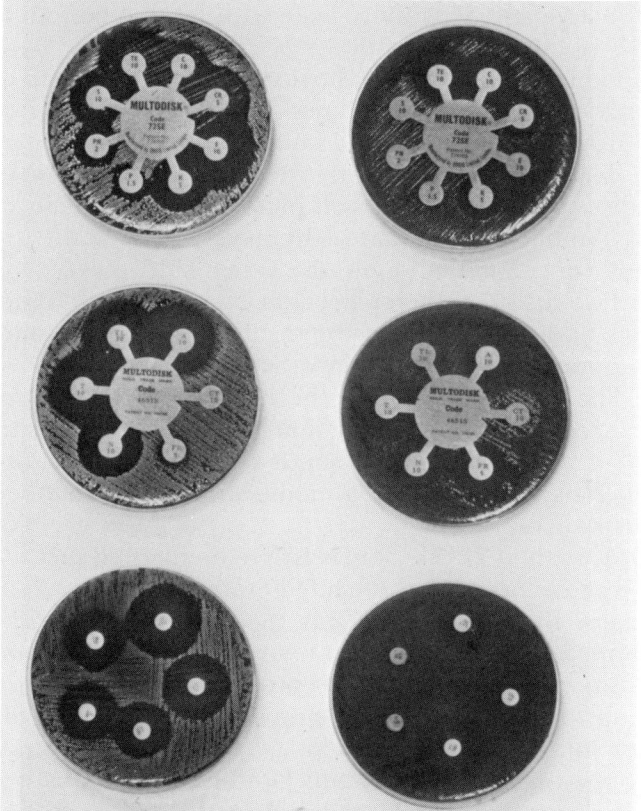

Fig. 4.9. Test for sensitivity to antimicrobial agents using paper discs. The organism on the right is more resistant than the organism on the left.

the suspension using a cotton wool swab, ensuring that the surface of the plate is evenly covered with the inoculum. The paper discs are laid carefully on to the agar taking care not to move the disc once it has touched the agar surface. Incubation of the plate is carried out for 18 hours at 37°C after which the zone sizes around the discs are measured and recorded. This method of testing is very quick, but has the disadvantage that no control organism is used. However, in the author's experience, interpretation is easy and, in general with the agents listed in Table 4.1, the author has found that a zone width of more than 8 mm from the edge of the disc may be taken to indicate that the organism is sensitive. The choice of agar used for the method may be left to the worker as there are many different specialized products available. However, as a guide, Mueller–Hinton agar (Mueller and Hinton, 1941) is a good all purpose agar and the author has found Diagnostic Sensitivity agar with lysed blood gives reliable results with isolates from reptiles.

The second method is that of Stokes (1968). This has an advantage over the previous test in that it allows the use of control organisms and it may be used either on isolated cultures or for a direct test on the specimen. The disadvantage of the technique is that a maximum of only four discs can be used on each plate. The specimen is inoculated in a broad band across the plate. On one side of this the first control organism is inoculated and on the other side the second control organism. Two discs are then placed on each side so that they overlap the controls and the unknown organism. In this way four separate discs are applied. After incubation the zone sizes are measured and recorded. The zones surounding the discs on the control organisms should be measured and agree with previous tests. If the same size as the control or a larger zone surrounds the test discs, the organism is reported as sensitive. Recently a modification to the method permits the use of six discs.

The third method is the Bauer–Kirby method (Bauer *et al*, 1966) which has been adopted in the United States of America. The method uses Mueller–Hinton agar and has the advantage of standardizing the inoculum. Large agar plates are poured and dried before use. The test organism is inoculated into tryptose phosphate broth and incubated for up to 5 hours until the growth is equal to the turbidity of the barium sulphate standard. This gives a concentration of organisms of approximately 10^8 per ml. Cotton wool swabs are used to inoculate the agar and discs are placed on the surface in a circle near the outside of the plate. Incubation is carried out overnight at 37°C after which the zone sizes are recorded. For interpretation the sizes

Table 4.1. Examples of sensitivity to antimicrobial agents of organisms isolated from clinical disease in reptiles

Case Number	Reptile	Infection	Organism	Ampicillin	Benzylpenicillin	Carbenicillin	Cephaloridine	Chloramphenicol	Chlortetracycline	Colistin	Erythromycin	Furazolidone	Gentamicin	Kanamycin	Lincomycin	Methicillin	Neomycin	Oxytetracycline	Streptomycin	Tetracycline	Tylosin	Sulphamethoxazole/Trimethoprim
7	Snake	"Mouth-rot"	*Proteus*	R	R	S	R	S	R	R	R	R	S	S	R	R	S	R	S	R	R	R
			Providencia	R	R	S	S	R	R	R	R	R	S	S	R	R	S	R	S	R	R	R
8	*Lacerta vivipara*	Conjunctivitis	*Aeromonas*	R	R	R	R	R	R	S	R	R	S	S	R	R	S	R	S	R	S	S
9	*Python reticulatus*	Tail nodule	*Acinetobacter*	R	R	S	S	R	R	R	R	R	S	S	R	R	S	S	S	S	R	S
10	*Iguana iguana*	Abscess	*E. coli*	R	R	S	R	R	R	R	R	S	S	S	R	R	S	R	R	R	R	S
			Citrobacter	R	R	S	R	R	R	R	R	R	S	S	R	R	S	R	S	R	R	R
11	*Testudo graeca*	Shell lesion	*Pseudomonas*	R	R	S	R	S	R	R	R	R	S	S	R	R	S	R	R	R	R	R

Key
R resistant   S sensitive

are checked against a standard graph showing the zone sizes for sensitive organisms.

All three methods described above have both disadvantages and advantages. The Bauer–Kirby method is not suited to small laboratories as the work involved in preparing the standard inocula is time consuming. However, if manpower is available, it is a very accurate method. Stokes' method is easy to carry out and can be used in the small laboratory, although if the organism is to be tested against a wide variety of agents, the number of plates used will be large. It is wise to confirm the sensitivity results on pure cultures of organisms isolated from the specimen.

For most laboratories the first method is recommended. The system has been used by the author for many years and has proved reliable and easy to carry out. Because no control organisms are included in the test, care must be taken to ensure that discs do not lose their potency. Discs not in use should be stored in a deep freeze. When required they must be warmed to 4°C before being placed on the agar surface. Interpretation of zone sizes with this method is also important. The author does not report any organisms as "moderately resistant" and this eliminates any doubt about the zone size due to the uncontrolled inoculum. With this method colonies should be dense but not confluent. The experienced worker quickly learns to interpret the zone sizes when the inoculum is either too weak or too concentrated. For the inexperienced person it is advisable for "practice" tests to be carried out with deliberately incorrect inoculum concentrations so that the difference in zone sizes can be noted. When reading the results of tests carried out directly on the specimen before the isolation of individual organisms particular care must be taken in assessing the zone size. More than one organism is likely to be present and the zone size must be measured from the edge of growth nearest the disc.

If possible all major groups of antimicrobial agents should be represented and the most widely used products included. The persons to whom the report is directed should be consulted in case they wish any particular agents to be used. The author performs tests for many veterinary surgeons and routinely 19 different agents are included in the tests. These are listed in Table 4.1. All 19 agents are used in every test and this allows the clinician a wide choice. It is not wise for the laboratory to make judgements as to the choice of agent. For example, streptomycin is often effective against *Aeromonas* spp., yet may prove toxic when administered parenterally (see Chapter 18).

The author has found that the pattern of antibiotic sensitivities of organisms isolated from reptilian infections broadly agrees with those obtained from other species (Owens *et al*, 1975). Many bacteria isolated from reptiles appear to be highly resistant to antibiotics but this observation may be due to the high proportion of *Pseudomonas* spp. isolated. Table 4.1 shows typical results obtained from clinical material.

There are two special considerations concerning methicillin and the sulphonamides. To obtain an accurate result for methicillin modified test methods are required. Barber (1964) described a technique using agar plates with 5% sodium chloride and with subsequent incubation at 37°C. An alternative method uses Diagnostic Sensitivity Test agar, with the addition of blood and incubation at 30°C (Annear, 1968). The latter is the easiest for a small laboratory as the medium can be used for all sensitivity tests and all that is required is an incubator set at 30°C. The sulphonamide group present a different problem. Their action is based upon antagonism to p-aminobenzoic acid which prevents the organism from utilizing this chemical. The presence of the acid in many culture media invalidates their use for sensitivity tests as false resistant strains may be reported. For this reason a medium free of the acid must be used and Mueller–Hinton agar is suitable.

Once all the tests are completed it is important that a report is issued promptly. To facilitate this a form should be designed so that the agents to which the organism is sensitive can be quickly indicated. It is bad practice to report results using the manufacturer's name for an agent; whenever possible the chemical name should be quoted.

The laboratory can often give advice on an antibiotic policy. The widespread use of antibiotics has lead to a situation where resistance is prevalent amongst certain organisms. This can render antimicrobial therapy useless. There are several factors contributing to the development of bacterial resistance (Linton, 1977). The appearance of new resistant strains is likely to be detected in the laboratory and can be monitored. Steps should be taken to avoid the risk of creating further resistant strains. First, care must be taken when making up, dispensing and administering antimicrobial agents; spillage must be avoided. Courses of treatment must be of sufficient duration to ensure total bactericidal or bacteriostatic effects and prophylactic administration should be discouraged whenever possible. Further, the prudent use of agents will ensure that those known to create resistance problems are kept as second line agents and only used when other drugs prove unsatisfactory. Finally, a few agents warrant being placed on a reserve list and only being used if no other is available. For example, chloramphenicol, which is an important drug in human medicine, should not, in the author's opinion, be used routinely in reptile work.

Interpretation of results

Once laboratory tests have been concluded the results must be assessed. This is particularly important when several bacterial isolates have been obtained from a specimen—a common occurrence in reptile work (see Chapter 6). The pathogenicity of certain species is well recognized, for example *Aeromonas* and *Pseudomonas* spp. (Cooper and Leakey, 1976), and in such cases interpretation is relatively straightforward. There are, however, many occasions when species of bacteria are isolated from reptiles but their significance is uncertain. For example, a young reticulated python (*Python reticulatus*) had a series of nodules along the spine. A biopsy was performed by a veterinary surgeon and culture of several sites yielded an *Acinetobacter* sp. which was sensitive to several agents (see Table 4.1). Two courses of oxytetracycline was administered and after 6 months specimens taken at a further biopsy did not yield any organisms. Since *Acinetobacter* sp. was isolated in pure culture from all specimens it was assumed that this organism was associated with the infection.

Mixed cultures obtained from specimens can be better interpreted if one has some knowledge of the organisms involved. For example, *Staphylococcus epidermidis* is often isolated from skin lesions and abscesses. In nearly all cases the bacterium is present with other, pathogenic, organisms and it can safely be assumed that the staphylococcus is a skin contaminant.

A further guide to the significance of particular organisms is the number isolated. By careful examination of the primary agar cultures an estimate can be made of the relative numbers of organisms present. The organism present in the greatest numbers is usually the major pathogen.

Results obtained by other laboratory techniques may help microbiological results. For example, histological examination can confirm the presence of organisms (see Chapter 3). Unfortunately, however, such results are often not available until the microbiological tests have been concluded and reported.

The interpretation of results obtained from *post mortem* material poses many problems. Some hours may elapse before the carcass can be examined and autolysis will reduce the chances of recovery of organisms. Enteric organisms can quickly become disseminated after death, resulting in their isolation from many sites including the lungs, liver and kidneys. It is therefore important, when dealing with *post mortem* material, to try to locate a focus of infection from which specimens can be examined; comparison with other sites will help ascertain which organisms are likely to be significant.

In cases of septicaemia, whether alive or dead, blood culture is desirable. The withdrawal of blood from live reptiles is discussed in Chapter 17. In the case of dead animals, the author opens the heart (as discussed earlier) and swabs are taken. The isolation of organisms in pure culture is strongly suggestive of pathogenicity although a long delay *post mortem* must again cast doubt on the significance of those bacteria usually associated with the alimentary tract.

A further problem encountered with reptiles is related to the food they eat. Snakes are often fed rodents which are themselves colonized by different micro-organisms. In two cases (both snakes) examined by the author, the organism *Bordetella bronchiseptica* was isolated from the heart and an abscess respectively. This organism is a commensal of many rodents and the fact that in each case the snakes had been fed rodents suggested that these were the source. In a third case, *Pseudomonas pseudomallei* was isolated from specimens taken from extensive scale-rot lesions (infectious dermal ulceration) in a boa constrictor (*Boa constrictor*). The pericardium was filled with oedematous fluid and this also yielded the organism. This bacterium is known to be a commensal of laboratory rats and the snake in question had been fed these animals. Why these rodent organisms had so successfully colonized the snakes is a matter for conjecture. Perhaps the reptiles were already debilitated and hence were rendered more susceptible to colonization.

H. Fungal Cultivation

Fungal infections are discussed in Chapter 7. The causal organisms require different media for cultivation. In general fungi grow slowly on culture plates and hence periods of up to 7 days or more may be required. It is essential that specimens are incubated at low temperatures—if possible, at 20°C, 25°C and 37°C. Material for incubation must be stab-inoculated as many fungi will not grow on the surface of agar. The most commonly used is Sabouraud Dextrose agar (Carlier, 1948) into which antimicrobial agents, for example, cycloheximide, penicillin and streptomycin (Georg *et al*, 1954) can be incorporated in order to inhibit the multiplication of bacteria. If cultures are to be incubated for long periods, it is preferable to prepare slopes in bottles to prevent drying of the agar.

III. Parasitological Techniques

Laboratory techniques play an important role in parasitology. It is not proposed to deal with techniques for the detection of ectoparasites—these are covered in Chapter 10—but brief mention will be made of the examination of material from reptiles for endoparasites.

Most investigations are carried out on faeces. It is important that fresh specimens are collected if successful identification of endoparasites is to be carried out. Faecal samples must first be carefully inspected and a note taken of their consistency and colour. In some cases, worms or parts of worms may be present which will permit a rapid identification. A permanent preparation of the parasite can be made, which is useful if the necessary reference books are not at hand. The worm may be fixed, cleared and mounted in glycerine jelly (Lambert, 1969). Andrews (1978) published details of several techniques for the relaxation and fixation of metazoan parasites from reptiles. This paper should be read by any person wishing to undertake detailed study of such parasites.

Parasite burdens are usually assessed by microscopical examination of the faeces for ova or other immature stages. The simplest method is to prepare a direct wet film of the specimen. A small amount of faecal material is emulsified in saline on a microscope slide. A coverslip must be carefully laid over the specimen, avoiding the formation of bubbles, and the slide viewed under a ×10 objective. Care must be taken not to place too much material on the slide so that the coverslip does not float. If preferred, a loopful of Lugol's iodine may be added to the preparation; this helps to emphasize the details of ova. A systematic search of the prepared slide should be made as it is easy to miss ova, especially if they are not present in great numbers. Once an ovum has been located, its individual features may be studied under high power. Whilst examining a wet preparation for ova other features can be noted. Protozoa may be present (see Chapter 8). Red blood cells may indicate haemorrhage in the lower intestine. Debris, such as fur, feather or vegetation may be seen—indicative of the diet fed.

Failure to demonstrate ova may be due to low numbers in the faeces. It may therefore be wise to carry out a concentration technique and two methods are possible. In the first, a 10% suspension of faeces is made in water so that there is 10 ml of suspension. This is passed through a sieve to remove pieces of debris before the addition of 2 ml of ether. The mixture is well shaken and topped up to 50 ml with water. The suspension is centrifuged for 1 minute and the supernatant discarded; the deposit is resuspended in 3 ml of water, before adding water to 50 ml. The suspension is centrifuged once more and the supernatant discarded. The deposit at this stage must be mixed with a little 35% zinc sulphate solution (adjusted to a specific gravity of 1·180), and transferred to a centrifuge tube. The tube should be filled to within 0·5 cm of its top and centrifuged for 2 minutes. Once the tube has come to rest, several loopfuls of the solution near the top of the tube may be placed on a slide and viewed.

An alternative concentration method is to emulsify a large portion of faeces in 10 ml of formol saline. This suspension is passed through a sieve, 3 ml of ether added and the whole mixture shaken vigorously. Centrifugation follows for 2 minutes after which it is necessary to loosen the fatty layer at the fluid's interface so that the supernatant and debris can be removed. Finally, the deposit is mixed in the residual fluid, placed on a slide and viewed under the microscope. This method also has the advantage that the formol saline will render the specimen non-infective and therefore safe to handle.

It is sometimes desirable to undertake a quantitative study of the faeces for the presence of ova. This is of particular use when performed before, during and after treatment as it can help monitor the success of therapy. However, it must be remembered that some species of intestinal parasite are more damaging to the infested animal when they are in the larval phase and therefore an ova count may not be of direct relevance. In addition, there is as yet little information on the significance of different egg counts in reptiles.

The quantitative technique used is that of McMaster (Ewing, 1974). Two grammes of faeces are crushed in 28 ml of water. One millilitre is added to 1 ml of Sheather's sugar solution and whilst keeping the resultant mixture agitated a McMaster counting chamber is filled. The chamber is left to stand for a few minutes to allow the ova to rise to the coverslip; the latter are then counted under the microscope. The number of ova counted in the chamber multiplied by 300 gives the count per gramme of faeces. This technique may also be combined with a salt flotation concentration by the following steps. Two grammes of faeces are ground up in 60 ml of saturated sodium chloride solution. The counting chamber is immediately filled with the suspension and a count made. The number of ova per gramme is obtained by multiplying the count by 100. Six millilitres of formol saline may be added to 54 ml of salt solution if it is wished to render the material non-infective.

With all the above methods for obtaining microscopical evidence of intestinal infestation, it can be helpful to add a loopful of Lugol's iodine to the deposits placed on the microscope slide in a similar way to that used for a wet preparation.

Parasites can also be detected in the blood and are discussed later.

IV. Haematological Techniques

Haematology is still in its infancy insofar as reptiles are concerned, due in some part to the problem of obtaining satisfactory samples.

Much is likely to be learnt of the haematological status of the reptile from a stained blood film. It will allow a qualitative assessment to be made and may also show the presence of parasites. Only a drop or two of blood is required to make a film. It is essential that the slides used are clean and grease-free. Practically it is of advantage to keep some slides stored in alcohol, and to wipe them dry immediately before use. A small drop of blood should be placed at one end of the slide. Using the edge of a second slide the drop is evenly spread along the first. The film can be dried in an incubator before fixing in methyl alcohol for 20 minutes. After fixation it may be stained using several different dyes. A very popular stain is Giemsa. The fixed film is placed into freshly diluted (10%) Giemsa stain and left for 45 minutes; the diluent is buffered at pH 7. After the staining time has elapsed the film must be washed in buffer and differentiated until the various cells are clear. After drying a permanent preparation is made using a xylol compatible mountant. Another method, using May Grunwald Giemsa stain, is a less lengthy technique. Films fixed as before are flooded with May Grunwald stain which has been freshly diluted in equal parts with buffered distilled water. After 5–8 minutes the film is transferred, without washing, to Giemsa stain diluted as before, where it is left for 15 minutes. The slide must be washed and differentiated in buffered water before mounting.

If a film has been prepared for the demonstration of parasites, it is sometimes desirable to remove the haemoglobin. For this purpose the slide should be immersed in distilled water until no more red haemoglobin leaves the film. Giemsa stain is then applied for at least 30 minutes. It is not necessary to differentiate the film after this time and it may be dried and mounted. It is possible to concentrate parasites in the specimen by haemolysing the blood and filtering (Bell, 1967).

The various stains used may vary from batch to batch when made up from powder and it is recommended that they be purchased in their liquid concentrated form. After dilution in buffer all unused stain must be discarded as it is essential that fresh solutions are used.

It is possible to perform cell counts from a blood film. The stains all differentiate the leucocytes easily and therefore an estimate of the relative numbers of the various types of cell can be made. However, difficulty may be encountered in identifying the various cell types and reference to published work is advisable—for example, the relevant section of Frye (1973), the chapter by Saint Girons (1970) and the thesis of Will (1977). If sufficient blood is available a number of other tests can be performed. Packed cell volume (PCV) can be measured using a standard microhaematocrit system and techniques used in fish (Hawkins and Mawdesley-Thomas, 1972) and birds (Hodges, 1977) can be employed to yield data on red and white cell counts and haemoglobin values. Other methods are discussed by Duguy (1970). Unfortunately electronic methods (for example, using the Coulter Counter) are unsuitable for use with reptile blood and time-consuming manual techniques must be employed.

There are several steps which can be taken to reduce the risk of error in haematological results. It is important that the sample used is truly representative and to ensure this, blood should be handled carefully. If it cannot be examined immediately, anticoagulated blood for cell counts must be stored at 4°C, although after 24 hours the results may be variable. The choice of anticoagulant agent is also important; EDTA is satisfactory for most haematological procedures (McDonald, 1976). Blood films can safely be prepared and stored after fixation, but for the best results they should be stained immediately after preparation. It may be possible to obtain sufficient blood for the preparation of a film from a needle prick: The first drop of blood must be discarded as it tends to have a high cell count. Any tendency to squeeze the pricked part to promote blood flow is to be discouraged as this may dilute the blood with serous fluid.

V. Biochemical Techniques

Biochemistry (clinical chemistry) is another field in which there is a paucity of data relating to reptiles. Nevertheless, it is likely to play an increasingly important role in diagnosis. Some techniques—for example, the estimation of serum calcium, phosphorus and magnesium—can be carried out using standard medical or veterinary methods. In the case of others one may be able to extrapolate from work with fish and here the bibliography by Hawkins and Mawdesley-Thomas

(1972) can prove useful. Reference should also be made to the work of Dessauer (1970).

VI. Conclusions

Many different methods of laboratory investigation have been described in this chapter. However, it should be recognized that it is only in the last few years that interest in the pathology of reptiles has developed to its present level. Because of this many techniques have yet to be adapted satisfactorily for use with reptilian samples. Much information has still to be collected and interpreted in order to establish values and to provide data on such subjects as normal bacterial flora. The accumulation of this knowledge will be a result of the co-operation between herpetologists, laboratory workers and veterinary surgeons. Laboratory personnel in particular play an important part. They must be prepared to apply many different tests to obtain a full result and must be wary of reaching incorrect conclusions because of inadequate examination of material.

References

Andrews, C. (1978). *Br. J. Herpet.* **5,** 735–739.
Andrews, R. D., Reilly, J. R., Ferris, D, H. and Hanson, L. E. (1965). *Bull. Wildl. Dis. Assoc.* **1,** 55–59.
Anğ, Ö., Özek, Ö., Cetin, E. T. and Töreci, K. (1973). *J. Hyg.* **71,** 85–88.
Annear, D. I. (1968). *Med. J. Aust.* **1,** 444–446.
Aronson, J. D. (1929). *J. infect. Dis.* **44,** 215–223.
Baker, F. J. (1967). "Handbook of Bacteriological Technique." pp. 24–25, 2nd Edition. Butterworth, London.
Barber, M. (1964). *J. gen Microbiol.* **35,** 183–190.
Bauer, A. W., Kirby, W. M., Sherris, J. C. and Turck, M. (1966). *Am. J. clin. Path.* **45,** 493–496.
Bell, D. (1967). *Ann. trop. Med. Parasit.* **61,** 220–223.
Borland, E. D. (1975). *Vet. Rec.* **96,** 401–402.
Breach, M. R. (1972). In "Microbiology of the Seventies." (F. J. Baker, ed.), pp. 108–119. Butterworth, London.
Carlier, G. I. M. (1948). *Br. J. Derm.* **10,** 61–63.
Chattopadhyay, B. and Pilford, J. N. (1976). *Med. Lab. Sci.* **33,** 191–194.
Clegg, F. G. and Heath, P. J. (1975). *Vet. Rec.* **96,** 90–91.
Cooper, G. N. (1957). *J. clin. Path.* **10,** 226–230.
Cooper, J. E. and Leakey, J. H. E. (1976). *Trans. R. Soc. trop. Med. Hyg.* **70,** 80–84.

Cooper, J. E., Needham, J. R. and Griffin, J. (1978). *Lab. Anim.* **12,** 91–93.
Cowan, S. T. (1974). "Cowan and Steel's Manual for the Identification of Medical Bacteria." Cambridge University Press, Cambridge.
Cowan, S. T. and Steel, K. J. (1966). "Manual for the Identification of Medical Bacteria." Cambridge University Press, London.
Cruickshank, R. (1969). "Medical Microbiology." E. and S. Livingstone, Edinburgh and London.
Curtis, M. A., Lapage, S. P., Bascomb, S. and Willcox, W. R. (1972). *In* "Microbiology of the Seventies". (F. J. Baker, ed.) pp. 96–107. Butterworth, London.
Dessauer, H. C. (1970). *In* "Biology of the Reptilia". (C. Gans, ed.). Vol. 3, pp. 1–72. Academic Press, London and New York.
Duguy, R. (1970). *In* "Biology of the Reptilia". (C. Gans, ed.). Vol. 3, pp. 93–110. Academic Press, London and New York.
Ehrlich, P. (1882). *D. med. Wschr.* **8,** 269–270.
Ewing, S. A. (1974). *In* "Veterinary Clinical Pathology". (E. H. Coles, ed.). p 476. W. B. Saunders, Philadelphia.
Ferris, D. H., Rhoades, H. E. and Hanson, L. E. (1959). *Cornell Vet.* **49,** 344–349.
Ferris, D. H., Rhoades, H. E., Hanson, L. E., Galton, M. and Mansfield, M. E. (1961). *Cornell Vet.* **51,** 405–419.
Fisk, A. (1940). *Brit. J. exp. Path.* **21,** 311–314.
Frye, F. L. (1973). "Husbandry, Medicine and Surgery in Captive Reptiles." V. M. Publishing Inc., Kansas.
Georg, L. K., Ajello, L., Papageorge, C. (1954). *J. Lab. clin. Med.* **44,** 422–428.
Gillies, R. R. and Dodds, T. C. (1968). "Bacteriology Illustrated." E. and S. Livingstone, Edinburgh and London.
Gochenour, W. S., Yager, R. H., Wetmore, P. W. and Hightower, J. A. (1953). *Am. J. publ. Hlth.* **43,** 405–410.
Gram, C. (1884). *Fortschr. Med.* **2,** 185–189. See for translation "Milestones in Microbiology". (T. D. Brock, ed.) (1961) pp. 215–218. Prentice-Hall, London.
Hawkins, R. I. and Mawdesley-Thomas, L. E. (1972). *J. Fish Biol.* **4,** 193–232.
Hewlett, R. T. and Nolan, H. (1896). *Brit. med. J.* **1,** 266–267.
Hodges, R. D. (1977). *In* "Comparative Clinical Haematology." (R. K. Archer and L. B. Jeffcott, eds.). pp 483–517. Blackwell Scientific Publications, Oxford.
Holt, P. E. (1979). *J. small Anim. Pract.* **20,** 353–359.
Holt, P. E. and Cooper, J. E. (1976). *Vet. Rec.* **98,** 156.
Holt, P. E., Cooper, J. E. and Needham, J. R. (1979). *J. small Anim. Pract.* **20,** 269–286.
Hynes, M. (1942). *J. Path. Bact.* **54,** 193–207.
Jensen, K. A. (1955). *Bull. int. Un. Tuberc.* **25,** 89–95.
Johne, A. (1885). *Fortschr. Med.* **3,** footnote p. 200.

Kopeloff, N. and Beerman, P. (1922). *J. Infect. Dis.* **31,** 480–482.
Lambert, R. A. (1969). "Parasitology: Identification of Helminths." Butterworth, London.
Leifson, E. (1936). *Am. J. Hyg.* **24,** 423–432.
Linton, A. H. (1977). *Vet. Rec.* **100,** 354–360.
McDonald, H. S. (1976). *In* "Biology of the Reptilia" (C. Gans and W. R. Dawson, eds.). Vol. 5A, pp. 19–126. Academic Press, London and New York.
Maurer, I. M. (1974). "Hospital Hygiene." Edward Arnold, London.
Mueller, J. H. and Hinton, J. (1941). *Proc. Soc. exp. Biol. Med.* **48,** 330–333.
Needham, J. R. (1974). *Med. Lab. Tech.* **31,** 141–143.
Needham, J. R. (1977). *J. Inst. An. Tech.* **28,** 179–181.
Needham, J. R. (1978). *Vet. Rec.* **102,** 286–287.
Needham, J. R. (1979). "Handbook of Microbiological Investigations for Laboratory Animal Health." Academic Press, London, New York and San Francisco.
Needham, J. R. (1981). "Animal Quality and Models in Biomedical Research" (A. Spiegel, S. Erichsen and H. A. Solleveld, eds.). Gustav Fischer Verlag, Stuttgart and New York.
Newsom, S. W. B. and Walsingham, B. M. (1974). *J. clin. Path.* **27,** 921–924.
Owens, D. R., Wagner, J. E. and Addison, J. B. (1975). *J. Am. vet. med. Ass.* **167,** 605–609.
Preston, N. E. and Morrell, A. (1962). *J. Path. Bact.* **84,** 241–243.
Robertson, M. (1916). *J. Path. Bact.* **20,** 327–349.
Saint Girons, M–C. (1970). *In* "Biology of the Reptilia". (C. Gans, ed.). Vol. 3, pp. 73–92. Academic Press, London and New York.
Sanford, J. (1976). *Vet. Rec.* **99,** 61–64.
Schiff, L. J., Barbera, P. W., Port, C. D., Yamashiroya, H. M., Shefner, A. M. and Poiley, S. M. (1972). *Lab. Anim. Sci.* **22,** 705–708.
Shotts, E. B., Gaines, J. L., Martin, L. and Prestwood, A. K. (1972). *J. Am. vet. med. Ass.* **161,** 603–607.
Stevens, M. (1977). *The Medical Technologist.* June, pp. 20–21, 24–25, 27–28.
Stokes, J. E. (1968). "Clinical Bacteriology." Edward Arnold, London.
Stuart, R. D. (1946a). *Glasg. Med. J.* **27,** 131–142.
Stuart, R. D. (1946b). *J. Path.* **53,** 343–349.
Stuart, R. D., Toshach, S. R. and Patsula, T. M. (1954). *Canad. J. publ. Hlth.* **45,** 73–83.
Verstraete, A. P. (1973). *Lab. Anim.* **7,** 189–193.
Vogel, H. (1958). *Am. Rev. Tuberc. pulm. Dis.* **77,** 823–838.
Wallach, J. D. (1977). *Int. Zoo Yb.* **17,** 170–171.
Will, R. (1977). "Hämatologische und serologische Untersuchungen bei Lacertiden (Reptilia Squamata)." Thesis, University of Hohenheim.
World Health Organization (1961). *Wld. Hlth. Org. Tech. Ref. Ser.* No. 210.

Infectious Diseases

5 Viruses

H F. CLARK

The Wistar Institute of Anatomy and Biology,
36th Street at Spruce, Philadelphia, USA

P. D. LUNGER

University of Delaware, Newark, USA

I. Introduction

Reptiles as hosts of virus infection are the least studied of the major classes of vertebrates. Impetus for the investigation of mammalian, avian, and fish virus diseases has arisen from the profound economic importance to agriculture and fisheries industries of many representative species. Intensive studies of viruses of certain amphibian species followed observation of association of herpesviruses with kidney tumours enzootic in high incidence in certain populations of North American leopard frogs (*Rana pipiens*) (Mizell, 1969). A presumptive role of virus in the aetiology of a lymphosarcoma common in certain European colonies of captive *Xenopus laevis* (Balls, 1965) further justified virological investigation of these amphibians.

Modern virological investigations require expensive cell culture procedures. Reptiles are of economic importance only in exceptional instances. Although numerous tumours of reptiles have been described, their incidence has largely been sporadic (Lucké and Schlumberger, 1949) and has not suggested infectious aetiology. The recent description of oncornaviruses associated with tumours of snakes (Zeigel and Clark, 1969; Clark *et al*, 1979a) has not stimulated intense interest in the biomedical community.

Nevertheless, cell cultures, both primary and as continuous cell lines, are very conveniently prepared from reptilian tissues (Clark, 1972; Clark *et al*, 1970). Modest studies of both diseased and apparently healthy reptiles have already led to identification of reptilian viruses representative of several major virus groups (Lunger and Clark, 1978; Ahne, 1977). The results of most of these studies are too preliminary to allow unequivocal association of virus with reptilian disease. It is, however, clear that reptiles are frequently hosts of virus infections. The acquisition of more complete knowledge of these virus–reptile host systems will be necessary to complete any total comprehension of virus–host cycles in vertebrate wildlife.

II. Viruses Circumstantially Associated with Reptilian Disease

A. Fer-de-lance Virus—Respiratory Disease

This virus was identified as the result of an epizootic that swept a snake farm in Zurich, Switzerland, in August of 1972 (Fölsch and Leloup, 1976). During the course of the epizootic, 128 of 431 fer-de-lance (*Bothrops atrox*) died. Mortality rates as high as 87 per cent were observed in individual animal rooms. Older *Bothrops* appeared particularly susceptible as 98 per cent of snakes more than 8 years in captivity died. None of 13 *Naja naja* or 2 *Elaphe longissima* died.

Clinical signs in this epizootic were marked. The initial stage of the illness, lasting 5 to 12 days, was characterized primarily by a loss of muscle tone leading the animals to assume prostrate, "stretched out" positions rather than their normally coiled posture. In the terminal stage of the disease, lasting only 1 or 2 days, snakes often showed abnormal activity. The pupils were greatly dilated and the mouth was often held open. Discharges from the mouth preceded terminal prostration.

Necropsy revealed a body cavity and lungs filled with fluid. An acute suppurative bronchopneumonia was present. Additionally, there was evidence of secondary spread of infection from the lungs to the liver, kidneys and, in females, to the reproductive organs.

In an attempt to isolate the causal agent of the respiratory disease, the lungs of four snakes with fatal infections were removed, triturated, and injected into embryonated eggs of the false water cobra *Cyclogras gigas*. Infected eggs died a few days later. Egg embryo suspension inoculated into gecko embryo (GE 2) and rattlesnake fibroma cell cultures incubated at 30°C caused cytopathic effect (CPE) characterized by massive syncytium formation (Clark *et al*, 1979). The cytopathic agent recovered from supernatant fluids of these cultures was designated fer-de-lance virus (FDLV).

FDLV replicated efficiently with varying degrees of CPE in each of nine reptilian cell lines tested. FDLV also readily infected mammalian (hamster, bovine, and human) cells incubated at 30°C but fish cell lines were not susceptible. In addition to the development of CPE, all infected cells haemadsorbed guinea-pig red blood cells very intensely, and chick red blood cells to a lesser extent. Virus replicate to the highest titre *in vitro* at incubation temperatures of approximately 23°C to 32°C. The upper temperature limit supporting virus replication varied according to host cell, but was in all cases less than 37°C.

FDLV was also adapted readily to growth in the allantoic cavity of the embryonated hen's egg; allantoic fluid yielded haemagglutinin (HA) titres as high as 1:512. Consistent infection of the hen's egg required incubation within a temperature range of 27°C to 32°C, with the highest titres obtained at 27°C. However, because of the difficulty in maintaining egg viability at 27°C, a standard incubation temperature of 30°C was finally adopted.

FDLV caused no overt disease or histologically detectable pathology when injected intracerebrally into newborn mice or by a variety of routes into adult mice. Attempts to evaluate the disease-inducing potential of FDLV in adult water snakes led to equivocal results, as a pre-existing background of FDLV infection was apparently present in the test animals (Leif, personal communication).

Electron microscopic observation of FDLV-infected cells in culture revealed pleomorphic, spheroidal or filamentous particles budding from plasma membranes or free as mature particles (Fig. 5.1–5.4). These exhibited typical myxovirus morphology, with a peripheral fringe of haemagglutinin and internal nucleocapsid strands of 150 to 160 nm in diameter. The size of released particles ranged from 146 to 321 nm in mean diameter, depending upon the host cell system and the cell incubation temperature (Lunger and Clark, 1979a, b).

That FDLV is a paramyxovirus was indicated by demonstrating that it possesses a single-stranded RNA genome with a sedimentation value of 50S. However, serological comparison of FDLV with known mammalian and avian paramyxoviruses indicated that this virus is antigenically distinct.

Further experiments are required in order to determine the role of FDLV in inducing the type of disease described in *Bothrops*. In particular, it will be important to those concerned with reptile husbandry to ascertain whether FDLV is a highly pathogenic virus capable alone of causing severe epizootics or whether it may be a

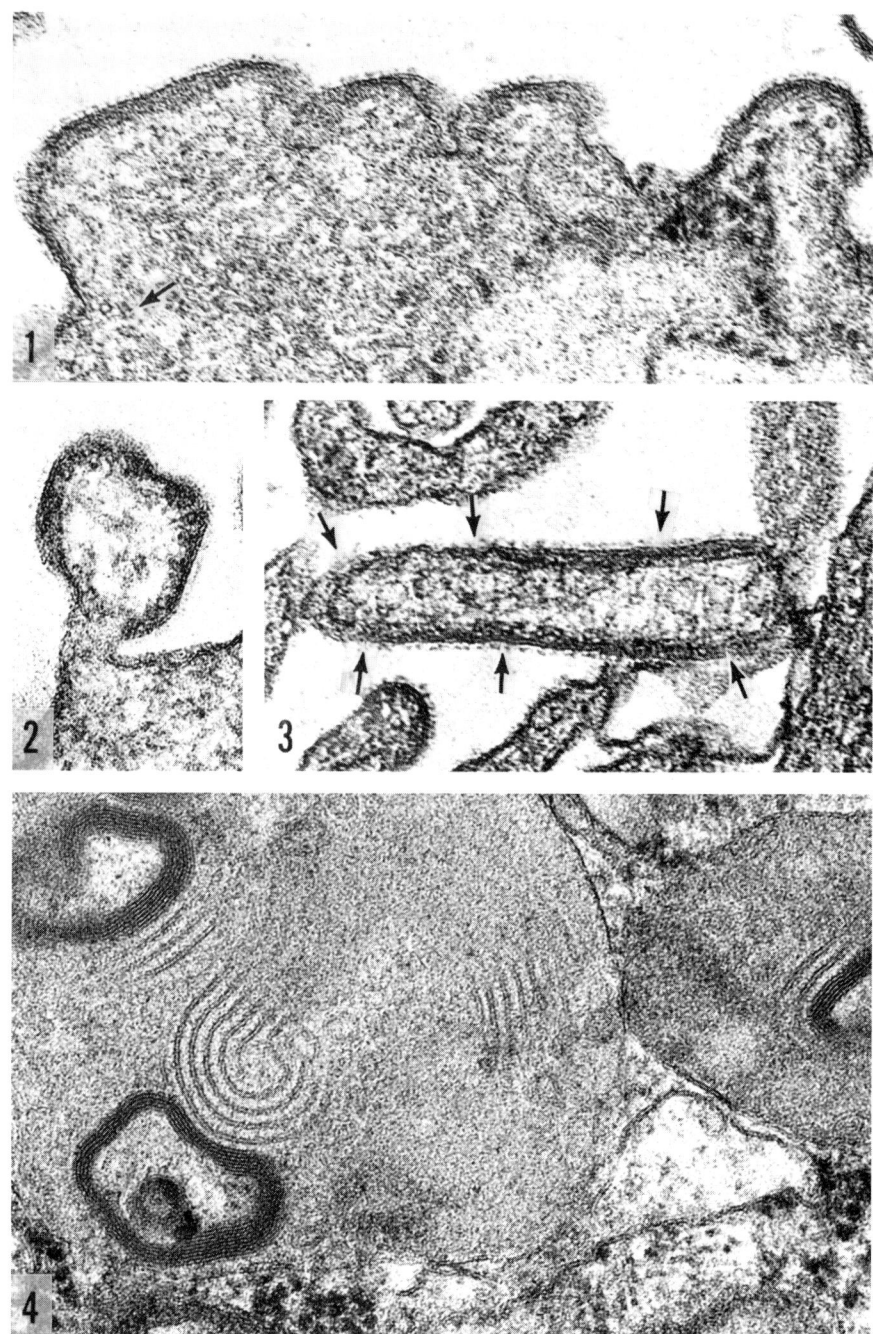

source of common latent infections leading to acute disease in animals subjected to other stress factors.

B. Green Sea Turtle Virus—Skin (and possibly Systemic) Disease

An enzootic disease of green sea turtles (*Chelonia mydas*), apparently caused by a virus, was described at a commercial sea turtle farm on Grand Cayman Island in the British West Indies (Rebell et al, 1975). Nine successively hatched groups of turtles developed spontaneously "gray-patch disease" which affected 90 to 100 per cent of animals in each group. The onset of disease was noted between 56 and 90 days after hatching. The disease was characterized by either circumscribed papular skin lesions or, more commonly, spreading grey skin patches with superficial epidermal necrosis. Turtles with extensive skin disease exhibited a mortality of 5 to 20 per cent. No explanation for the observed mortality or pathological description of fatally infected animals has been reported.

Histopathological examination of sections of papules and grey-patch lesions revealed similar features. Cells of the upper and middle layers of the epidermis frequently contained nuclei with basophilic inclusion bodies and marginated chromatin. Electron microscopic examination of skin lesions in thin section revealed intranuclear enveloped particles 160 to 180 nm in diameter each containing a characteristic electron-dense core. Immature non-enveloped nucleocapsids measuring 105 to 120 nm in diameter were also observed in infected nuclei.

Lesion impressions or scraping extracts negatively stained with

---

Fig. 5.1. FDLV-infected rattlesnake fibroma cells. Large regions of the cell surface show peripheral "spines" and subadjacent plasmalemmal thickening. The cytoplasm in these zones often contains large accumulations of nucleocapsid strands seen as tubules in cross section (arrow). ($\times 100\,000$)

Fig. 5.2. FDLV-infected rattlesnake spleen cells. A spheroidal particle in the process of budding. Nucleocapsid cross sectional profiles are subadjacent to the presumptive viral envelope. ($\times 100\,000$)

Fig. 5.3. FDLV-infected rattlesnake fibroma cell. Rod-shaped or filamentous particles (arrows) are commonly observed. ($\times 100\,000$)

Fig. 5.4. FDLV-infected rattlesnake fibroma cell. Viral-induced, membrane-bound, cytoplasmic inclusion bodies contain multilamellar configurations in a granular matrix. ($\times 100\,000$)

phosphotungstic acid and examined by electron microscopy similarly exhibited both naked nucleocapsids and fully enveloped virus particles. The morphological appearance of the virions and their intranuclear site of development are both characteristic of the herpesvirus group.

Experimental transmission of the disease was accomplished by inoculating lesion extracts on to the scarified flippers of normal 6- to 8-week old turtles. Lesions developed along scratch lines within three weeks in 49 of 50 animals. The histopathological appearance of the lesions was identical to that noted in the natural disease. Herpes-like virions were detected by electron microscopic examination of the experimentally induced skin lesions.

Experimental manipulation of ambient water temperature was shown to have a profound effect on the pattern of gray-patch disease incidence (Haines and Kleese, 1977). Spontaneous development of disease was monitored in 3-week old turtles subjected to a variety of water temperature regimens. Animals in water abruptly heated from 25°C (control temperature) to 30°C or in water gradually heated to 30°C and maintained at 30°C showed hastened onset and increased severity of disease. Animals more gradually and transiently warmed to 30°C, and those maintained at 25°C throughout the experiment had more moderate disease.

Isolation of the presumptive causal agent of grey-patch disease was recently announced (Koment and Haines, 1977). It was also reported to replicate rapidly at an incubation temperature of 25°C in an epithelioid cell line derived from the skin of *C. mydas*. The virus was reported to induce cytopathology characteristic of the herpesvirus group and to be immunologically distinct from catfish herpesvirus and herpes simplex virus (human) but no further characterization was recorded.

The green sea turtle virus presents an experimental system of special interest, as it is the only virus of reptiles reported to date to have been successfully used in experimental transmission of naturally occurring reptilian infectious disease. However, this conclusion, to be definitively accepted, must be confirmed by experimental induction of disease with virus propagated and cloned for genetic homogeneity in cell culture. Precise determination of the optimum temperature for virus growth *in vivo* and *in vitro* would also provide invaluable information on the relative role of virus temperature requirements and host–animal stress factors in the observed effects of high ambient temperatures on enhancement of clinical disease. It will be of great interest to those wishing to control this disease to determine the extent of natural latent virus infection so that the relative roles of induction of masked infection and of virus spread from infected animals and the contaminated environment may be properly assessed.

C. Erythrocyte Virus of Australian Geckos—Anaemia

The disease caused by this intra-erythrocytic virus of reptiles causes what was undoubtedly the first reptilian virus disease to be studied, but its aetiology was not realized until 1960. A protozoan genus and species, *Pirhemocyton tarentolae*, were originally created to describe the presumed causal agent associated with inclusions in erythrocytes of geckos (*Tarentola mauritanica*) affected with a disease characterized by progressive anaemia (Chatton and Blanc, 1914). Several other species of *Pirhemocyton* were subsequently described from other reptiles, based only upon similar microscopic evidence (Stehbens and Johnston, 1966). It was demonstrated that infection could be transmitted by experimental inoculation of whole (but not lysed and filtered) blood from infected animals (Dodin and Brygoo, 1956), but otherwise the nature and life history of the "protozoan parasite" were never characterized.

The viral nature of the disease previously attributed to *Pirhemocyton* was indicated by electron microscopic examination of erythrocytes of an infected Australian gecko *Gehyra variegata* (Stehbens and Johnston, 1966). This lizard exhibited inclusions with a morphology typical of that described for *Pirhemocyton* when examined at the light microscopic level. However, electron microscopic examination revealed no protozoan parasites. Rather, it was shown that the observed inclusions represented virus "assembly pool" or "factory" areas. Within these areas were numerous uniform bodies of 220 nm mean diameter, hexagonal or pentagonal in cross-sectional appearance, and present in various stages of maturation. The outer shell of these bodies consisted of two unit membranes; a dense core composed of granular or fibrillar material (presumably nucleic acid) was also commonly present. All morphological features of the individual bodies as well as the synthetic "factory" are compatible with the presumptive identification of those bodies as viruses of the iridovirus group. This virus group includes representatives isolated from a variety of species of amphibians, as well as from insects and mammals (Kelly and Robertson, 1973).

This virus of reptilian erythrocytes has not yet been isolated. However, numerous reports of the presence of "*Pirhemocyton*" suggest that it is widespread in feral reptiles.

D. Virus of Pacific Pond Turtles—Hepatitis

This virus was detected in each of two Pacific pond turtles (*Clemmys marmorata*) suffering a fatal systemic disease within a few weeks of their collection from a creek in California, USA (Frye et al, 1977). Each animal, when examined immediately after death, exhibited only a "slightly swollen" liver and spleen. However, histopathological examination revealed the presence of acute hepatic necrosis. Intranuclear inclusions and marginated chromatin were seen in many hepatocytes and, less commonly, in cells of the kidney and spleen.

Electron microscopic studies of liver and spleen revealed the presence of icosahedral intranuclear particles 100 nm in diameter, either empty or containing a dense core. Mature enveloped particles 140 nm in diameter were seen in the cytoplasm and in intracellular locations. The morphology and intracellular maturation pattern of these particles was typical of herpesviruses. Their isolation has not been reported.

III. Viruses Associated with Reptilian Tumours

A. Sarcoma-associated Viruses

The snake oncornavirus isolated as a result of studies on a sarcoma of the Russell's viper (*Vipera russelli*) (Zeigel and Clark, 1969, 1971) was the first oncornavirus identified from an ectothermic vertebrate, and remains the best characterized. Until its isolation, the tumour-associated RNA viruses (oncornaviruses, in the family Retroviridae) were known only from mammals and birds. The phylogenetic extension of host range of this class of viruses to reptiles was a major argument used in proposal of a hereditary viral "virogene" theory of integrated cancer virus genomes which possibly explains the widespread spectrum of vertebrate cancer (Huebner and Todaro, 1969).

Since the isolation of the first Russell's viper virus, several related oncornaviruses have been isolated from *V. russelli* (Andersen, 1977) and a single, very distantly related, oncornavirus has been isolated from the corn snake (*Elaphe guttata*) (Clark et al, 1979a). One other oncornavirus of an ectothermic vertebrate, the virus of lymphosarcoma of northern pike, has been described for fish (Papas et al, 1976). However, the detection of several oncornaviruses in the course of very limited studies of snakes suggests a special concentration in this suborder of vertebrates.

1. *Russell's Viper Oncornaviruses*

(a) *Isolation* The original Russell's viper oncornavirus was isolated as a result of study of an adult female animal resident in the Buffalo, New York Zoological Gardens (Zeigel and Clark, 1969). The animal was killed because it was declining in condition and an unsightly swelling of approximately two years' duration made it unsuitable for exhibition. Necropsy examination revealed the presence of a large (117·5 g), spherical mass attached only to mesentery anterior to the heart in the body cavity. No other tumours were seen. Histological examination indicated that the tumour was an oedematous myxofibroma. Although neoplasia of other visceral organs was not observed, intravascular masses of "dense" cells, possibly representing metastatic emboli, were observed in the liver, spleen, kidney, and pancreas (Zeigel and Clark, 1971). Electron microscopic examination revealed that these intravascular "dense" cell masses exhibited many ultrastructural features in common with fibroma cells.

Cell cultures were established from tissues of the tumour and of other major visceral tissues. A continuous cell line was established only from spleen cell culture (cell line VSW—*Vipera* spleen warm). The morphology of VSW cells resembles that of the tumour cells at both a light-microscopic and fine-structural level of morphology. VSW cells were first examined by electron microscopy at the 48th cell passage level; at this time, large numbers of both intracytoplasmic and released typical "Type-C" virions were observed. No virions were ever seen in electron microscopic studies of tumour tissue or of intravascular metastatic cells *in situ*.

The morphology of viper virus from VSW cells (VV-VSW) is very similar to that of mammalian and avian oncornaviruses. Typical stages of maturation by budding from plasma membranes are observed (Fig. 5.5 and 5.6). Mature virions are 108 nm in diameter and possess a dense core 45 nm in diameter. Because of the relatively small size of the core, VV-VSW appears to bear a closer morphological affinity to avian than to mammalian oncornaviruses.

In order to assess the effect of viper virus infection and possible "transformation" upon the phenotype of VSW cells, VSW cells were compared with cells of a virus-free cell line (VH2) established from the heart of a tumour-free Russell's viper (Clark *et al*, 1973). VSW cells had a less differentiated cytoplasm and a higher nuclear: cytoplasmic cell ratio than VH2 cells. VH2 cells were more tolerant than VSW cells to extremes of incubation temperature and to

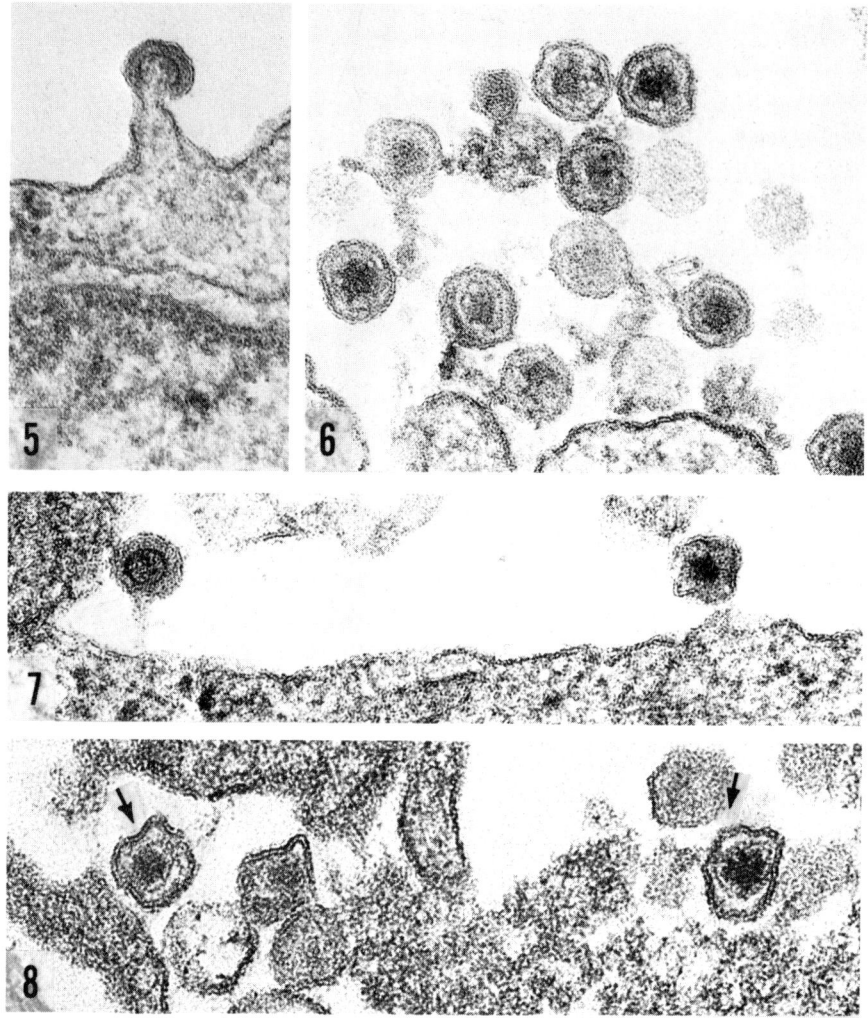

Fig. 5.5. VSW cell. A Type-C particle budding from the plasmalemma. (×100 000)

Fig. 5.6. VSW cell. Released Type-C virions in the extracellular space. (×100 000)

Fig. 5.7. Viper heart (VH2 cell line) cell. "Immature" (left) and "mature" or released (right) Type-C particles. (×100 000)

Fig. 5.8. Viper heart cell. Released Type-C virions (arrows) in the extracellular space. (×100 000)

treatment with dextran sulphate. VH2 supported the replication of a wider spectrum of superinfecting viruses. Karyotypic alterations were much more marked in VSW cells.

Subsequent to the above-mentioned study, the production of C-type virus (VV-VH2) was observed by electron microscopic study of VH2 cells (Andersen, 1977). This virus is morphologically indistinguishable from VV-VSW (Fig. 5.8 and 5.9). Its appearance was not marked by any obvious phenotypic alteration in VH2 cells. A third, morphologically identical virus (VV-VH3) was subsequently detected in a cell line (VH3) established from another tumour-free Russell's viper. As in the case of VH2 cells, early passage VH3 cell cultures were free of virus based upon fine-structural examination or by assay of sedimentable DNA polymerase activity.

(b) *Biological properties* Early attempts to infect mammalian, avian or fish cell lines or available reptilian cell lines or primary reptile cell culture systems with VV-VSW met with consistent failure (Clark, unpublished). However, VV-VSW was found to infect cells of a rattlesnake (*Crotalus horridus*) fibroma cell line (Orr *et al*, 1972) established from a virus-free tumour of a timber rattlesnake. Repeated passage of VV-VSW-inoculated cells was necessary before released VV could be detected by either electron microscopic examination or by examination for sedimentable DNA polymerase activity (Andersen, 1977). Cytopathic effects associated with VV-VSW infection were absent or minimal. Subsequently it was demonstrated that early passage heart and kidney cell cultures of *C. horridus* could also be infected with either VV-VSW, VV-VH2 or VV-VSW previously cultivated in rattlesnake fibroma cells (VV-VSW[RF]). Infection of rattlesnake cell cultures with VV-VH2 or VV-VSW(RF) was accompanied by development of severe cytopathic effects, not noted in the case of VV-VSW. This observation may be related to the fact that VV-VSW is a glycoprotein-deficient "defective" virus (see later).

The oncogenic potential of viper oncornaviruses is not known. Injection of VSW cells into a few adult geckos (*Gekko gecko*) did not produce tumours. Viper oncornaviruses have not been injected experimentally into *V. russelli*.

(c) *Biochemical, biophysical and immunological properties* VV-VSW resembles mammalian and avian oncornaviruses in possessing a 60–70S RNA genome and exhibiting a virion buoyant density of 1·16 g/ml (Gilden *et al*, 1970). The VV-VSW virion RNA has been reported to be smaller than that of representative mammalian leukaemia viruses

(Maruyama et al, 1971); this observation may indicate a deletion responsible for the inability to code for high molecular weight glycoprotein.

As is characteristic of oncornaviruses, VV-VSW possesses an RNA-dependent DNA polymerase. The enzyme has been recorded to possess a significantly higher specific activity than that of feline, murine and hamster oncornaviruses (Hatanaka et al, 1970). Various authors have reported different temperature optima for activity of the VV-VSW DNA polymerase. Twardzik et al (1973) recorded a temperature optimum of 40–45°C for the endogenous reaction; Menko et al (1976) reported a broad temperature optimum of from 32°C to >40°C. More recent experiments, in which 60-minute assays were carried out under linear reaction conditions, have indicated that the optimum temperature for the endogenous reaction is 34°C (Andersen, 1977), a low temperature more appropriate to the ectothermic vertebrate origin of the virus. In the same series of experiments, an elevated optimum temperature of 42°C was demonstrated for an exogenously templated reaction. The DNA product of VV-VSW DNA polymerase has been reported to hybridize with homologous viral RNA but not with RNA of several mammalian oncornaviruses (Hatanaka et al, 1971).

The original analysis of VV-VSW structural polypeptides separated on columns of Biogel A-5 in the presence of 6 M guanidine hydrochloride revealed six protein peaks (Nowinski et al, 1973). Subsequent analysis of VV-VSW using the Laemmli (1974) polyacrylamide gel electrophoresis system led to identification of four major polypeptides with molecular weights of 24, 19, 13, and 12 thousand daltons (Andersen, 1977). VV-VSW is defective in that it lacks, or possesses in very low concentration only, a high molecular weight glycoprotein. Viper viruses of VH2 and VH3 cell origin resemble VV-VSW in their complement of major polypeptides and in their deficiency in glycoprotein. However, VV-VSW propagated in rattlesnake fibroma cells acquires a typical high molecular weight glycoprotein, suggesting an endogenous helper virus function in rattlesnake cells.

VV-VSW appears to be antigenically distinct from avian and murine leukaemia viruses; antisera to the latter did not react in complement-fixation tests with either whole or ether-disrupted viper virus (Gilden et al, 1970). Furthermore, antisera to the purified DNA-polymerase antigens of a broad spectrum of avian and mammalian oncornaviruses did not react with the DNA polymerase of VV-VSW (Benveniste and Todaro, unpublished).

(d) *Intramitochondrial virion replication* A unique aspect of oncornavirus replication in VSW and VH2 cells is the apparent production of intramitochondrial virions (IMV). Lunger and Clark (1973) noted that fine-structural examination of VSW cells revealed not only "C-type" virus maturation at typical plasmalemmal and vacuolar membrane sites but also virion-like structures within mitochondria. Although morphological and biochemical evidence of intramitochondrial replication of certain avian Type-C viruses has been reported (Mach and Kará, 1971), only the viper system is characterized by intramitochondrial structures with the appearance of complete virions.

Viper IMV (Fig. 5.9–5.12) are approximately 106 nm in diameter with a dense 75 nm core surrounded by an intermediate layer. Peripheral to the intermediate layer is a trilaminar envelope derived from cristal membranes.

IMV maturation stages differ somewhat from those of Type-C virus maturing at plasma membranes (Lunger and Clark, 1973). A thin crescent-shaped density appears adjacent to the inner face of the inner mitochondrial membrane and sequentially develops a C-shape and then a spherical configuration with distinct core and peripheral regions. The final stage of maturation is the enclosure of this particle within a membrane derived from inner mitochondrial membrane. Although the final stage is not identical to Type-C mature-released virions, the general mature virion structure and formative stages suggest that it is Type-C virion. Further strong circumstantial evidence for this conclusion is (1) the constant association of IMV with simultaneous production of typical Type-C virus from plasma membranes, and (2) the induction of IMV formation in cultured rattlesnake cells following experimental infection with released viper Type-C virions (Andersen, Lunger and Clark, manuscript in preparation). IMV have not been detected in control rattlesnake, Tokay gecko, leopard gecko, iguana, box turtle, or mammalian or avian cells.

Normally propagated VSW and VH2 cells exhibit IMV in approximately 4 per cent of mitochondrial thin section profiles (Lunger and Clark, 1974). This prevalence is increased if VSW cells are incubated at 35°C rather than 30°C or are super-infected with rabies virus. Treatment of VSW cells with ethidium bromide also led to enhanced IMV prevalence (Klietmann *et al*, 1977; Lunger *et al*, 1977), despite the fact that this drug specifically inhibits certain mitochondrial biosynthetic processes.

The significance of this unique intramitochondrial infection is unclear. There is no evidence that IMV are released. Egression of

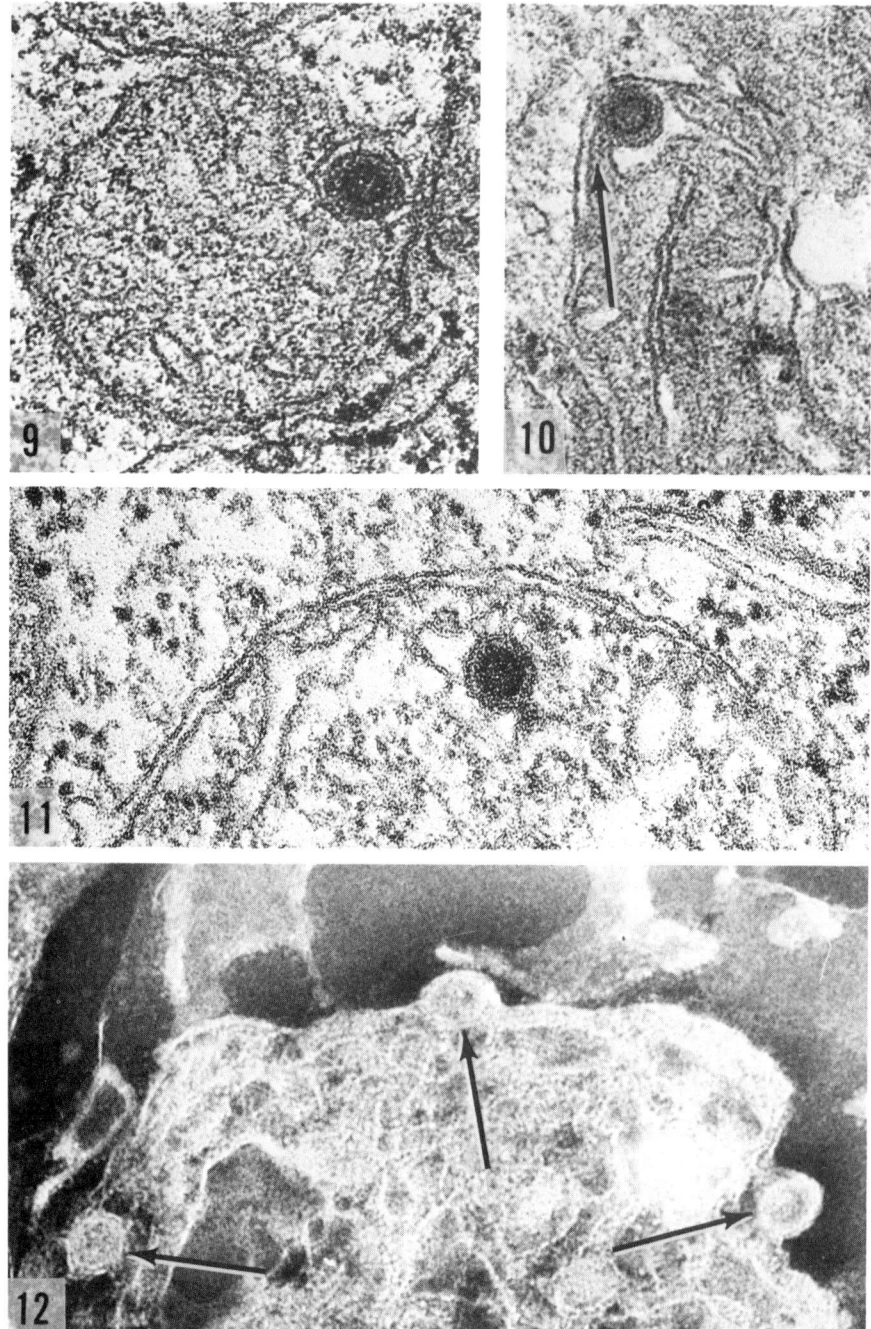

virus from mitochondria has not been seen by electron microscopic examination. No evidence of cardiolipin, a substance in high concentration in inner mitochondrial membranes, has been found in released viper virions (Malhotra, Andersen and Clark, unpublished). The effect of IMV on mitochondria is also unclear. Infected mitochondria often are swollen and exhibit cristal disorganization. Mitochondria from VSW cells contain a several-fold excess of DNA when compared with mitochondria of IMV-free viper cells; VSW cell mitochondrial DNA also contains an excess of catenated dimers (Klietmann et al, 1977). Further study of the effect of IMV upon mitochondrial physiology would seem to be justified as an approach to evaluating the role of virus:mitochondrial interaction in oncogenesis.

(e) *Type-A particles* Type-A particles are not strictly identified but are assumed to be in some way related to oncornavirus synthesis in homeothermic vertebrates. Type-A particles have recently been detected in VSW cells (Fig. 5.13). These particles are 60 to 70 nm in total diameter and frequently exist as juxtanuclear aggregations. Particles have been seen in approximately 0·5 per cent of VSW cells; the prevalence is elevated following growth of cells in eithidium bromide. It is thought that these particles may represent an accumulation of viral by-products in degenerating cells (Lunger and Clark, 1977).

2. *Corn Snake (Elaphe) Oncornavirus*

The first direct electron microscope observation of Type-C virus associated with tumour tissue in a reptile resulted from examination of a corn snake (*Elaphe guttata*) tumour (Lunger *et al*, 1974). The host

---

Fig. 5.9. VSW cell. The intramitochondrial virus (IMV) illustrated here is situtated in its typical peripheral location within the mitochondrion. (×100 000)

Fig. 5.10. VSW cell. The arrow in this figure indicates the close topographical relationship between the IMV investing membrane and cristal membranes. (×100 000)

Fig. 5.11. VSW cell. On occasion, as illustrated here, IMV is situated in other than peripheral locations. (×100 000).

Fig. 5.12. A portion of a negatively stained, purified mitochondrion derived from VSW cells. Arrows indicate structures thought to represent IMV at the organelle periphery. (×100 000)

animal, a 125 cm-long female, had been in a private collection for 13 years, during ten of which it was in a community cage with five other corn snakes from southern New Jersey. One of the companion snakes had died three years earlier with a similar disease. The animal examined had developed a dorsal subcutaneous swelling about one year previously. This was surgically removed two weeks before the animal was killed, but another subcutaneous swelling had rapidly reappeared.

The subcutaneous mass was determined histologically to be an embryonal rhabdomyosarcoma. No other tumours were observed. Fine-structural study of the sarcoma revealed typical Type-C virus both extracellularly and budding from plasma and vacuolar membranes. Particles were approximately 110 nm in total diameter with a condensed nucleoid about 50 nm in diameter. Like viper oncornaviruses, their morphological appearance resembled that of avian rather than mammalian, leukaemia viruses. Occasional C-type virions were also observed in the spleen of the tumour-bearing snake; in parallel studies no C-type virus could be found in the spleens of two tumour-free control corn snakes.

Attempts to establish cell lines from the corn snake tumour and several visceral organs were unsuccessful as were attempts to infect virus-free *Vipera*, *Gekko*, *Eublepharis*, and hamster kidney cell lines with tumour suspension. Subsequently it was demonstrated that, like viper Type-C viruses, the virus of the corn snake sarcoma could be successfully cultivated in either rattlesnake fibroma or early passage rattlesnake heart or kidney cells (Clark *et al*, 1979a). Infection of rattlesnake cells was detected by both electron microscopic examination and detection of sedimentable DNA polymerase within four to ten cell passages after inoculation of tumour suspension (Fig. 5.14 and 5.15).

The isolated virus, designated corn snake retrovirus (CSRV), has an RNA genome and a buoyant density of 1·16. It possesses an RNA-dependent DNA-polymerase with a specific activity 10- to 20-fold less than that of viper oncornavirus. The polypeptide composition of CSRV also differs from that of VV. Unlike VV, CSRV possess a major glycoprotein with a molecular weight of 72 000; nonglycosylated proteins of 12 000, 13 000, 16 000 and 24 000 molecular weight are also found in CSRV. Preliminary antigenic comparisons of CSRV with VV, performed by double immunodiffusion in agar gel, indicate that at least two components of each virus share common antigenic determinants, while other antigens of each virus are clearly distinct.

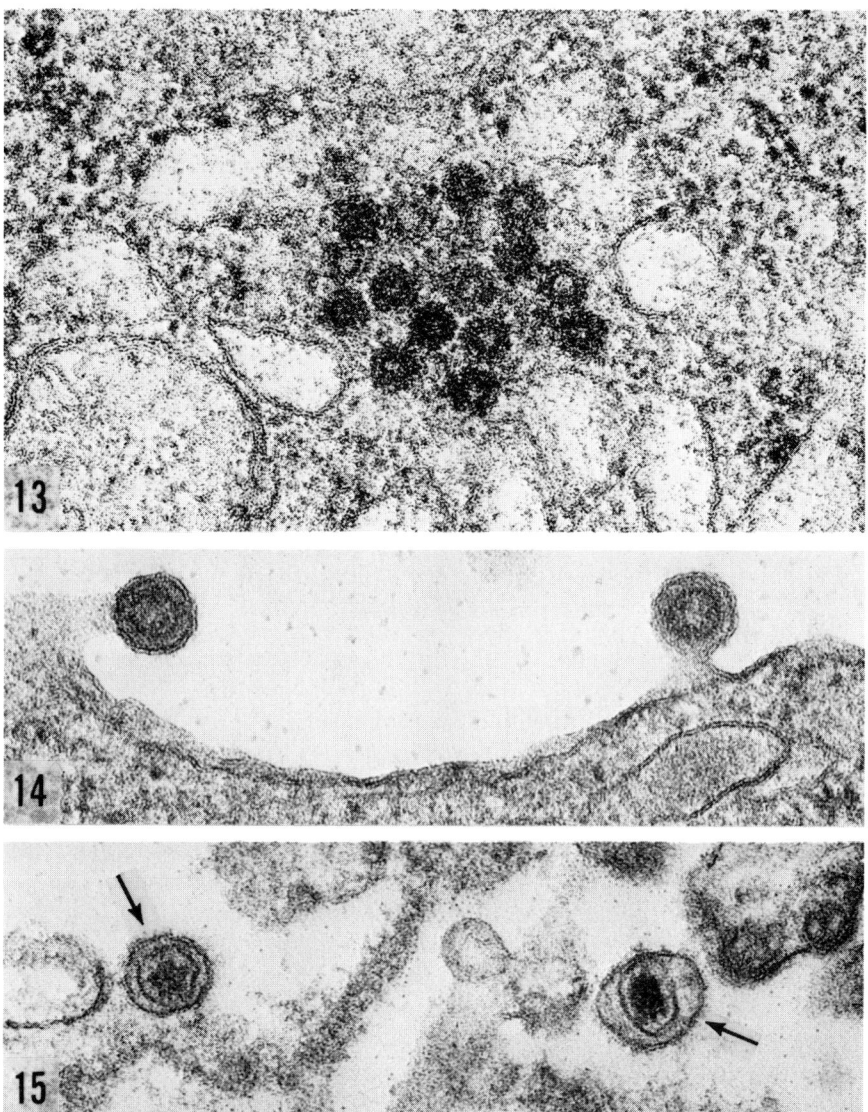

Fig. 5.13. VSW cell. An aggregation of intra-cytoplasmic Type-A particles, which individually measure 60–70 nm in diameter, and display an electron lucent centre. (×100 000)

Fig. 5.14. Two corn snake retroviruses (CSRV) budding from a rattlesnake fibroma cell. (×100 000)

Fig. 5.15. Two released CSRV (arrows) from a rattlesnake fibroma cell culture. (×100 000)

B. Green Lizard Papilloma-associated Virus

Although papilloma (wart)-like lesions have frequently been described in reptiles, clear-cut evidence of virus associated with such lesions has only been reported in one instance. Raynaud and Adrian (1976) examined benign papillomas of the green lizard (*Lacerta viridis*) electron microscopically. Viruses were confined to the highly keratinized regions of the papillomas. Examination of only three animals revealed mixed virus infections in these lesions: particles with the morphological appearance of herpesviruses, papovaviruses, and reoviruses were seen. None of these viruses has been cultivated; hence the morphological identification must be considered presumptive only. However, the very frequent association of papillomas with mammalian papoviruses justifies further searching for a viral aetiological agent of these tumours in reptiles.

IV. Viruses Non-pathogenic for Reptiles, in which Reptiles may play a Reservoir Role

A. Togaviruses

Numerous togaviruses (formerly arboviruses) have either been isolated from reptiles or experimentally injected into reptiles, especially snakes. As these viruses typically persist in alternate arthropod (primarily mosquito) and vertebrate host cycles in nature, and there is evidence of widespread involvement of representatives of all major vertebrate classes in the vertebrate host cycle, few can truly be considered exclusive viruses of reptiles. There is also little evidence that these viruses cause significant disease in reptiles. Interest in reptilian infections has usually centred on the theory that reptiles, because of their relatively slow rates of metabolic processes (including those processes leading to clearance of viraemia), may be particularly important long-term or over-wintering reservoir hosts. These studies have been reviewed recently (Lunger and Clark, 1978).

Attempts to establish a significant role by reptiles as hosts of togaviruses have included both field surveys for existence of infection in wild reptile populations and laboratory studies involving experimental infection. Field studies on the incidence of natural reptile infections have been based most convincingly upon isolation of virus, but the greatest mass of data obtained has consisted of antibody surveys of sometimes equivocal validity.

1. *Evidence of Natural Infection in Reptiles*

Infection of reptiles with togaviruses has traditionally been investigated by means of serological surveys which involve the testing of sera of wild-caught animals for the presence of antibodies detected by the haemagglutination inhibition (HI) or virus neutralization (VN) tests. The finding of antibodies with VN activity may be considered a specific indication of previous infection with the homologous virus. However, it is possible that reptilian sera may occasionally give false positive results in the HI test. This problem has been reviewed by several authors (Hayes *et al*, 1964; Lee, 1968; Yuill *et al*, 1971).

Serological evidence of togavirus infection has been reported from approximately 25 species of snakes, 14 species of lizards, 12 species of turtles and one crocodilian (Lunger and Clark, 1978; Hoff and Trainer, 1973). Reports of evidence of infected reptiles include studies from diverse regions of North and South America, Europe, Asia, and Australia. Infection of reptiles with togaviruses is obviously not a rare event.

Reports of isolations of togaviruses from wild-caught reptiles are much less common than the detection of anti-viral antibody. By far the most successful attempts to recover virus from wild reptiles resulted from studies of snakes collected in the Western United States and Western Canada. Gebhardt *et al* (1964) reported successful isolation of western equine encephalitis virus (WEEV) from as many as 44 per cent (37/84) of snakes collected in Utah in the months of May to July. Snakes of three genera yielded virus isolates: garter snakes (*Thamnophis sirtalis* and *T. elegans*), gopher snakes (*Pituophis catenifer*), and blue racers (*Coluber constrictor*). In the course of this study, baby snakes born in captivity to wild-caught mothers were also tested for the presence of virus. Four of 15 pools containing bloods of 15 baby snakes each yielded WEE virus, indicating that vertical transmission of this virus may play a role in its maintenance in nature.

Burton *et al* (1966) reported the isolation of WEEV from nine of over 200 garter snakes collected in Saskatchewan between April and September. However, only two of the nine isolates were recovered from the initial blood sample taken after capture; other isolates were recovered at bleedings long after (162 to 168 days) an initial negative blood sample. It was concluded that viraemia with WEEV may normally be a cyclical phenomenon in this geographic area.

The only isolates of togavirus reported from chelonians were recovered from the species *Terrapene carolina* and *Malaclemys terrapin* collected in New Jersey, USA (unpublished data of Goldfield and

Sussman, 1964, cited by Hoff and Trainer, 1973). Two isolates of Japanese encephalitis virus were recovered in a survey of 747 snakes collected in Korea; both isolates were obtained from the snake *Elaphe rufodorsata* (Lee *et al*, 1972). The latter are the only actual isolations reported from reptiles collected outside the North American continent.

2. *Experimental Infections of Reptiles*

Because of the postulated potential role of reptiles as reservoir hosts of togaviruses, capable of causing serious disease in man and domestic animals, togaviruses represent the only group of viruses utilized extensively in experimental infections of reptiles (Lunger and Clark, 1978). Investigators have explored the susceptible reptile host range of togaviruses, the duration and effect of ambient temperature upon viraemia (in order to determine reptilian suitability as reservoirs), and the consistency of induction of immune response (in order to assess the reliability of serological surveys as true indicators of the incidence of past infection).

Experimental studies have included only a few viruses, the great majority using the alphaviruses of western and eastern equine encephalitis (WEEV and EEEV, see later). In addition, Doi *et al* (1968) injected the flavivirus, Japanese encephalitis virus (JEV), into lizards of the species *Tachydromus tachydromoides* and observed the development of viraemia present from 3 to 18 days post infection (p.i.) followed by little detectable antibody response. Lee (1968) injected JEV into several species of Korean colubrid snakes. Viraemia, irregular in nature and sometimes lasting up to at least 44 days p.i., was induced in 11 of 27 animals. Subsequently a very poor antibody response was again noted.

Tick-borne encephalitis virus was injected in high concentration into lizards of the genus *Lacerta* by Gresiková and Albrecht (1959). A viraemia present between days 3 and 7 p.i. was induced and virus was recovered from brain tissue. When similar experiments were repeated using a lower-titred inoculum in the green lizard *Lacerta viridis* only, a very low-titred viraemia and no other signs of infection were noted (Rehacek *et al*, 1962). The latter results led to a conclusion that these lizards could not be efficient natural reservoir hosts of the virus. Aspöck and Kunz (1971) inoculated sand lizards (*Lacerta agilis*) and grass snakes (*Natrix natrix*) with Tahyna and Calovo togaviruses and failed to demonstrate any evidence of infection in either species.

The exquisite sensitivity of many species of American reptiles to alphaviruses WEEV and EEEV was first suggested by the work of Rosenbusch in Argentina (1942). The lizard *Tupinambis teguixin* and two vipers of the genus *Bothrops* exhibited virus infection in the brain at intervals from 13 to 39 days after infection with EEEV. Two of the infected snakes died with clinical signs of encephalitis; this is the only report claiming induction of disease in togavirus-infected reptiles.

Numerous subsequent reports have indicated a uniform susceptibility of reptiles to infection with EEEV. Karstad (1961) reported that each of 56 experimentally inoculated reptiles (snakes, lizards, turtles, and alligators collected in Georgia, USA) responded to virus inoculation with viraemia in high titre and/or development of high levels of virus-specific antibody. Craighead *et al* (1962) reported uniformly successful experimental infection of several species of Panamanian lizards with development of viraemia. Hayes *et al* (1964) infected many species of snakes and turtles with EEEV and reported evidence of infection in approximately 50 per cent of the animals. Garter snakes (*Thamnophis* sp.) were especially susceptible. One garter snake and three spotted turtles (*Clemmys guttata*) inoculated with virus and maintained under conditions designed to simulate over-wintering each maintained viraemia for at least six months p.i.

The most detailed studies of experimental togavirus infection of reptiles have been performed with reptiles collected in the Western United States and experimentally infected with WEEV. In the original experimental studies of Thomas *et al* (1958) three garter snakes were allowed to be bitten by WEEV-infected *Culex tarsalis* mosquitoes and four were inoculated directly with WEEV. Each of the seven snakes developed viraemia of up to 36 days' duration, often in high titre. It was demonstrated in several subsequent studies that garter snakes either inoculated directly with virus (Thomas and Eklund, 1960; Gebhardt and Hill, 1960), or infected by *C. tarsalis* mosquito bites (Thomas and Eklund, 1962) in the autumn and then allowed to hibernate, would exhibit viraemia with high frequency the following spring and early summer. The post-hibernation viraemia was demonstrated to last as long as 70 days; infection of *C. tarsalis* mosquitoes feeding on these viraemic snakes was demonstrated.

The time interval between infection of snakes and initiation of hibernation was found to be of critical importance to the establishment of over-wintering infection in another experimental study (Gebhardt *et al*, 1973). Snakes entering hibernation up to 11 days after inoculation with WEEV circulated virus after hibernation whereas those entering hibernation 19 days or more after onset of infection did not maintain infection after hibernation.

The *C. tarsalis* mosquito and garter snake combination was shown to present an exquisitely efficient potential for virus transmission. In one study of eight snakes, each bitten by only a single infected mosquito, four snakes developed viraemia (Gebhardt et al, 1966). Conversely, *C. tarsalis* mosquitoes were shown to be infected (31 per cent infection rate) following feeding on snakes with viraemic titres as low as 2.7×10^2 pfu/ml (Gebhardt et al, 1966). These experiments indicate that garter snakes in Western North America are presently by far the best documented potential natural reptilian hosts of a human pathogenic virus.

Other reptiles may be equally efficient hosts of WEEV. Twenty-seven of 28 Texas tortoises (*Gopherus berlandieri*) were shown to develop viraemia of up to 105 days' duration after experimental inoculation with WEEV, provided that they were maintained at ambient temperatures of at least 20°C (Bowen, 1977). High ambient temperatures were shown to reduce the duration but led to elevation in the titre of the viraemia. It was suggested that these tortoises also may be significant natural reservoir hosts of this virus.

V. Viruses Restricted to Reptiles, of Unknown Disease-producing Potential

Several viruses have been isolated from apparently healthy reptiles or observed (by electron microscopy) in reptile tissues in the absence of disease. These include the *Iguana* herpesviruses, the herpesvirus observed in the venom of elapid snakes, and the rhabdoviruses isolated from *Ameiva* lizards. Although these viruses have not been associated with disease in reptiles, all evidence indicates that each specifically infects reptiles and is not related to viruses of man or domestic animals. The *Iguana* herpesvirus was the first exclusively reptilian virus to be biologically characterized and is the only reptilian virus conclusively shown to be experimentally infectious for reptiles.

A. *Iguana* Herpesvirus

The iguana virus was first detected when spleen, kidney, and heart explant cell cultures, derived from a normal adult male green iguana (*Iguana iguana*) from the Buffalo Zoo and incubated at 30°C, underwent spontaneous cell degeneration (Clark and Karzon, 1972). The CPE was characterized by multi-nucleated giant cell (syncytium) formation and the presence of intranuclear eosinophilic inclusion bodies; CPE progressed and led to total destruction of cell monolayers. A similar type of cell degeneration was observed in cultures of a second green iguana subsequently removed from the same cage in the Buffalo Zoo.

Transmission of supernatant fluids from degenerating iguana cell cultures to cultures of the box turtle cell line TH-1 incubated at 30°C or 36°C led to induction of giant cell-type CPE. The agent transferred was named iguana virus. The virus was subsequently shown to grow slightly more efficiently in cell lines developed from *Iguana iguana*, but it could not be cultivated in several cell lines derived from *Gekko gecko*, *Vipera russelli* or *Podocnemis unifilis* or in primary cell cultures of *Caiman* or *Python* origin. Likewise, the virus did not replicate in cell lines of amphibian (*Rana* or *Bufo*), avian, or mammalian derivation.

Incubation temperature has a marked effect on the replication of iguana virus in cell culture. Iguana virus CPE progressed at similar rates in cultures incubated at 30°C and 36°C, but was delayed at 23°C. Thus, iguana virus is the first virus of exclusively ectothermic origin shown to replicate efficiently at temperatures as warm as homeothermic vertebrate body temperature. Nevertheless, the pattern of virus maturation differed at 30°C and 36°C. At 30°C (and at 23°C), released virus titres were approximately 1 per cent of those of cell-associated virus. At 36°C, although high-titred virus was detected intracellularly, no released virus was observed.

The type of CPE induced was also markedly affected by temperature. At 36°C CPE was composed almost exclusively of syncytia containing up to several hundred nuclei; at 30°C the CPE was a mixture of individually rounded and pyknotic cells and small giant cells usually containing less than ten nuclei. In TH-1 cells only, unique crystalline-appearing hexagonal eosinophilic cytoplasmic inclusions were seen within syncytia developing at 36°C but not at lower temperatures.

The induction of syncytial CPE characterized by eosinophilic intranuclear inclusions suggested that iguana virus might be a herpesvirus. Further data agreeable with this hypothesis were demonstration of a mean size between 100 and 220 nm by filtration, of ether sensitivity, and presumptively of a DNA nucleic acid type by inhibition of replication with 5′-bromodeoxyuridine.

The herpesvirus nature of iguana virus was confirmed by electron-microscopic studies (Zeigel and Clark, 1972). Nucleocapsids of typical herpesvirus morphology were observed in various stages of maturation within infected cell nuclei. Acquisition of one or two membranes by egress of capsids through the nuclear membrane was sometimes observed. Membrane-bound released virions 165 to 300 nm in diameter were also seen. Negative-contrast examination of preparations stained with phosphotungstic acid revealed naked capsids 115 nm in diameter composed of hollow capsomers 13 nm in length and 9·5 nm in width. The virion is apparently composed of 162 capsomers, as typical of herpesvirus.

Although iguana virus is a typical herpesvirus, it has been shown to be antigenically unique and not related to known herpesviruses of mammalian or ectothermic vertebrate origin (Clark and Karzon, 1972). Thus it was of special interest to determine whether iguana virus would induce acute disease or only latent infection in reptiles. A tendency towards induction of "masked" or latent unexpressed infection is a characteristic of many viruses of the herpesvirus group.

Iguana virus was injected into 12 young green iguanas by a variety of routes (Clark and Karzon, 1972). Seven of these animals died between 2 and 14 days after infection but the deaths could not be attributed to iguana virus, as no virus was recovered from any visceral organs by inoculation of organ suspensions on to susceptible cell cultures. The five remaining virus-inoculated animals were killed 15 days post-infection; these animals were tested for infection both by inoculation of organ suspensions into susceptible cell cultures and by cultivation of their liver and kidney cells as explants. Although only a single organ suspension (of spleen) yielded iguana virus, four of five animals revealed evidence of infection by spontaneous syncytial type cytopathic degeneration of their cultured cells. Infected animals included individuals held at either 23°C or 30°C, and inoculated via the intracerebral, the subcutaneous, or the oral route. None of five uninoculated controlled iguanas tested by identical methods showed any evidence of presence of a cytopathic virus. This experiment provided strong evidence for the existence in iguanas of a true latent herpesvirus infection, in which mature infectious virions are not normally present but are synthesized (or "unmasked") experimentally by *in vitro* cell culture. Since transmission in nature requires infectious virus, it must be assumed that, in parallel with known mammalian herpesvirus systems, latent infection *in vivo* must be unmasked by stress conditions often enough to maintain the infectious cycle in nature. Whether production of infectious virus *in vivo* may be associated with disease remains unknown.

Following a similar experimental design a variety of reptiles and amphibians, including two other species of lizard, three species of snakes, two species of turtle, one crocodilian, and two species of anurans were inoculated with iguana virus and tested 14 to 16 days later for infection detectable by cell culture of organ explants. Virus was recovered only from heart cell culture of a single Tokay gecko and from a spleen cell culture of one of two box turtles. Again no evidence of disease was noted in any of these animals. Thus it appears that *Iguana iguana* is the most likely natural host of this virus, justifying for the present the trivial name "iguana virus".

B. Cobra Venom Herpesvirus

This virus was discovered accidentally in the course of the study of the structure of the murine Rauscher leukaemia virus partially digested by treatment with "a crude enzyme preparation of snake venom" (Padgett and Levine, 1966). In this laboratory study, venom from either the Indian cobra *Naja naja* or the banded krait *Bungarus fasciata* was incubated with the mouse oncornavirus. Morphological forms unlike those previously associated with oncornaviruses, but similar to capsids of herpesviruses, 98 to 120 nm in diameter, were seen scattered throughout the virus preparations. These were assumed to be the substructure of the mouse virus unmasked by digestion with venom enzymes. It was claimed that the venom preparations were themselves free of virus.

However, in a subsequent study of three preparations of Indian cobra venom from diverse sources (including the preparation used in the above-mentioned study) and another preparation of banded krait venom, herpesvirus-like structures were seen in all (Monroe *et al*, 1968). The viruses were observed in reconstituted lyophilized venom preparations by either phosphotungstic acid negative-staining or by thin-sectioning of pellets obtained by high speed centrifugation of venom suspensions. Viruses were from 100 to 125 nm in diameter and possessed a capsomeric substructure characteristic of herpesvirus. All were membrane-free and thus immature forms. Attempts to cultivate virus from cobra venom in reptilian cell culture have been unsuccessful to date.

The exact source of the herpesvirus present in such high concentration in at least some venoms of elapid snakes is unknown. However, no report of examination of venom gland tissues for characteristic inclusions of herpesvirus infection or for virus particles has been reported. It is of interest to note that the cytomegalovirus was originally called salivary gland virus. It is interesting to speculate that herpesviruses seen in snake venom may indicate an expanded phylogenetic extension of the host range of this virus subgroup.

C. *Ameiva* Lizard Rhabdoviruses

Two antigenically distinct viruses, designated Marco and Chaco viruses, were isolated from lizards (*Ameiva ameiva*) collected at Belem, Brazil, by injection of lizard tissues into newborn mice. These isolates were originally assumed to be togaviruses (Causey *et al*, 1966). Because neither further isolates nor antibodies could be found in an extensive survey of other homeothermic and ectothermic vertebrates in the region, it was assumed that lizards represent the primary hosts of these viruses.

Recent electron microscopic studies have revealed that both Chaco and Marco viruses possess typical rhabdovirus morphology (F. Murphy and T. Monath, unpublished). The viruses have been propagated in both mammalian and reptilian cell cultures, but are otherwise uncharacterized. Their pathogenic potential in reptiles is unknown.

VI. Summary

It is clear from the limited studies described that reptiles harbour a variety of viruses causing varying patterns of expressed or latent disease paralleling the situation recognized in other vertebrate groups. It is extremely likely that reptiles host a much greater number of viruses than those so far isolated, but the economic cost of modern virological techniques will undoubtedly preclude a rapid expansion of knowledge in this area.

No reptilian virus has yet met rigid criteria for demonstration of an aetiological role in disease, i.e., the typical disease has not been re-created by injection of isolated and repeatedly cloned virus into susceptible experimental animals. The virus of the green sea turtle and FDLV appear to be the best candidates for early fulfilment of these requirements. Similarly, it is likely that the oncornaviruses isolated from snakes have some oncogenic potential. However, the demonstration of that potential may require a study involving the inoculation and maintenance for long periods of large numbers of expensive and potentially dangerous venomous reptiles.

The role in reptilian disease of most of the other viruses described is uncertain. The most frequently isolated reptilian viruses are togaviruses which probably rarely cause any disease in reptiles. Definitive interpretation of the role of reptiles as reservoir hosts of these mammalian pathogens is not yet possible. It does appear that in at least one area, the Western United States and Canada, the garter snake has the potential for efficiently maintaining western equine encephalitis virus in the ecosystem. It would be surprising if parallel opportunities do not exist elsewhere.

Finally, viruses and cell cultures of reptile origin may provide particularly useful research tools for elucidating basic mechanisms of virus-cell interaction. Almost all strictly reptilian viruses have optimum temperatures well below those of homeothermic vertebrate viruses. It has been shown with certain viruses of fish that such low temperature viruses grown in mammalian cells held at low temperature can provide a unique model for studying virus macromolecular processes (Clark and Soriano, 1974). Also, almost all viruses of ectothermic vertebrates are presumed to be multi-cistronic temperature-sensitive mutants. For this reason they may present particularly useful vehicles for recombinant DNA research, since their likelihood of infecting man appears especially remote.

Cell cultures of reptilian origin have been the subject of several investigations indicating incubation temperature effects on chromosomal alteration (Huang and Clark, 1967; Cohen and Clark, 1968; Cohen *et al*, 1972). Cell cultures of *Gekko gecko* have been used to further knowledge of the transforming capacity of the primate virus SV40 (Clark *et al*, 1972). The usefulness of viruses and cells of reptiles in interpreting basic principles of viral infection applicable to man may finally lead to a thorough study of the effect of those viruses on reptiles themselves.

References

Andersen, P. R. (1977). Studies on reptilian type-C oncornaviruses. Thesis, University of Delaware.
Ahne, W. (1977). *In* "Krankheiten der Reptilien". (H. Reichenback-Klinke, ed), pp 13–30. G. Fischer, Stuttgart and New York.
Aspöck, H. and Kunz, C. (1971). *Zbl. Bakt.*, I. Abt. Orig. **216**, 1–8.
Balls, M. (1965). *Ann. N.Y. Acad. Sci.* **126**, 256–273.
Bowen, G. S. (1977). *Amer. J. trop. Med. Hyg.* **26**, 171–175.
Burton, A. N., McLintock, J. and Rempel, J. G. (1966). *Science* **154**, 1029–1031.
Causey, O. R., Shope, R. E. and Bensabath, G. (1966). *Amer. J. trop. Med. Hyg.* **15**, 239–243.
Chatton, E. and Blanc, G. (1914). *Compt. Rend. Soc. Biol.* **77**, 496.
Clark, H F. (1972). *In* "Growth, Nutrition and Metabolism of Cells in Culture". (G. Rothblat and V. J. Cristofalo, eds.), Vol. 2, pp 287–325. Academic Press, New York and London.
Clark, H F. and Karzon, D. T. (1972). *Infect. Immun.* **5**, 559–569.

Clark, H F. and Soriano, E. Z. (1974). *Infect. Immun.* **10**, 180–188.
Clark, H F., Cohen, M. M. and Karzon, D. T. (1970). *Proc. Soc. exp. Biol. Med.* **133**, 1039.
Clark, H F., Jensen, F. and Defendi, V. (1972). *Int. J. Cancer* **9**, 599–607.
Clark, H F., Cohen, M. M. and Lunger, P. D. (1973). *J. natn. Cancer Inst.* **51**, 645–657.
Clark, H F., Andersen, P. R. and Lunger, P. D. (1979a). *J. gen. Virol.* **43**, 673–683.
Clark, H F., Lief, F. S., Lunger, P. D., Waters, D., Leloup, P., von Fölsch, D. W. and Wyler, R. W. (1979b). *J. gen. Virol.* **44**, 405–418.
Cohen, M. M. and Clark, H F. (1968). *Cytogenetics* **7**, 16.
Cohen, M. M., Clark, H F. and Jensen, F. (1972). *Int. J. Cancer* **9**, 618–625.
Craighead, J. E., Shelokov, A. and Peralta, P. H. (1962). *Am. J. Hyg.* **76**, 82–87.
Dodin, A. and Brygoo, E. R. (1956). *Bull. Soc. Pathol. Exotique* **49**, 807.
Doi, R., Oya, A. and Telford, Jr., R. S. (1968). *Jap. J. med. Sci. Biol.* **21**, 205–207.
von Fölsch, D. W. and Leloup, P. (1976). In "Erkrankungen der Zootiere". Verh. Ber. XVIII Int. Symp. Erk. der Zootiere, Insbruck: Akademie Verlag, Berlin.
Frye, F. L., Oshiro, L. S., Dutra, F. R. and Carney, J. D. (1977). *J. Am. vet. med. Ass.* **17**, 882–884.
Gebhardt, L. P. and Hill, D. W. (1960). *Proc. Soc. exp. Biol. Med.* **104**, 695–698.
Gebhardt, L. P., Stanton, G. J., Hill, D. W. and Collett, G. C. (1964). *New Eng. J. Med.* **271**, 172–177.
Gebhardt, L. P., Stanton, G. J. and St. Jeor, S. C. (1966). *Proc. Soc. exp. Biol. Med.* **123**, 233–235.
Gebhardt, L. P., St. Jeor, S. C. Stanton, G. J. and Stringfellow, D. A. (1973). *Proc. Soc. exp. Biol. Med.* **142**, 731–733.
Gilden, R. V., Lee, Y. K., Oroszlan, S. and Walker, J. L. (1970). *Virology* **41**, 187–190.
Gresiková, M. and Albrecht, P. (1959). *J. Hyg. Epid. Micr. Immunol.* **3**, 258–263.
Haines, H. and Kleese, W. C. (1977). *Infect. Immun.* **15**, 756–759.
Hatanaka, M., Huebner, R. J. and Gilden, R. V. (1970). *Proc. natn. Acad. Sci. U.S.A.* **67**, 143–147.
Hatanaka, M., Huebner, R. J. and Gilden, R. V. (1971). *Proc. natn. Acad. Sci. U.S.A.* **68**, 10–12.
Hayes, R. O., Daniels, J. B., Maxfield, H. K. and Wheeler, R. E. (1964). *Amer. J. trop. Med.* **13**, 595–606.
Hoff, G. and Trainer, D. O. (1973). *J. Herpetol.* **7**, 55–62.
Huang, C. C. and Clark, H. F. (1967). *Canad. J. Genet. Cytol.* **9**, 449–461.
Huebner, R. J. and Todaro, G. J. (1969). *Proc. natn. Acad. Sci. U.S.A.* **64**, 1087–1094.
Karstad, L. (1961). Reptiles as possible reservoir hosts for eastern encepha-

litis virus. Paper presented at 26th North American Wildlife Conference, Washington, D.C.
Kelly, D. C. and Robertson, J. S. (1973). *J. gen. Virol.* **20,** 17–41.
Klietmann, W., Andersen, P. R., Lunger, P. D., Clark, H F. and Nass, M. M. K. (1977). *Molec. Cell. Biochem.* **14,** 129–133.
Koment, R. W. and Haines, H. G. (1977). A new reptilian herpesvirus isolated from the green sea turtle, *Chelonia mydas*. Paper presented at the Annual Meeting of American Society for Microbiology.
Laemmli, U. K. (1974). *Nature* **227,** 680–685.
Lee, H. W. (1968). *Seoul J. Med.* **9,** 157–161.
Lee, H. W., Min, B. W. and Lim, Y. W. (1972). *J. Korean Med. Assoc.* **15,** 69–74.
Lucké, B. and Schlumberger, M. G. (1949). *Physiol. Rev.* **29,** 91–216.
Lunger, P. D. and Clark, H F. (1973). *J. natn. Cancer Inst.* **50,** 111–117.
Lunger, P. D. and Clark, H F. (1974). *J. natn. Cancer Inst.* **53,** 533–540.
Lunger, P. D. and Clark, H F. (1977). *J. natn. Cancer Inst.* **58,** 809–811.
Lunger, P. D. and Clark, H F. (1978). *Adv. Virus Res.* **23,** 159–204.
Lunger, P. D. and Clark, H F. (1979a). *J. comp. Path.* **89,** 265–279.
Lunger, P. D. and Clark, H F. (1979b). *J. comp. Path.* **89,** 281–291.
Lunger, P. D., Hardy, W. D., and Clark, H F. (1974). *J. natn. Cancer Inst.* **52,** 1231–1235.
Lunger, P. D., Klietmann, W. and Clark, H F. (1977). *Acta virol.* **21,** 375–382.
Mach, O. and Kára, J. (1971). *Folia biol. Praha* **17,** 65–72.
Maruyama, H. B., Hatanaka, M. and Gilden, R. V. (1971). *Proc. natn. Acad. Sci. U.S.A.* **68,** 1999–2001.
Menko, A. S., Sokol, F., Clark, H F. and Tan, K. B. (1976). *Arch. Virol.* **50,** 125–135.
Mizell, M. (1969). "Biology of Amphibian Tumours." Springer-Verlag, New York.
Monroe, J. H., Shibley, G. P., Schidlovsky, G., Nakai, T., Howatson, A. F., Wivel, N. W. and O'Connor, T. E. (1968). *J. natn. Cancer Inst.* **40,** 135–145.
Nowinski, R. C., Fleissner, E. and Sarkar, N. H. (1973). *In* "Perspectives in Virology VIII". (M. Polland, ed.), pp 31–59. Academic Press, New York and London.
Orr, H. C., Harris, Jr., H. C., Bader, A. V., Kirschstein, R. L. and Probst, P. G. (1972). *J. natn. Cancer Inst.* **48,** 259–264.
Padgett, F. and Levine, A. S. (1966). *Virology* **30,** 623–630.
Papas, T. S., Dahlberg, J. E. and Sonstegand, R. A. (1976). *Nature* **261,** 506–508.
Raynaud, M. M. A. and Adrian, M. (1976). *C. R. Acad. Sci. Paris* **283,** 845–847.
Rebell, H., Rywlin, A. and Haines, H. (1975). *Am. J. vet. Res.* **36,** 1221–1224.
Rehacek, J., Nosek, J. and Gresiková, M. (1962). *In* "Biology of Viruses of the Tick-Borne Encephalitis Complex". (H. Libikova, ed.), pp 392–393. Academic Press, New York and London.

Rosenbusch, F. (1942). *Proc. 6th Pac. Sci. Cong.* **5,** 209–214.
Stehbens, W. E. and Johnston, M. R. L. (1966). *J. Ultrastruct. Res.* **15,** 543–554.
Thomas, L. A., Eklund, C. M. and Rush, W. A. (1958). *Proc. Soc. exp. Biol. Med.* **99,** 698–699.
Thomas, L. A. and Eklund, C. M. (1960). *Proc. Soc. exp. Biol. Med.* **105,** 52–55.
Thomas, L. A. and Eklund, C. M. (1962). *Proc. Soc. exp. Biol. Med.* **109,** 421–424.
Twardzik, D. R., Papas, T. S. and Portugal, F. H. (1973). *J. Virol.* **13,** 166–170.
Yuill, T. M., Brandt, W. E. and Buescher, E. L. (1971). *J. Immunol.* **106,** 1413–1415.
Zeigel, R. F. and Clark, H F. (1969). *J. natn. Cancer Inst.* **43,** 1097.
Zeigel, R. F. and Clark, H F. (1971). *J. natn. Cancer Inst.* **43,** 309.
Zeigel, R. F. and Clark, H F. (1972). *Infect. Immun.* **5,** 570–582.

6 Bacteria

J. E. COOPER

*Royal College of Surgeons of England,
Lincoln's Inn Fields, London, England*

I. Introduction

Bacteria appear to play a very important role in reptilian diseases, both as primary pathogens and as secondary invaders. They are commonly isolated in localized infections but are also often involved in epizootics characterized by a bacteraemia and septicaemia. The significance of bacteria in diseases of reptiles has been emphasized by many authors, amongst them Brogard (1980), Cooper (1978), Jackson (1976), Marcus (1971, 1980), Mayer and Frank (1974), Page (1966) and Reichenbach-Klinke and Elkan (1965). More detailed reports of disease outbreaks have been described by other authors and are discussed later. Bacteriological techniques are covered in Chapter 4 and the Actinomycetes, which strictly are bacteria, are primarily discussed with fungi in Chapter 7.

II. Normal Flora

An important consideration in the investigation of bacterial diseases in reptiles is that of the normal flora of these animals. Relatively little work has been done on this subject (Yates *et al*, 1976). The available literature refers largely to studies on gut flora, with particular reference to *Salmonella* spp. For example, Tan *et al* (1978) investigated the intestine of the household lizards *Gekko gecko*; the cultures included Gram-positive bacteria, such as *Staphylococcus aureus*, *S. epidermidis* and *Streptococcus faecalis*, and such Gram-negative organisms as *Escherichia coli*, *Salmonella typhimurium* and *Pseudomonas aeruginosa*. The extent to which such a survey reflects the "normal" bacterial flora is debatable since the species in question lives in close contact with man and many of the organisms isolated were possibly acquired from human sources and environment. Nevertheless, the findings show that reptiles can harbour a wide range of organisms, amongst them both human and reptilian potential pathogens. Müller (1972) studied the faecal flora of several species of snake and found that *Rettgerella rettgeri* was the most commonly cultured organism (37% of isolates); other species identified were *Proteus vulgaris* (31%), *P. mirabilis* (29%) and *Morganella morganii* (4%). *Salmonella* and *Arizona* spp., *Edwardsiella tarda* and "Gram-positive and oxidase-positive cocci" were also isolated from a small number of snakes. Page (1961) suggested, on the basis of "limited surveys", that *Pseudomonas, Proteus, Klebsiella, Escherichia, Micrococcus* and *Corynebacterium* spp. were the normal inhabitants of the oral cavity of healthy king snakes and that "Gram-negative organisms far outnumber Gram-positive organisms in this cavity". Similar findings were reported in garter snakes by Mergenhagen (1956). There appears to have been very little work on the gut flora of chelonians, crocodilians or the tuatara but Schad *et al* (1964) demonstrated *Lampropedia* spp. in the gut (and within colonic nematodes) of *Testudo graeca* and suggested that these might be part of the normal flora of this and other herbivorous reptiles. Gordon *et al* (1979) investigated apparently normal American alligators, *Alligator mississippiensis* and isolated *Aeromonas hydrophila* from the oral cavity of 85%, from the external jaw area of 50% and from the internal organs of 70%; they suggested that it was a ubiquitous and non-pathogenic organism under normal circumstances. The author's own investigations have shown a predominance of Gram-negative organisms, particularly *E. coli, Proteus* spp., *Aeromonas* spp. and *Pseudomonas aeruginosa* in faeces, cloacal swabs and gut contents of snakes, lizards and chelonians in captivity. Similar organisms have also usually been cultured from the skin and external orifices although whether such bacteria represent a resident flora or merely faecal contamination is unknown. Gram-positive bacteria, such as *S. aureus*, have been isolated relatively infrequently though they are not uncommonly seen in keratin overlying the epidermis in histological sections (Fig. 6.1). They were also reported, together with Gram-negative bacteria, from "clinically normal snakes and lizards" by Burke (1978). Müller (1972) considered the skin of snakes to be a common source of *E. tarda, Salmonella* and *Arizona* spp. but this has not been the author's experience. Jackson and Fulton (1970) described the surface microflora of chelonians as being "rich in members of the family Enterobacteriaceae".

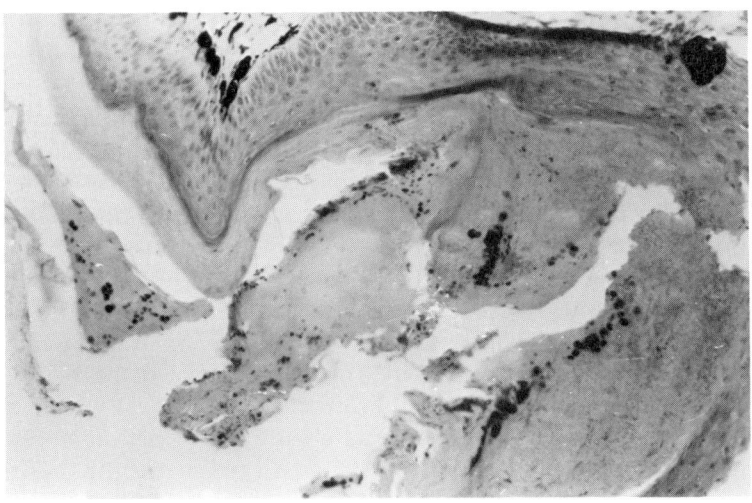

Fig. 6.1. A section of skin from a common iguana (*Iguana iguana*), stained with Gram stain. Many clusters of Gram-positive cocci are present in the keratin overlying the epidermis. (×100)

It will be apparent that relatively little is known of the normal bacterial flora of reptiles and nothing about the role or persistence of this flora. It has even been suggested that the bacterial flora is affected by changes in ambient temperature (Nicholson *et al*, 1976). In the case of the anaerobic organisms only one study has been traced (Mayer and Frank, 1977) and work is long overdue on this topic.

III. Pathogenicity

The special anatomy and physiology of reptiles influence understanding and interpretation of bacterial infections. For example, the presence of a cloaca, into which faeces, urates and gonadal products all empty, renders sampling of any one component difficult. From the physiological point of view, ectothermy (poikilothermy) presents problems of interpretation. The pathogenesis of bacterial infections in mammals is relatively well understood but in ectothermic vertebrates, where the body temperature can fluctuate widely, the whole concept of host–parasite relationship is less clear. For example, will a rise in temperature from 10°C to 15°C favour pathogenic bacteria, which can multiply quicker at the latter, or will the increased rate of antibody response in the reptile favour successful control of the infection? These and other questions cannot yet be answered and, as subsequent parts of this chapter will illustrate, few relevant investigations have yet been carried out.

Other factors are also likely to determine whether or not a bacterium produces disease. It is a well recognized fact in fish that environmental stress (for example, exposure to toxic chemicals, certain metabolites and temperature changes) can, if it coincides with the presence of pathogenic micro-organisms, result in infectious disease (Snieszko, 1974). Probably a similar situation occurs in reptiles: the author, for example, has encountered sudden outbreaks of *Pseudomonas* infections in reptile collections where the organism has been known to be present for a long period without any evidence of disease. In such cases the stressor(s) involved is often unclear though it is noteworthy that changes of temperature—such as a sudden hot day in summer—or a new member of staff may be associated with the outbreak. Similarly, it has been postulated that aeromoniasis in free-living alligators may be associated with stress factors such as trapping and with increased water temperatures (Gordon *et al*, 1979). Another important factor may be the number of organisms in the reptile's environment and the role of hygiene in reducing such challenges is discussed later in the chapter. Keymer (1978b) suggested that the higher incidence of bacterial infections in terrapins, as opposed to tortoises, might be because the warm wet conditions under which the former are kept might favour bacterial multiplication. There have been detailed studies on the ecology of some fish pathogens and similar work is needed in the case of reptiles.

Although various organisms can be part of the normal bacterial flora, the portal of entry of pathogens must be considered. In the case of gut flora, it is assumed that the bacteria pass through the mucosa and can thence enter the bloodstream or other abdominal organs. It is unclear whether prior damage to the mucosa is necessary. The entry of infectious agents through the damaged skin is well recognized. The intact reptile skin is well protected by thick keratin but any breach of this defence can result in the development of local or generalized infections. For example, local abscessation may follow a single tick bite while a bacterial septicaemia can be the sequel of mite infestation (Camin, 1948). Organisms may also be ingested and in this context it is noteworthy that lizards in particular may eat such insects as cockroaches, which are known to harbour a variety of pathogens (Elkan and Cooper, 1976). Abscesses are not uncommon in the buccal cavity and gular region of reptiles and it is possible that in such instances potentially pathogenic organisms have been ingested and, perhaps, passed through an abrasion or empty tooth socket during mastication. Bacterial infections of the female reproductive tract and eggs may be due to an ascending infection (via the cloaca), haematogenous spread or, possibly, spread of infection from the ovary or oviduct (Holt, 1979).

The ability of a reptile to combat a bacterial infection is not inconsiderable. Although relatively little is known of the inflammatory process in reptiles, histological investigation of lesions reveals a well developed inflammatory reaction which may involve eosinophils, heterophils or lymphocytes. Local infections, such as abscesses, tend to become "walled off" by fibrous tissue and the pus produced in such cases is usually laminated, suggesting a slow inflammatory response with long-term invasion and death of leucocytes. Little is known of the fate of organisms in the blood but bacteria can often be seen within the cytoplasm of both circulating and tissue monocytes, suggesting that phagocytosis plays a role. Humoral antibodies are also likely to be involved (see Chapter 15). Antibacterial activity is a well recognized feature of skin secretions of amphibians, for example *Rana ridibunda* (Cevikbas, 1978) but similar studies on reptiles appear not to have been carried out. There is evidence of bactericidal activity in some snake venoms, for example *Crotalus* spp. (Glaser, 1948), but this is unlikely to play any significant role in the prevention or control of bacterial disease.

It will be apparent from the foregoing that the distinction between infection and disease in a reptile is not always clear cut. A snake may be infected with *Aeromonas* bacteria in its gut but not suffering from clinical aeromoniasis. It is important that the two are differentiated whenever the role of bacteria in reptiles is being discussed.

Although Koch's postulates have rarely been fulfilled in reptilian disease, there are several bacteria that are universally recognized as potential pathogens. The vast majority are Gram-negative bacilli such as *Aeromonas* spp. and *Pseudomonas* spp. In the author's experience broth cultures of these organisms will, if injected intra-peritoneally into snakes (mainly *Psammophis* spp.) cause death within 48 hours in 80 per cent of animals and similar pathogenicity has been reported by other workers, for example Shotts *et al* (1972). Keydar *et al* (1971) described experiments in which they were able to cause disease and death in snakes with as few as 2×10^4 *P. aeruginosa* given by injection and also by feeding the snakes mice infected with *P. aeruginosa*. The role of other bacteria, such as *E. coli*, *Proteus* and *Enterobacter* spp., is less clear though many people, amongst them the author, have incriminated them in both local and generalized disease. Keymer

(1978a), writing about tortoises, stated that "bacteria such as coliform organisms *Proteus* spp. and *Pseudomonas aeruginosa* are of doubtful pathogenicity". This may have been so in his series but would not appear to be generally true. *Salmonella* spp. have frequently been isolated from reptiles or their faeces and are of great significance in that they may pose a zoonotic threat to humans; there is little evidence that they produce clinical disease in the reptiles themselves (see later). *Mycobacterium* spp. have long been recognized as a cause of disease in reptiles and usually produce characteristic tubercles; carriage of the organisms does not appear to have been reported. Other bacterial genera and species have been reported as the cause of, or associated with, reptilian disease including staphylococci, streptococci, clostridia and leptospires. *Serratia marcescens*, for long not considered a pathogen, has been isolated from abscesses (Boam *et al*, 1970) and a number of other organisms have been incriminated as the causes of localized or generalized infections.

IV. Types of Bacterial Disease

The classification of bacterial diseases of reptiles poses problems since there is as yet little information on the relative pathogenicity of the different species of bacteria or the spectrum of diseases which they produce. As a result, any breakdown on the basis of causal organisms is, with a few exceptions such as tuberculosis, impracticable and probably irrelevant. For this reason bacterial diseases will be categorized in this chapter according to the tissues which they involve and whether the infection is of a localized or generalized nature. The main headings are:

    Localized infections:
        abscesses:
        dermatitis:
        stomatitis:
        cloacitis:
        ocular infections:
        other infections:
    Generalized infections:
        septicaemia:
        tuberculosis:
        salmonellosis:
        leptospirosis:
        other infections:

There is much overlap but these divisions facilitate discussion.

Much of the information in the succeeding few pages is based upon published work or experience of disease in captive reptiles. However, several of the conditions discussed have been reported, albeit rarely, in free-living or recently captured specimens—for example, dermatitis and stomatitis (Pitman, 1974) and cloacitis (Cooper, 1973).

A. Localized Infections

1. *Abscesses*

Abscesses are common in all four orders of reptiles. Although usually subcutaneous (Fig. 6.2) they can also involve internal organs and may

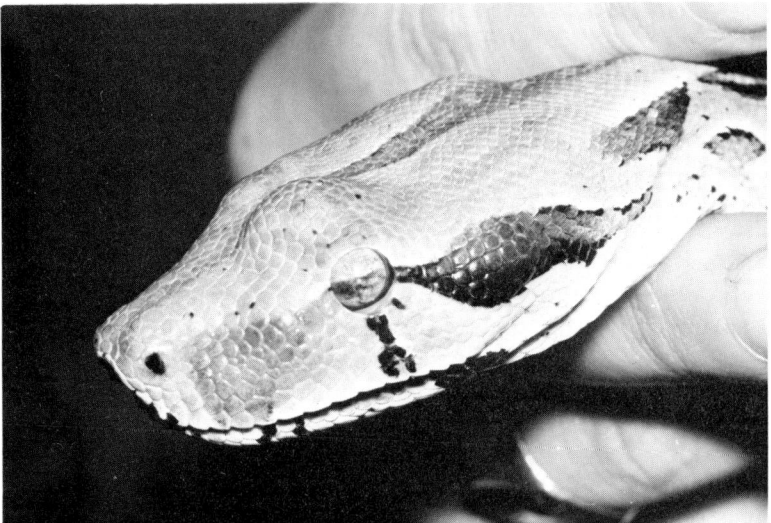

Fig. 6.2. A boa constrictor (*Boa constrictor*) with a subcutaneous swelling above its left eye. This swelling was examined under general anaesthesia and proved to be a chronic abscess. It was removed surgically.

be multiple, suggesting haematogenous dissemination of pyogenic organisms. The bacteria most commonly isolated from abscesses are Gram-negative bacilli, often in mixed culture, but it is unclear in many cases as to whether these were the initial cause or subsequent invaders. Gram-positive cocci may also be present and are particularly well demonstrated, usually in large clusters, with a Gram stain.

A useful stain for demonstrating Gram-negative organisms in histological sections is that of Brown and Brenn (Holt et al, 1979). *Dermatophilus congolensis* was isolated from an abscess in the lizard *Amphibolurus barbatus* in Australia (Simmons et al, 1972) and then successfully transmitted to two species of lizard and a sheep. Boam et al (1970) attributed abscesses in four iguanid lizards to *Salmonella marina* (1), *Serratia marcescens* (2) and a *Micrococcus* sp. (1). Tumour-like lesions in the lizards *Anolis equestris* and *Sauromalus varius* were described in the 1930's by Duran-Reynals and Clausen (1937) and Conti and Crowley (1939) respectively. The cause of the former appeared to be a bacterium named *Serratia anolium* while the latter was designated *Bacterium sauromali*. The lesions in both cases resembled chronic abscesses. Subsequent studies on *S. anolium* showed that similar lesions could be produced in other lower vertebrates (reptiles, amphibians and fish) but not in rabbits, guinea-pigs or mice (Clausen and Duran-Reynals, 1937). A most interesting discovery was that while only localized lesions were produced in lower vertebrates kept at room temperature, a higher temperature (37°C) resulted in more generalized lesions and, usually, death.

Although some abscesses in reptiles contain serous or mucous fluid the majority are characterized by the presence of solid (or semi-solid) caseous pus. Often, as was mentioned earlier, there is a laminated appearance (Fig. 6.3). Subcutaneous abscesses usually manifest themselves as discrete swellings under the skin which are hard to the touch and which rarely ulcerate until very large. Most abscesses have a fibrous capsule which, on histological section, is seen to surround a layer of leucocytes, especially eosinophils and heterophils.

Individual abscesses usually appear to cause little or no discomfort to the reptile. However, in certain sites they may hamper movement and are often aesthetically unpleasant. Added to this, there is evidence that infection may spread, especially in the case of bone abscesses which are usually poorly encapsulated; in iguanas, *Iguana iguana*, for example, infection can spread up the vertebral column from a bone abscess in the tail and may even produce lesions in the peritoneal cavity and viscera.

Differential diagnosis of abscesses includes haematomas, fungal and parasitic granulomas, and neoplasms. In the case of lesions adjacent to skeletal structures—for example, on the ramus of the jaw—it is essential to carry out radiography to ascertain whether there is bone involvement, *before* attempting treatment. Aspiration of pus is sometimes possible, using a wide-bore needle; a direct smear will reveal dead or dying leucocytes and bacteria and the latter can

6   BACTERIA   173

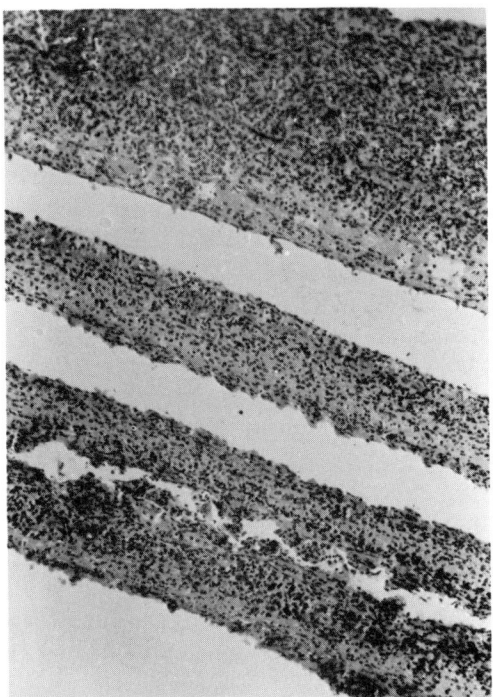

Fig. 6.3. Part of the wall of a chronic abscess from a Greek tortoise (*Testudo graeca*). The layers of necrotic debris, containing a mixture of inflammatory cells and blood, are clearly seen; they have become separated during processing. (×150)

often be cultured. Alternatively, if there are multiple lesions, a small sample (for example, on a digit) can be excised and examined histologically.

Abscesses are best treated surgically. There are different techniques but in the author's experience optimum results are obtained if the whole lesion is removed, together with its capsule and overlying epithelium, rather than by merely "shelling-out" the pus. Following removal the area should be irrigated with an appropriate antibiotic or antiseptic and then sutured. There is some evidence that a course of parenteral antibiotics can be helpful in preventing recurrence.

In the case of internal abscesses surgical removal is again possible and is probably the only solution. The diagnosis can be made as a result of palpation, radiography or laparotomy.

Bone abscesses may respond to antibiotic therapy following sensitivity tests. If the abscess is on a digit or the tail, however, it is usually wiser to amputate the affected appendage.

Micro-abscesses are not uncommonly seen during the course of histological examination. Usually they occur in the liver and consist of a central area of necrosis surrounded by mixed (sometimes pyknotic) inflammatory cells. Larger abscesses and granulomas may be seen in other organs, for example, the thyroid.

2. Dermatitis

The role of bacteria in initiating skin infections is not known but there is no doubt that they will rapidly colonize and accelerate the effects of skin lesions. For example, skin abrasions, due to "grab-sticks" or other mechanical appliances, often become infected and a wide range of bacteria can be cultured and seen in histological sections in such cases. Skin lesions in captive reptiles may also follow exposure to suboptimal temperature or humidity and these too quickly become infected. Pockets of keratin appear to be particularly common sites for bacterial multiplication (Zwart and van Ham, 1980).

The term "scale-rot" is commonly used in herpetological circles to refer to a wide range of skin lesions, mainly in snakes and lizards. More exact terms are necrotic dermatitis and ulcerative dermal necrosis (Jackson, 1976). The condition varies enormously in its severity. In mild cases there may only be areas of discoloured scales, representing necrosis of the outer layers of keratin. More severe cases show extensive erosion or ulceration and there may be exudate. The latter is often termed "pus" but is usually a mixture of tissue fluid, which has leaked through the wound, and assorted blood and epithelial cells. Nevertheless, bacteria can usually be cultured in profusion from such lesions and the presence of many eosinophils and heterophils in histological sections would suggest a response to bacterial invasion.

Treatment of reptiles with "scale-rot" consists of cleaning the affected area, preferably with a suitably diluted broad spectrum disinfectant, and removal of loose necrotic debris. In mild cases this is often sufficient but more severe lesions need topical and/or systemic antibiotic therapy following a sensitivity test. In addition, extra vitamins appear to aid healing while fluid therapy (glucose-saline subcutaneously) may be necessary to counteract dehydration. It is always essential to ensure that an affected reptile is kept in a clean environment in order to reduce the risk of secondary infection. Water containers are a potential source of infection and it is wise to prevent the patient from bathing: treatment of the water—for example with hydrochloric acid or chlorine (McPherson, 1963)—will reduce the bacterial count. Alternatively a surgical adhesive drape (Op-Site: Smith and Nephew Ltd) may be used to cover the wound. Healing of all skin lesions is slow and an area of scar tissue or abnormal scalation may remain after clinical recovery.

Skin lesions may be due to organisms other than bacteria; fungi and helminth parasites are two particular examples. Differential diagnosis is not always easy since bacteria can frequently be isolated from any skin lesion; a small biopsy is often useful in such cases.

Dermatitis occurs in crocodilians and chelonians as well as the Squamata. In chelonians the horny shields may become pitted, ulcerated or raised due to an underlying purulent exudate. Again fungi can be involved and a careful diagnosis must be carried out. A condition called "septicemic cutaneous ulcerative disease of turtles" was described by Kaplan in 1957 and the causal organism appeared to be *Escherichia* (now *Citrobacter*) *freundii*. Affected animals show clinical signs of anorexia and weakness and there are skin haemorrhages. Pathological lesions include necrotic foci in the liver and other organs. Treatment has been recommended using chloramphenicol (Kaplan, 1958) but prevention is preferable, by improved hygiene and prompt attention to skin wounds through which *C. freundii* may gain access.

A similar condition was described in a colony of turtles (mixed species) by Jackson and Fulton (1970) who felt that there might be a synergistic relationship between *Citrobacter* and *Serratia*, the latter facilitating the entry of the former through the skin.

Wallach (1975) incriminated a chitinolytic bacterium, *Beneckea chitinovora* (*Bacillus chitinovorus*), in a condition of turtles characterized by discolouration, ulceration and erythema of the "shell". He was able to reproduce the disease by inoculating the carapace and plastron of apparently healthy turtles. Iodine was recommended for treatment and as preventive measures Wallach advocated a two-week isolation period for new turtles, sufficient space to reduce shell injury and an embargo on feeding crustaceans (which may harbour *B. chitinovora*) to turtles. Although similar lesions have been seen in turtles (terrapins) in Britain, *B. chitinovora* has not been isolated.

3. *Stomatitis*

Perhaps the best known disease of reptiles, at least to herpetologists, is "mouth-rot" or "canker" (Fig. 6.4). However, like "scale-rot", these terms can cover a wide range of conditions. The true aetiology of

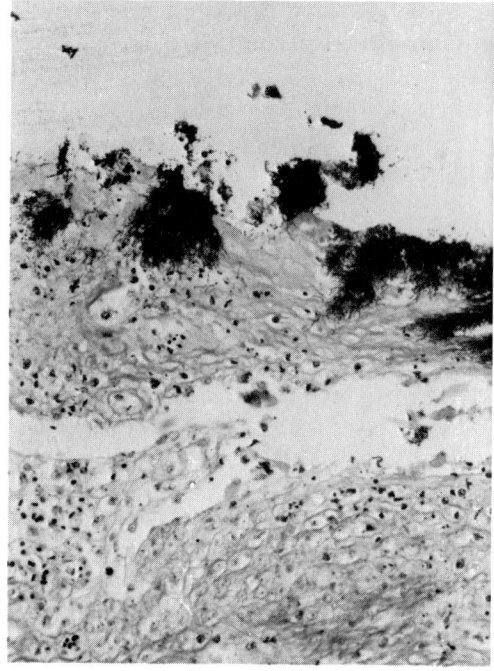

Fig. 6.4. Necrotic debris on the tongue of a tortoise (*Testudo graeca*) with stomatitis. Brown and Brenn stain shows many Gram-negative bacilli (Holt *et al*, 1979). (×160)

infectious lesions of the mouth and upper alimentary tract is uncertain although it is well recognized that trauma can predispose to a bacterial infection of the lips and rostrum, especially if the reptile persistently damages itself on the glass of its enclosure in captivity. A similar situation may occur in the mouth; for example, the author has frequently observed small haemorrhages and ulcerations in the mouths of snakes used for venom production. In this case the damage is inflicted during the "milking" procedure and bacteria subsequently gain entry.

Another cause of stomatitis may be an underlying deficiency, perhaps of vitamin A or C (Wallach, 1969). For example, snakes often develop "mouth-rot" when they are debilitated or not feeding, even in the absence of obvious traumatic injuries.

The bacteria involved in stomatitis vary and often it is difficult to incriminate a particular organism because of the large numbers of species cultured in the laboratory. *Pseudomonas* and *Aeromonas* spp. are regular isolates but many others, including Gram-positive cocci, may be demonstrated. Occasionally yeasts are seen in impression smears. Page (1961) incriminated *Aeromonas* spp. and was able to reproduce the disease by oral administration of an *Aeromonas* sp. designated SA-5.

Therapy consists of debridement, antiseptics, antibiotics or sulphonamides and supportive care. Various antibacterial and antiseptic agents have been recommended, amongst them sulphadimidine, merthiolate, benzalkonium chloride and hydrogen peroxide (Marcus, 1971) and a selection of antibiotics (Burke, 1978). A technique found useful by the author is daily irrigation with streptomycin sulphate, using a syringe and narrow-gauge needle (25–27 gauge). The antibiotic not only destroys the organisms but also helps to dislodge necrotic debris. Supportive treatment includes fluids, vitamins (orally or by injection) and, where necessary, force-feeding with an oesophageal tube. If the lesions are severe there may be bone involvement or extensive necrosis of underlying muscle; systemic antibiotics will be needed if the reptile's life is to be saved. In the case of chronic granulomatous or ulcerative lesions, surgery may be necessary, including the use of cryosurgery (Green *et al*, 1977). Addison and Jacobson (1974) reported the use of an autogenous vaccine (a *Pseudomonas aeruginosa* bacterin) which appeared to aid healing in a case of chronic stomatitis in a reticulated python (*Python reticulatus*). More such studies with control animals would be welcome.

Prevention of stomatitis is not easy. Burke (1978) claimed that "many snake mouths . . . are devoid of readily recoverable bacteria" and suggested that trauma to the mouth coupled with environmental sources of bacteria might be involved in some cases. It would seem advisable to reduce the risk of such trauma, to ensure hygiene is practised and to provide a balanced diet. Early detection is important and a useful routine is to check the mouths of incoming reptiles for lesions and to perform a similar examination regularly thereafter. Early lesions should be swabbed and treated with an appropriate antibiotic or sulphonamide.

4. *Cloacitis*

Cloacitis is relatively common in reptiles. Often there is a predisposing cause such as a cloacal calculus or the injudicious use of a metal probe for sexing snakes. The clinical signs range from a mild oedema and ulceration of the cloacal lips to a massively swollen cloaca and associated blood-stained droppings. The area appears sensitive to the touch and there may be signs of dehydration. Clinical examination plays an important role in the diagnosis of this condition and palpation of the cloacal area should be an integral part of the investigation of any sick reptile (Cooper, 1973).

Treatment should not be undertaken until an examination has confirmed whether or not there is a calculus present; if there is, it must be removed manually or surgically. Antibiotic therapy should, wherever possible, follow a sensitivity test and the appropriate agent can either be instilled daily into the cloaca or, if the infection is severe, administered parenterally. *E. coli*, *Aeromonas* spp. and *Pseudomonas* spp. are common isolates in cloacitis although a *Staphylococcus* sp. has been reported (Cooper, 1973). The bacterial flora of the cloaca appear not to have been investigated in reptiles but it would seem that such organisms, together with those in the faeces, are the likely isolates.

5. *Ocular Infections*

These are covered separately in view of their relative prevalence. Infections of the eye are often seen in all three common orders of reptiles, ranging from mild conjunctivitis to panophthalmitis.

True conjunctivitis, often associated with keratitis, occurs in lizards, crocodilians and chelonians. In snakes there is a protective spectacle overlying the eye but infection can occur under it—so called "subspectacle abscess" or "conjunctivitis". The portal of entry of infection in the case of true conjunctivitis/keratitis is probably the surface of the eye itself; for example, following physical damage. Conjunctivitis may also be a feature of respiratory infections and, occasionally, stomatitis. The affected eyes show discharge and the lids may adhere. In the case of subspectacle abscesses the infection is believed to be blood-borne, though it is of interest to note that often only one eye is involved. This may support the hypothesis of Marcus (1971) that exudate from buccal lesions (for example, in necrotic stomatitis) may obstruct the duct of the Harderian gland and cause distension of the subspectacle space. The main clinical feature is a distended discoloured spectacle—which must not, however, be confused with the opacity of the spectacles in a snake which is about to slough.

Various bacteria are isolated from conjunctivitis and subspectacle abscesses—again usually Gram-negative bacteria—but their exact role is uncertain. In the case of conjunctivitis there is often a response to a tetracycline or chloramphenicol eye ointment. Chelonians with mild conjunctivitis following hibernation often recover spontaneously and there is doubt as to whether the condition is infectious. Another complicating feature in chelonians (and possibly other reptiles) is a vitamin A deficiency and it is the author's policy to administer this vitamin intramuscularly when an eye infection is suspected in tortoises, terrapins or turtles. Subspectacle abscesses should be treated surgically (Wallach, 1969), by incising the spectacle and flushing out the purulent exudate. The use of a streptomycin or neomycin solution in such cases has proved particularly successful in the author's experience.

Occasionally the spectacles of snakes become distended for other reasons and this is important in differential diagnosis. Sloughing has been mentioned; developmental abnormalities are another (rare) possibility (Cooper, 1975). A group of captive-bred young Haitian boas (*Epicrates striatus*) at one zoological collection in Britain developed bilaterally symmetrical distended spectacles; the fluid beneath was clear and no bacteria could be cultured from it. The aetiology was never determined but the eyes gradually returned to normal over a ten-week period. During this time the animals remained healthy and continued to feed well.

More extensive eye infections may follow conjunctivitis but are usually a sequel to injury and may on occasion arise as a result of a blood-borne infection. Lambiris (1976) attributed 12 of his 19 cases in snakes to "nematode infection" but provided no pathological data to support this diagnosis. In generalized ophthalmitis the whole eye becomes filled with purulent material and the only practical solution is surgical enucleation. Satisfactory techniques were described by Lambiris (1976) and Zwart *et al* (1973). Failure to remove the eye promptly can result in spread of infection to the brain.

6. *Other Infections*

Localized bacterial infections may also occur elsewhere in reptiles. Wounds, in particular, commonly become infected (Fig. 6.5). An infection of the venom glands due to *P. aeruginosa* was described in snakes by Keydar *et al* (1971) who reported a response to polymyxin B sulphate.

Infections of internal organs are often manifestations of more generalized bacterial disease but according to Will (1975), bacteria are commonly the cause of liver disease. Respiratory infections have long been recognized in reptiles and were reviewed by Murphy (1973a); they frequently overlap with, or are manifestations of, septicaemic conditions. Affected animals may show clinical signs

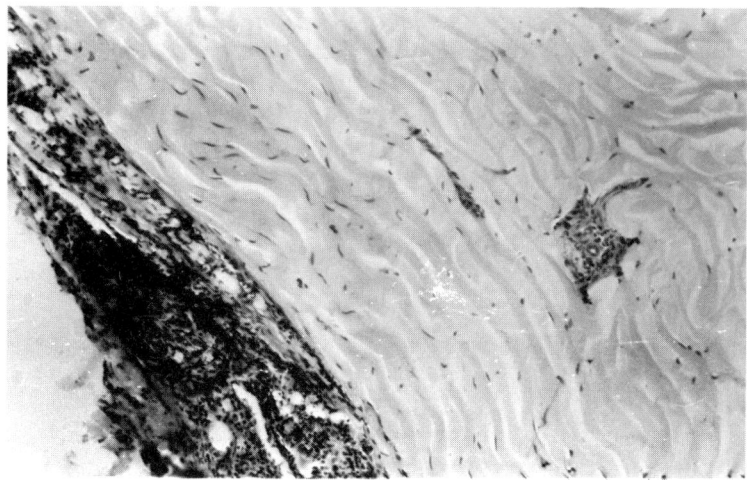

Fig. 6.5. Myositis in a common iguana. Normal muscle occupies much of the picture but on the left hand side there is degenerate muscle heavily infiltrated with mixed inflammatory cells. A prolific growth of *Pseudomonas aeruginosa* was cultured from this lesion. (×150)

ranging from mild nasal discharge to marked dyspnoea. Various drugs have been recommended for treatment and some of these are discussed in more detail under "Septicaemia" and in Chapter 18.

Reproductive infections are becoming increasingly recognized on account of the interest in captive breeding. The most common condition encountered by the author, mainly in snakes and chelonians, is an oviductitis/peritonitis which closely resembles "egg peritonitis" of poultry. There are no specific clinical signs other than lethargy and anorexia. At *post mortem* examination, there is a purulent exudate within the oviduct and, often, in the peritoneal cavity. The colour of the exudate is frequently yellow and histopathological examination confirms the presence of yolk. The cause of such conditions may be a ruptured egg or one that fails to enter the oviduct. *E. coli* is the most common bacterial isolate.

Infected eggs are not uncommonly encountered in reptiles and may need to be removed surgically. In severe cases they are discoloured and associated with purulent material within the oviduct. Gram-negative bacilli are the usual isolates but their origin is unclear. It is possible that the infection is introduced by the male at mating. One very sexually active male royal python (*Python regius*), which had previously been treated for extensive abscesses associated with an *Aeromonas* sp., mated repeatedly with a female of the same species;

she later needed surgery for the removal of 24 infected eggs. Both *Aeromonas* and *Pseudomonas* spp. were isolated from the eggs and the snake died a few days post-operatively from a bacterial septicaemia. Holt (1979) described infected eggs in a spur-thighed tortoise (*Testudo graeca*). A *Pseudomonas* sp. and a *Proteus* sp. were isolated and the tortoise died of a *Pseudomonas* infection.

B. Generalized Infections

1. *Septicaemia*

Septicaemic diseases of reptiles have been recognized for many years and again it is usually the Gram-negative organisms, especially *Aeromonas* and *Pseudomonas* spp., that are involved. It is worthy of note that, although a number of authors describe *A. hydrophila* as the species of *Aeromonas* most commonly involved in this and other bacterial infections, often the biochemical tests do not entirely conform with such an identification. It is probably best to refer to an "*Aeromonas* sp." and then to list the organism's characteristics.

Reptiles with a septicaemia may show no premonitory signs—and just be found dead—or may exhibit clinical features ranging from lethargy to inco-ordinated "convulsing". An affected snake often writhes and contorts (Jackson, 1974) or, especially if there is lung involvement, opens its mouth and gapes. Heywood (1968) described a more chronic form in boas; the animals showed respiratory signs and stomatitis and died after 5–6 weeks. Chelonians may also show respiratory signs but a particularly common feature is red discolouration (vascular congestion and haemorrhage) of the plastron (Holt, 1979). *Post mortem* findings likewise vary enormously. In classical cases there is marked congestion of the internal organs, the liver is discoloured and the lung oedematous and pneumonic. Petechial haemorrhages may be widespread. Where the condition has resulted from an oviduct infection or a ruptured internal abscess, there is peritonitis and adhesion of serosal surfaces. Histopathological findings in all these cases are similar to those in septicaemic conditions in other vertebrates. A feature which may be of significance is a lowered packed cell volume (PCV) and excessive quantities of haemosiderin in liver and other organs (Cooper and Leakey, 1976). Such changes are also a feature of fish which are sick or in poor condition (Bowser, 1973; Houston and DeWilde, 1972).

The difficult cases to interpret are those where a reptile dies unexpectedly and a bacterium is isolated in pure culture from heart blood and other tissues but where pathological lesions are minimal or non-existent. The author's interpretation of such cases is that the organism has killed the host by inducing a toxaemia or peracute septicaemia; however, this is as yet unproven and further work is needed on the significance of such bacteraemias in reptiles. In this context, it should be noted that Fölsch and Leloup (1976) attributed a fatal infection in snakes to a paramyxovirus, the pathogenicity of which was "enhanced" by *Pseudomonas* infection (see Chapter 5).

Septicaemia can follow a localized infection or be the result of pathogenic bacteria entering a natural or surgical wound. In free-living reptiles a significant factor can be eutrophication of lakes; for example, Shotts *et al* (1972) reported deaths amongst fish, turtles and alligators associated with a build-up of *Aeromonas* spp.

Septicaemia can occur in captive reptiles with no evidence of underlying factors. In such cases it is possible that certain stressors, coupled with a build-up of organisms in the reptile's environment, may be responsible. For example, in an epizootic in snakes in Kenya (Cooper and Leakey, 1976) the susceptibility of snakes being regularly "milked" for venom, as opposed to non-venomous species kept undisturbed, suggested that the stress of handling and venom collection may have been an important factor.

Diagnosis of a septicaemia is based largely upon *post mortem* findings. However, the clinical signs may be helpful, especially if a bacterial infection has already been diagnosed in other reptiles in the collection. In cases with respiratory signs purulent material may be present in the buccal cavity or trachea and this should be cultured. Blood samples from affected reptiles will also yield bacteria while Giemsa-stained smears may reveal bacilli both free in the plasma and phagocytosed in mononuclear cells. In some cases there may be evidence of a leucocytosis—for example, as has been demonstrated in experimental *Aeromonas* infection in alligators (Glassman and Bennett, 1978)—but more work is needed on this subject.

Treatment also poses problems. Often the condition is peracute and the reptile is dead before therapy can be initiated. Perhaps the best chance of successful treatment is when an outbreak occurs in a collection and the causal organism is identified early; antibiotic sensitivity tests should be carried out and appropriate therapy of reptiles at risk commenced, preferably by injection. Often, however, the causal organisms are sensitive to only a few antibiotics (see Chapter 4) and these may include potentially toxic compounds such as neomycin and streptomycin. Gentamicin and carbenicillin have both been used successfully by the author, apparently without harmful side effects, but are expensive. There is also the question of encouraging bacterial resistance, a problem that is particularly relevant in the case of *Pseudomonas* and which has been discussed by medical authors (Lowbury *et al*, 1972). In a number of outbreaks of bacterial septicaemia in reptiles at the Nairobi Snake Park, oxytetracycline therapy was started before sensitivity results were available and it was interesting to note the high proportion of apparent recoveries, even in cases where this antibiotic was later shown to be ineffective *in vitro*. This strongly suggests that the organism can be sensitive *in vivo* when it is not so on the laboratory bench. Temperature may play a role in treatment; Marcus (1971) stated that it was important to keep snakes at an ambient temperature above 22°C when treating pneumonia with tetracycline. In this context, it should be noted that Vaughn *et al* (1974) showed that lizards inoculated with *Aeromonas hydrophila* tended to maintain themselves at a higher temperature than uninoculated controls.

Regardless of whether antibiotic therapy is carried out, hygienic precautions must be instigated. Sick reptiles should be isolated and tended separately. Those that die must be removed promptly and the cage thoroughly cleaned and disinfected. The choice of a disinfectant is important, especially when dealing with *Pseudomonas* spp. which are notoriously resistant to standard agents and, indeed, may multiply in certain dilute disinfectants. The author's personal approach is to use either 1% formalin—which must be adequately rinsed off before reptiles are reintroduced—or boiling water. In either case, the longer the exposure to the disinfecting agent the better.

Prevention of bacterial septicaemia is based largely upon hygiene and other managemental factors. Of particular importance are the control of mites, the quarantining (isolation) of incoming reptiles and prompt attention to wounds and local lesions in established stock. The snake mite *Ophionyssus natricis* can serve as an important vector of bacteria (Camin, 1948) and all new stock should be sprayed with a suitable parasiticide, such as trichlorphon. One outbreak of an *Aeromonas* infection at a zoological collection was brought to a sudden end by mite control and rigorous attention to hygiene (Heywood, 1968).

In the case of captive aquatic reptiles hygiene is equally important. Studies on free-living species have shown that such factors as eutrophication of lakes and low oxygen tension will result in a build-up of organisms and predispose to infections (Shotts *et al*, 1972). Water in vivaria must therefore be kept clean and this can be aided by oxygenation. In the case of disinfection advantage may be taken of the work carried out on fish pathogens; several disinfectants have been recommended (Ministry of Agriculture, 1978).

Insofar as quarantine is concerned, incoming reptiles should be isolated for at least two weeks. During this time they must be observed carefully and examined weekly. They should also be treated for mites, as outlined above. If facilities permit, bacteriological culture should be carried out on faeces (or cloacal swabs) in order to ascertain which bacteria are being carried. Elimination of pathogens from the intestinal tract is not easy, but some success has been achieved in the eradication of *Pseudomonas* spp. by the daily oral administration of high doses of neomycin for ten days (Cooper, unpublished data).

Reptiles are more likely to succumb to bacterial infections when they are debilitated or suffering from intercurrent disease. Adequate care of such reptiles is vital. Skin wounds can serve as a portal of entry for pathogenic bacteria and in such cases both a clean cage and regular attention to the wound are recommended. Local lesions, such as abscesses, may give rise to a septicaemia and therefore treatment should be carried out at an early stage.

An approach to preventive medicine that has attracted relatively little attention in reptiles is vaccination (immunization). It could play a helpful role in the protection of reptiles against both generalized and local infections. Unfortunately there is little information available on the immune response in reptiles and it is not known whether humoral antibodies, or cellular immunity, or both, play any part in protecting them from bacterial infections. From the practical point of view, attempts to protect snakes against *Pseudomonas* and *Aeromonas* infections have proved disappointing: trials were carried out in Kenya using either killed vaccines or hyperimmune sera (Cooper and Leakey, 1976). However, there was evidence of protection when experimental snakes were inoculated simultaneously with serum and broth culture of the organisms.

More research on vaccination in reptiles is long overdue and may result from current interest in the immune responses of lower vertebrates (Salanitro and Minton, 1973). In recent years an encouraging development has been the production of *Pseudomonas* vaccines for use in human patients with burns (Miler *et al*, 1977; Jones *et al*, 1978) and it is possible that this work may have applications in lower vertebrate disease. It should be noted that such research is not new: interesting work on protecting animals against *Aeromonas* infection, the cause of "red leg" in frogs, was carried out 45 years ago (Borden, 1936).

Other bacterial diseases of reptiles may progress to a septicaemia and examples were given earlier in this chapter. Septicemic cutaneous ulcerative disease of turtles was discussed under "Dermatitis".

2. *Tuberculosis*

Mycobacterial infections have been recognized in many species of reptile but appear to be particularly prevalent in snakes (Cowan, 1968). The organisms isolated differ from their avian and mammalian counterparts and a number of different species are involved. For example, *Mycobacterium chelonei* is the common cause in chelonians while the main isolate from tuberculosis in snakes is usually *M. thamnopheos*.

Reptiles have also been used as experimental models for mycobacterial infections—for example, anole lizards (*Anolis carolinensis*) in studies on *Mycobacterium ulcerans*, a cause of cutaneous lesions in man (Marcus *et al*, 1975).

There appear to be no specific clinical signs in reptilian tuberculosis. Some reptiles become lethargic and lose weight but, in the majority, a diagnosis of tuberculosis is only made at *post mortem* examination. Lesions usually consist of caseous nodules in internal organs and on histopathological examination these are found to be tubercles. Acid-fast organisms can often be demonstrated within the tubercles and elsewhere in the body. It appears that pulmonary tubercles are a feature of chelonians and cutaneous and visceral (liver and spleen) lesions characteristic of lizards, snakes and crocodilians (Rhodin and Anver, 1977).

No reports of treatment of reptilian tuberculosis have been traced. However, following a case the cage should be thoroughly disinfected and, in view of the resistance of *Mycobacterium* spp., advice sought on suitable disinfectants.

3. *Salmonellosis*

The association of reptiles with *Salmonella* spp. has attracted particular attention because of the potential danger to humans of such infections (see later). The isolation of *Arizona* spp. from these animals is also a matter for some concern (Kennedy, 1973; Mayer and Frank, 1974) and the two genera will be considered together in this chapter. In fact, reptiles only rarely show pathogenic lesions associated with salmonellae; in the vast majority of cases the organisms are excreted in the faeces and the reptile appears clinically healthy. Diagnosis in such cases is based upon bacteriological culture (see Chapter 4).

Although clinical signs and pathological lesions are rare in reptilian salmonellosis, they do occur. For example, Keymer et al (1968) described a catarrhal colitis in the turtle *Eretmochelys imbricata* infected with a new species, *Salmonella regent*, and Marcus (1971) reported enteritis and septicaemia as possible manifestations of reptilian salmonellosis.

The treatment of reptiles infected with *Salmonella* spp. is rarely successful although Marcus (1977) discussed the use of neomycin, oxytetracycline and other antibiotics and Weber (1973) described the apparently successful use of oral oxytetracycline to eradicate *Salmonella* spp. from a group of tortoises (mainly *Testudo* spp.). However, the moral justification for treating an infected reptile can be questioned. It is probably preferable to destroy affected animals or, if they are valuable specimens in a collection, to ensure that they are isolated and every effort made to limit direct contact between them and man (see later).

4. *Leptospirosis*

Leptospira spp. have been isolated from snakes and serological evidence of such infections has been reported by a number of authors. Abdulla and Karstad (1962) experimentally infected reptiles with *L. pomona* and were able to show that snakes could be infected from one another by contact. Leptospires do not appear to be associated with clinical signs or pathological lesions in reptiles (Marcus, 1971).

Glosser et al (1974) detected antibodies to *L. interrogans* in 91 per cent of 46 terrapins (*Pseudomonas scripta elegans*) and were able to culture the organism from some of the turtles using hamsters as test animals.

5. *Other Infections*

Infections associated with other species of bacteria are also encountered from time to time. For example, Keymer (1978b) reported *Erysipelothrix insidiosa* infection of the spleen in a snapping turtle (*Chelydra serpentina*). The author has diagnosed clostridial infections in captive terrapins which he attributes to dirt (and hence low oxygen tension) in the water. There are usually no clinical signs, the terrapins being found dead. At *post mortem* examination there is advanced putrefaction and gas is present: Gram-positive spore-bearing bacilli are seen in large numbers in the tissues. *Clostridium novyi* has been reported to cause lethargy, anorexia and septicaemia in chelonians and was discussed, together with other diseases, in a review paper by

Murphy (1973b). Botulism appears to have been reported once in reptiles, in marine turtles (Smith, 1977).

Coxiella burnetii is not a bacterium but should be mentioned briefly. In a recent paper Yadav and Sethi (1979) reported its isolation from a monitor (*Varanus indicus*), tortoise (*Kachuga* sp.) and Indian python (*Python molurus*). In addition, antibodies were detected in the sera of "water snakes" (*Natrix natrix*). None of the reptiles showed clinical signs of disease.

V. Zoonoses

A number of the bacterial infections of reptiles are capable of causing disease in man and can therefore be termed zoonoses. Of these *Salmonella* spp. are undoubtedly the most important and many cases of salmonellosis in man have been attributed to reptiles, especially chelonians (Lamm *et al*, 1972). In a recent survey in Britain 163 faecal samples from imported tortoises (*Testudo* spp.) yielded 63 isolates of salmonellae and 62 (38%) of the samples were positive (Savage and Baker, 1980). Other reptiles kept as pets may also prove a source of infection including lizards (Hoff and White, 1977). Useful summaries of the situation are given by Orton *et al* (1972), Marcus (1977) and Keymer (1978a, b). *Edwardsiella tarda* has been incriminated in enteric infections, meningitis and wound infections of humans (Bockemühl *et al*, 1971) and the possible role of reptiles in transmitting this organism was outlined by Müller (1972). Mycobacteria of reptilian origin occasionally cause disease in man, including abscesses (Inman *et al*, 1969) and, rarely, thyroiditis (Rodgers *et al*, 1975). It is also postulated (Marcus *et al*, 1976) that reptiles may be natural reservoirs for the human pathogen, *Mycobacterium ulcerans*.

Other organisms, however, should also be considered a potential threat and chief amongst these are the *Pseudomonas* spp. The author has been unable to locate any references to the transmission of pseudomonads from reptiles to man (or vice versa) but, in view of the variety of infections in man which can be associated with *Pseudomonas*, care should be taken. Some indication of the wide host range is given in the review paper by Lusis and Soltys (1971). A similar situation applies to *Aeromonas*, which can be a cause of disease in man (Shilkin *et al*, 1968; Shotts *et al*, 1972) while *Proteus* spp. are probably also potentially hazardous.

Prevention of zoonotic infections depends upon adequate hygiene and prompt diagnosis of disease in reptiles. The hands should be washed after working with reptiles and neither eating nor smoking should be permitted in close proximity to the animals. Marcus (1977) outlined many precautions to reduce the risk of transmission of salmonellosis from reptiles, amongst them noting that small children should not handle reptiles and vivaria should not be cleaned in areas where human food is kept. Boycott *et al* (1953) warned that a risk could also exist where a tortoise shares the use of a lawn with children or other pet animals. There has been some interest in the treatment of turtle eggs with antibiotics in order to eradicate *Salmonella–Arizona* organisms; Sieberling *et al* (1975) reported good results by dipping the eggs in oxytetracycline or chloramphenicol.

Every effort must be made to obtain a definitive diagnosis when a reptile is sick or dies. Microbiological examination is of the greatest importance and should, whenever possible, also be a feature of the routine screening of animals in quarantine. However, it should be noted that one negative culture of faeces or vivarium water for *Salmonella* means nothing; repeated cultures should be carried out. The prevalence of *Salmonella* spp. may be higher in some species than others; for example, Kaura *et al* (1970) reported a 99·5 per cent carriage rate in certain lizards in India.

The role of reptiles as reservoirs of infection for other animals cannot be discussed in detail but it will be apparent from the foregoing pages that a number of organisms might be transmitted in this way. For example, Simmons *et al* (1972) postulated that lizards might serve as a source of *Dermatophilus congolensis* for sheep and cattle in Australia and Anver *et al* (1976) later isolated the same organism from a different species of lizard imported from Thailand. Transfer of bacterial infections may also be important in zoological collections, especially in mixed displays (Jackson and Jackson, 1971) and the trend towards such exhibits will hopefully prompt more detailed research on bacterial infections of reptiles.

References

Abdulla, P. K. and Karstad, L. (1962). *Zoonoses Res.* **1**, 295–306.
Addison, J. B. and Jacobson, E. R. (1974). *J. Zoo Anim. Med.* **5**, 10–11.
Anver, M. R., Park, J. S. and Rush, H. G. (1976). *Lab. Anim. Sci.* **26**, 817–823.
Boam, G. W., Sanger, V. L., Cowan, D. F. and Vaughan, D. P. (1970). *J. Am. vet. med. Ass.* **157**, 617–619.
Bockemühl, J., Pan-Urai, R. and Burkhardt, F. (1971). *Path. Microbiol.* **37**, 393–401.
Borden, A. G. (1936). "The Effect of a Nonspecific Vaccine on the Immunity

of Mice to *Pneumococcus* Type I and *Proteus hydrophilus*". M. Sc. Thesis. University of Connecticut.
Bowser, P. R. (1973). *J. Wildl. Dis.* **9,** 115–119.
Boycott, J. A., Taylor, J. and Douglas, S. H. (1953). *J. Path. Bact.* **65,** 401–411.
Brogard, J. (1980). "Les Maladies Bactériennes et Virales des Reptiles Étude Bibliographique." Association des Élèves, E.N.V.T., France.
Burke, T. J. (1978). *In* "Zoo and Wild Animal Medicine". (M. E. Fowler, ed.). pp 134–137. W. B. Saunders & Co., Philadelphia.
Camin, J. (1948). *J. Parasit.* **34,** 345–354.
Cevikbas, A. (1978). *Toxicon.* **16,** 195–197.
Clausen, H. J. and Duran-Reynals, F. (1937). *Am. J. Path.* **13,** 441–451.
Conti, L. F. and Crowley, J. H. (1939). *J. Bact.* **37,** 647–653.
Cooper, J. E. (1973). *J. Herpetol.* **7,** 316–317.
Cooper, J. E. (1975). *Vet. Rec.* **97,** 130–131.
Cooper, J. E. (1978). Bacterial diseases. Paper presented at Wildlife Disease Association Conference, Colorado, USA.
Cooper, J. E. and Leakey, J. H. E. (1976). *Trans. R. Soc. trop. Med. Hyg.* **70,** 80–84.
Cowan, D. F. (1968). *J. Am. vet. med. Ass.* **153,** 849–859.
Duran-Reynals, F. and Clausen, H. J. (1937). *J. Bact.* **33,** 369–379.
Elkan, E. and Cooper, J. E. (1976). *J. comp. Path.* **86,** 337–347.
Fölsch, D. W. and Leloup, P. (1976). *Tierärztl. Prax.* **4,** 527–536.
Glaser, H. S. R. (1948) *Copeia* 1948, 245–247.
Glassman, A. B. and Bennett, C. E. (1978). *Ga. J. Sci.* **36,** 61.
Glosser, J. W., Sulzer, C. R., Eberhardt, M. and Winkler, W. G. (1974). *J. Wildl. Dis.* **10,** 429–435.
Gordon, R. W., Hazen, T. C., Esch, G. W. and Fliermans, C. B. (1979). *J. Wildl. Dis.* **15,** 239–243.
Green, C. J., Cooper, J. E. and Jones, D. M. (1977). *Vet. Rec.* **101,** 529.
Heywood, R. (1968). *Cornell Vet.* **58,** 236–241.
Hoff, G. L. and White, F. H. (1977). *J. Herpetol.* **11,** 123–129.
Holt, P. E. (1979). *J. small Anim. Pract.* **20,** 353–359.
Holt, P. E., Cooper, J. E. and Needham, J. R. (1979). *J. small Anim. Pract.* **20,** 269–286.
Houston, A. H. and De Wilde, M. A. (1972). *J. Fish Biol.* **4,** 109–115.
Inman, P. M., Beck, A., Brown, A. E. and Stanford, J. L. (1969). *Arch. Dermatol.* **100,** 141–147.
Jackson, C. G. and Fulton, M. (1970). *J. Wildl. Dis.* **6,** 466–468.
Jackson, C. G. and Jackson, M. M. (1971). *J. Wildl. Dis.* **7,** 130–132.
Jackson, O. F. (1974). *Vet. Rec.* **95,** 11–13.
Jackson, O. F. (1976). *In* "A Manual of the Care and Treatment of Children's and Exotic Pets". (A. F. Cowie, ed.) pp 19–37. British Veterinary Association, London.
Jones, R. J., Roe, E. A. and Gupta, J. L. (1978). *Lancet* **ii,** 401–403.
Kaplan, H. M. (1957). *Proc. Anim. Care Panel* **7,** 273–277.

Kaplan, H. M. (1958). *Proc. Anim. Care Panel* **8,** 101–106.
Kaura, Y. K., Sharma, V. K. and Singh, I. P. (1970). *Res. vet. Sci.* **11,** 390–392.
Kennedy, M. E. (1973). *Can. J. comp. Med.* **37,** 325–326.
Keydar, Y., Eyland, E., Mendelssohn, H. and Marder, U. (1971). *Salamandra* **7,** 101–116.
Keymer, I. F. (1978a). *Vet. Rec.* **103,** 548–552.
Keymer, I. F. (1978b). *Vet. Rec.* **103,** 577–582.
Keymer, I. F., Ridealgh, D. and Fretwell, G. (1968). *J. Path. Bact.* **96,** 215–217.
Lambiris, A. J. L. (1976). *Zoologica Africana* **11,** 293–297.
Lamm, S. H., Taylor, A., Gangarosa, E. J., Anderson, H. W., Young, W., Clark, M. H. and Bruce, A. R. (1972). *Am. J. Epidemiology* **95,** 511–517.
Lowbury, E. J. L., Babb, J. R. and Roe, E. (1972). *Lancet* **ii,** 941–945.
Lusis, P. I. and Soltys, M. A. (1971). *Vet. Bull.* **41,** 169–177.
Marcus, L. C. (1971). *J. Am. vet. med. Ass.* **150,** 1626–1631.
Marcus, L. C. (1977). "Current Veterinary Therapy VI". (R. W. Kirk, ed.). pp 199–800. W. B. Saunders, Philadelphia.
Marcus, L. C. (1980). In "Reproductive Biology and Diseases of Captive Reptiles". (J. B. Murphy and J. T. Collins, eds.). pp 211–221. Society for the Study of Amphibians and Reptiles, Ohio.
Marcus, L. C., Stottmeier, K. D. and Morrow, R. H. (1975). *Am. J. trop. Med. Hyg.* **24,** 649–655.
Marcus, L. C., Stottmeier, K. D. and Morrow, R. H. (1976). *Am. J. trop. Med. Hyg.* **25,** 630–632.
Mayer, H. and Frank, W. (1974). *Zbl. Bakt. Hyg.* **1,** *Abt. Orig.* **A229,** 470–481.
Mayer, H. and Frank, W. (1974). "Erkrankungen der Zootiere". Verh. Ber. XIX Int. Symp. Erk. der Zootiere, Poznań. pp 93–98. Akademie Verlag, Berlin.
McPherson, C. W. (1963). *Lab. Anim. Care* **13,** 734–744.
Mergenhagan, S. E. (1956). *J. Bact.* **71,** 739.
Miler, J. M., Spilsbury, J. F., Jones, R. J., Roe, A. E. and Lowbury, E. J. L. (1977). *J. Med. Microbiol.* **10,** 19–27.
Ministry of Agriculture, Fisheries and Food (1978). "Disinfectants in Fish Farming". Fisheries Notice No. 59, Lowestoft, England.
Müller, H. E. (1972). *Zentbl. Bakt. Parasitkde.* **222,** 487–495.
Murphy, J. B. (1973a). *Br. J. Herpet.* **4,** 317–321.
Murphy, J. B. (1973b). *Hiss News-Journal* **1,** 77–81.
Nicholson, J., Marion, K. and Gauthier, J. (1976). *J. Alabama Acd. Sci.* **47,** 120.
Orton, W. T., Henderson, W. G. and Ball, D. (1972). *Community Medicine* **127,** 89–92.
Page, L. A. (1961). *Cornell Vet.* **51,** 258–266.
Page, L. A. (1966). *Bull. Wildl. Dis. Assoc.* **2,** 111–126.

Pitman, C. R. S. (1974). "A Guide to the Snakes of Uganda". Revised edition. Wheldon and Wesley, Codicote, England.
Reichenbach-Klinke, H. and Elkan, E. (1965). "The Principal Diseases of Lower Vertebrates". Academic Press, New York and London.
Rhodin, A. G. J. and Anver, M. R. (1977). *J. Wildl. Dis.* **13,** 180–183.
Rodgers, B. M., Wolfe, W. and Detmer, D. E. (1975). *J. Pediatr. Surg.* **10,** 827–829.
Salanitro, S. K. and Minton, S. A. (1973). *Copeia* 1973, 504–515.
Savage, M. and Baker, J. R. (1980). *Vet. Rec.* **106,** 558.
Schad, G. A., Knowles, R. and Meerovitch, E. (1964). *Can. J. Microbiol.* **10,** 801–804.
Shilkin, K. B., Annear, D. I. and Rowett, L. R. (1968). *Med. J. Aust.* **1,** 351–353.
Shotts, E. B., Gaines, J. L., Martin, L. and Prestwood, A. K. (1972). *J. Am. vet. med. Ass.* **161,** 603–607.
Sieberling, R. J., Neal, P. M. and Granberry, W. D. (1975). *Appl. Microbiol.* **30,** 791–799.
Simmons, G. C., Sullivan, N. D. and Green, P. E. (1972). *Aust. vet. J.*, **48,** 465–466.
Smith, L. D. S. (1977). Personal Communication with Rebell, G. *In* "Botulism. The Organism. Its Toxin. The Disease". p 208. C. C. Thomas, Illinois.
Snieszko, S. F. (1974). *J. Fish Biol.* **6,** 197–208.
Tan, R. J. S., Lim, E-W. and Ishak, B. (1978). *Res. vet. Sci.* **24,** 262–263.
Vaughn, L. K., Bernheim, H. A. and Kluger, M. J. (1974). *Nature* **252,** 473–474.
Wallach, J. D. (1969). *J. Am. vet. med. Ass.* **155,** 1017–1034.
Wallach, J. D. (1975). *J. Zoo Anim. Med.* **6,** 11–13.
Weber, A. (1973). *Kleintier Praxis* **18,** 48–50.
Will, R. (1975). *Zbl. Vet. Med.* B **22,** 626–634.
Yadav, M. P. and Sethi, M. S. (1979). *J. Wildl. Dis.* **15,** 15–17.
Yates, B., Marion, K. R. and Gauthier, J. J. (1976). *J. Alabama Acad. Sci.* **47,** 120–121.
Zwart, P. and van Ham, B. (1980). *In* "The Care and Breeding of Captive Reptiles". (S. Townson, N. J. Millichamp, D. G. D. Lucas and A. J. Millwood, eds.). pp 81–85. British Herpetological Society, London.
Zwart, P., Verwer, M. A. J. de Vries, G. A., Hermanides-Nighoh, E. J. and de Vries, H. W. (1973). *J. small Anim. Pract.* **14,** 773–779.

7 Fungi and Actinomycetes

P. K. C. AUSTWICK

Nuffield Institute of Comparative Medicine, Zoological Society of London, Regent's Park, London, England
Present address: Aerobiology Unit, Cardiothoracic Institute, Brompton Hospital, Frimley, Surrey, England

I. F. KEYMER

Zoological Society of London, Regent's Park, London, England
Present address: Veterinary Investigation Centre, Norwich, Norfolk, England

I. Introduction

The increasing recognition of fungi and actinomycetes as important causes of disease in man and domesticated animals has brought with it the realization that non-domesticated species can also be affected by pathogenic fungi both in the wild and in captivity. Most of the observations in this field have been made in mammals and the unravelling of the epidemiology of, for example, animal ringworm transmissible to man (e.g. *Trichophyton mentagrophytes* and *T. verrucosum* infection) has provided a great deal of information relevant to the control of these diseases. There has been no such stimulus to investigations of fungal diseases in the lower vertebrates for as yet no transmission to man has been demonstrated. Very much more work has been carried out in invertebrate mycopathology, more especially of insects, nematodes and protozoa with particular emphasis on control and host–parasite relationships, but happily this now has considerable relevance to reptilian disease (see later).

The reptiles have received some attention in respect of their viral, bacterial and protozoal infections (see Chapters 5, 6 and 8) but very little specifically on their mycoses. Estimates of the incidence of fungal disease range from the 0.4 per cent found by Ippen (1967) in reptiles examined *post mortem* to the 3·2 per cent reported by Keymer (1978a) in a necropsy survey of turtles and terrapins, but it is likely that many cases go unrecognized.

This chapter attempts to bring together all the published literature on reptile mycosis and, at the same time, introduces new data from the records of the Pathology Department of the Zoological Society of London during the period 1966–1978 inclusive. To faciliate reference this information has been presented in the form of three major tables dealing respectively with the mycoses of the respiratory and alimentary tracts, of the skin, orifices and limbs, and with the actinomycoses (Tables 7.1, 7.2, 7.3). This last group of diseases should really be included in bacterial infections (see Chapter 6), as there is no doubt that actinomycetes are filamentous bacteria, but for the time being tradition has meant their inclusion among the mycoses. As much detail as is either available or considered useful for future investigators has been included and the arrangement is designed to give easy access to the information under host species which are grouped in each table under their appropriate order.

A list of the fungi causing or associated with the infections is given in Table 7.4.

II. Historical

Reptilian fungal disease was reported as early as 1890 by Blanchard who found superficial excrescences which contained the conidia of *Fusarium urticearum* on the skin of a lizard (*Lacerta viridis*). But it was not until 1912 that the term "mycosis" appeared under reptiles in the reports of H. E. Plimmer (1912), then pathologist at the London Zoo. Succeeding pathologists at this establishment began to mention reptile mycosis regularly from the time of A. E. Hamerton who was appointed in 1926 and examination of these reports shows a consistent pattern of chronic nodular pneumonia, of visceral mycetomata and of cutaneous and subcutaneous disease associated with fungi. Hamerton (1929–41) enlisted the help of J. T. Duncan of the London School of Hygiene and Tropical Medicine to identify the fungi he isolated and so a number of generic determinations are available from that time. In fact some 18 of the 51 reports listed in Tables 7.1–7.3 were made by Hamerton, but he was well aware of the problems of diagnosis in mycotic disease when he wrote (1929):

"A variety of moulds have been isolated from cutaneous and visceral lesions in reptiles. In the absence of animal inoculation tests which in the case of many fungi are impracticable it is difficult to assign a pathogenic role to fungi recovered from animals after death. The constant association of a particular species or genus of fungus with a definite disease would, however, be significant."

Despite the growing interest in medical and veterinary mycology since 1950, it is only in the last 20 years that sufficient reports of reptilian mycoses have emerged to provide a basis for a systematic treatment of mycopathology in this group. Commencing with the report from the Brookfield Zoo in Chicago of mycosis in giant tortoises by Georg *et al* (1962) and the pioneering studies of Elkan (1962), a body of knowledge has built up which enables a fairly clear picture of the range of mycoses in reptiles to be represented and compared with those of mammals. Inevitably, most accounts describe cases from zoological collections, but there is some evidence that certain infections were contracted before capture and perhaps developed more rapidly under the stress conditions produced by confinement.

The literature on reptilian mycoses and the new 1966–78 data from the London Zoo cover some 60 titles describing 100 cases of fungal and actinomycete infection. The treatment, however, varies widely so that in only 42 per cent of the cases was the organism isolated and identified to species level and in only 49 per cent was any pathological examination made of the affected tissue. None of the fungi reported is an obligate parasite and most are relatively common soil saprophytes, so that the inclusion of a report in the tables does not necessarily imply pathogenic involvement and in some cases may only represent superficial contamination of the lesion or specimen. It is relevant here to note that 9 species were only isolated from the viscera, 4 only from the skin and a further 4 (including *Aspergillus fumigatus* and *Candida albicans*) from both sites. In those specimens handled personally care has been taken to indicate the possibility of secondary growth, e.g. that of *Aspergillus niger* on airway mycelial plaques of *Paecilomyces farinosus* in an American alligator (Jones, 1978).

Accounts in which "mycosis" in reptiles was not specified further have been excluded from this review, but when the host species and affected organ have been given then the record seemed worthy of inclusion.

III. Mycotic Infections

A. Respiratory Tract Mycoses

Most of the reported systemic mycoses in reptiles have involved the respiratory tract, primarily the lungs (33 out of 50 reports), and the lesions described in the majority of cases have been granulomatous, with the characteristic development of nodules and the formation of plaque lesions on the mucosa. Accompanying them has always been some degree of pneumonic consolidation and necrosis. The chronic nature and extent of the pulmonary lesions suggests that they have mostly developed over a long period of time and because of apparent inactivity were not noted clinically until the disease was in an advanced stage. The pathology of these lesions has been discussed in more detail under the heading of pathogenesis.

One feature of the *Metarhizium anisopliae* infection in a Mississippi alligator (Jones, 1978) was the presence of numerous large raised yellowish lesions on the mucosa of the larynx, trachea and bronchi, apparently arising from the lodgement of infected fragments from the lungs (Figs. 7.1, 7.2 and 7.9). Granulocytes and round cells were present with deep invasion by wide hyphae, some of which were sporulating beneath the surface. Associated granulating lesions have often been found in other organs, especially the liver, kidneys and spleen.

B. Alimentary Tract Mycoses

The upper alimentary tract in reptiles seems as prone to candidosis as it is in mammals, although there are few cases reported and these are not yet substantiated by histopathological confirmation (Thoday, 1975; Elkan, 1962). The stomach ulcers from which *Fusarium solani* was isolated in a radiate tortoise (Borst *et al*, 1972) and those associated with *Mucor circinelloides* infection in a Nile crocodile, show that the gastric mucosa is also susceptible to fungal invasion, in the latter case associated with debilitation (Jones, 1978) (Fig. 7.7).

Infections of the liver, kidneys and spleen are mainly described as chronic and granulomatous, usually associated with extensive pulmonary lesions. The nodular lesions generally show strong fibrous capsules and caseating centres. *Metarhizium anisopliae* and *Paecilomyces lilacinus* have both been observed directly in such lesions and it is of interest that the original isolate of *P. viridis* came from generalized visceral mycosis in a chameleon (Segretain *et al*, 1964).

C. Skin Mycoses

Fungal infection of the skin and its appendages is frequently said to be a major problem in captive reptiles but attempts to qualify these statements from the literature have largely failed because of the lack of specific information. Hunt (1957) considered that 1·0% of mortality in testudines was associated with shell "mycosis" and Frye (1973) suggested that this condition is both common and infectious. Certainly the 14 publications found describing "mouth-rot" (Mundfäule) would indicate that this type of infection is an important disease but the relative roles of bacteria (Burtscher, 1931), fungi and perhaps protozoa have yet to be elucidated. The terms "fungus", "shell-rot", "vent-slime", "sore-eyes", and "mycosis" have not been acceptable diagnostic criteria in this review unless accompanied by detailed descriptions of the associated organisms and normally evidence of actual infection of the tissues. Even the record of *Coniothyrium fuckelianum* invading the shell of a Greek tortoise, although personally verified, seemed only to have been the colonization of the keratin following previous damage (Goodwin, 1976). Almost one half of the reports involved members of the genera *Fusarium*, *Geotrichum* and *Trichosporon* or were mucoraceous or dematiaceous fungi but all the identified species are common saprophytes, so that their role in the disease processes and especially skin infections requires careful investigation. *Geotrichum candidum* and *Trichosporon cutaneum* are common alimentary tract commensals in animals (especially amphibia, Austwick unpublished) but they are also clearly occasionally pathogenic.

Dermatophilosis due to *Dermatophilus congolensis* has provided one of the main epidemiological surprises because it raises the possibility that reptiles could be acting as a reservoir for this obligate actinomycete along with the many species of wild mammal that have been found infected. As yet dermatomycosis caused by the ringworm fungi *Trichophyton* and *Microsporum* has not been observed in reptiles although the soil-inhabiting *Trichophyton terrestre* has been obtained from the normal scales of a boa constrictor (Austwick, unpublished). *Saprolegnia* spp. deserve special mention because of their frequent association with skin lesions in aquatic animals, especially fish, but their presence in the hind-limb lesion of a terrapin seen in this series showed only superficial invasion (Keymer, 1978b). Nodular subcutaneous lesions were described in 13 cases, in which the most interesting and well-recorded was that in a corn snake (Elkan, 1974; Keymer, 1976). This animal had had a single subcutaneous tumour removed two years before numerous similar lesions appeared, from which a *Chrysosporium* sp. was isolated. Further complications arise in that skin lesions of suspect viral (Smith and Coates, 1938) or neoplastic (Billups and Harshbarger, 1976) origin may become invaded by fungi (Blažek *et al*, 1968) and it is essential that this type of lesion is studied mycopathologically.

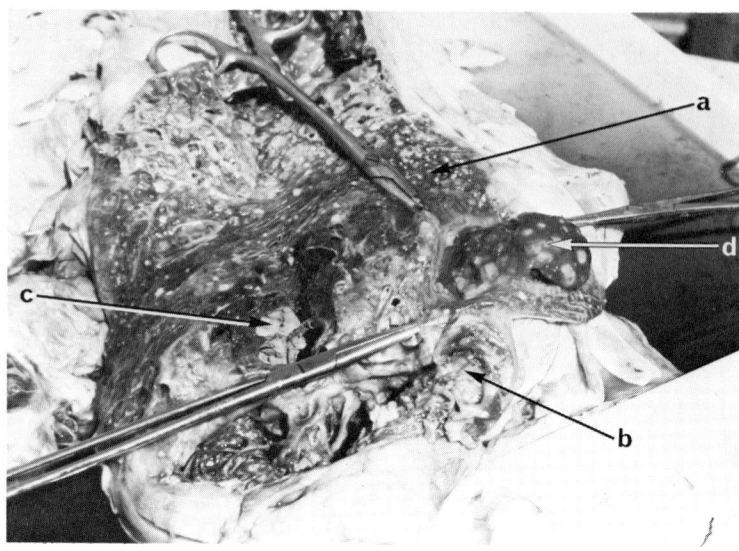

Fig. 7.1. Lung of Mississippi alligator with *Metarhizium anisopliae* infection. Lesions (a) miliary nodules (b) plaque over epithelium (c) green sporulating colony on plaque (d) mycetoma filling airway comprising caseous foci within reddish mucoid material.

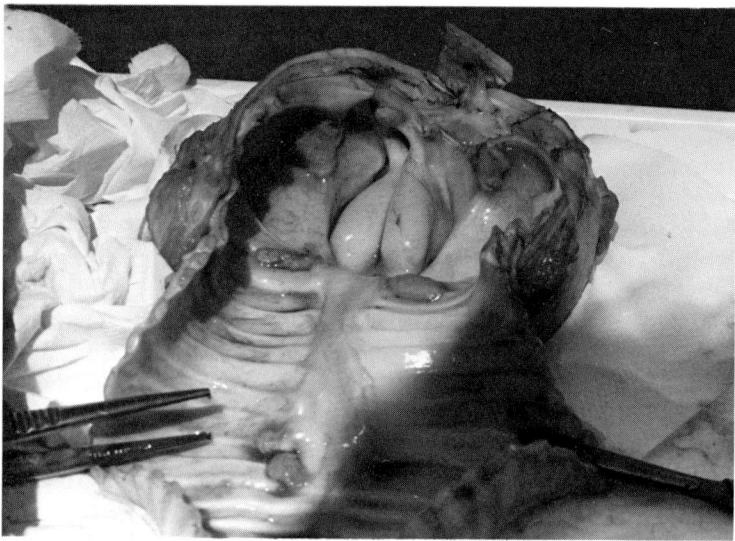

Fig. 7.2. Larynx of Mississippi alligator with raised plaque lesions. *Metarhizium anisopliae* infection.

7 FUNGI AND ACTINOMYCETES   199

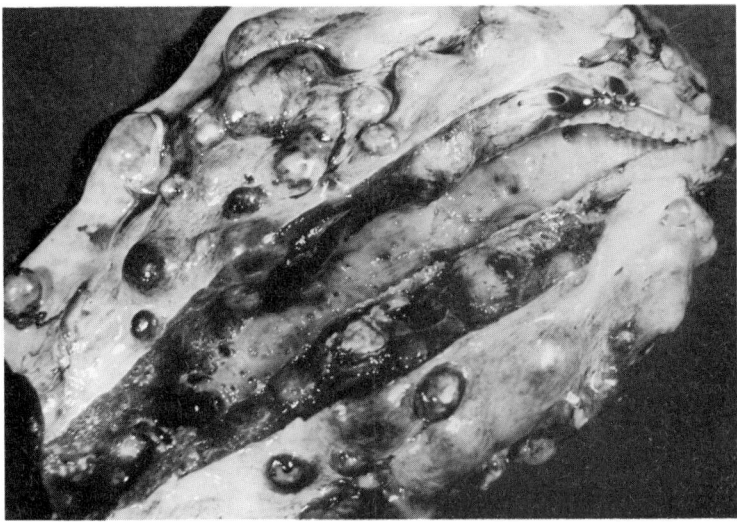

Fig. 7.3. Lung lobe of loggerhead turtle showing nodular pneumonia, interstitial haemorrhage and caseation of large granulomata. *Paecilomyces lilacinus* isolated.

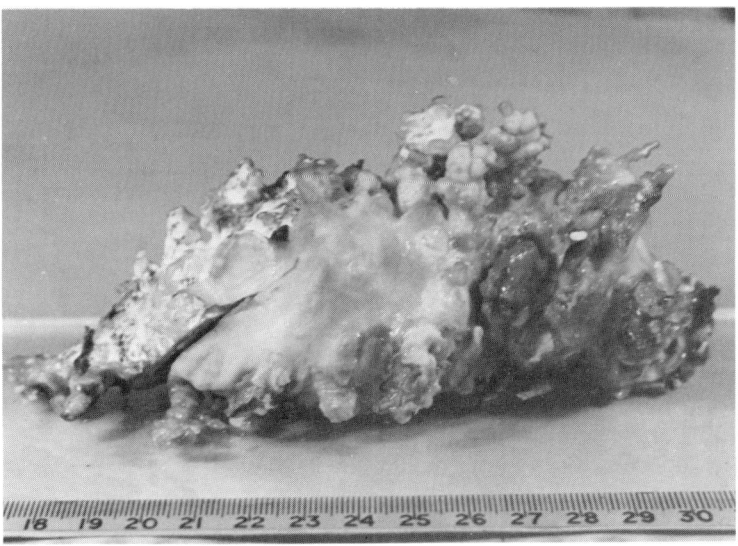

Fig. 7.4. Hyphal mat cast of airway of Mississippi alligator showing prolongations into bronchioles and surface mucus. *Paecilomyces farinosus* infection.

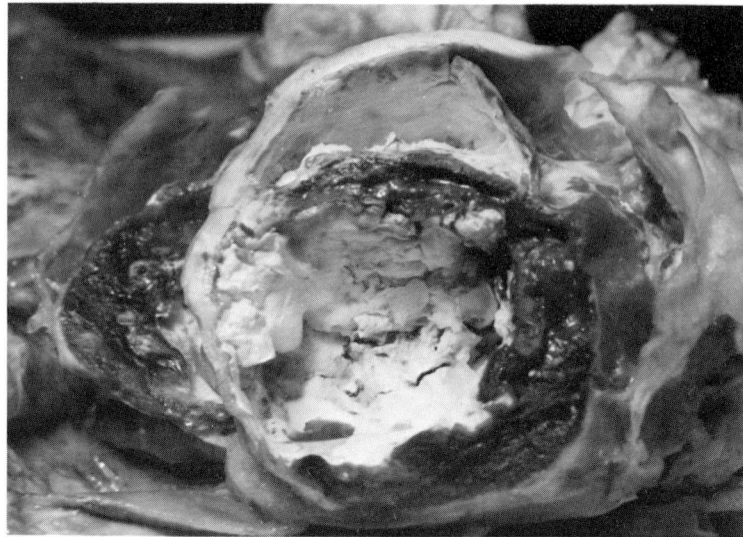

Fig. 7.5. Section through firm bulla in lung of Mississippi alligator showing multiple development of hollow sporulating colonies of *Paecilomyces farinosus* forming hyphal cast of airway.

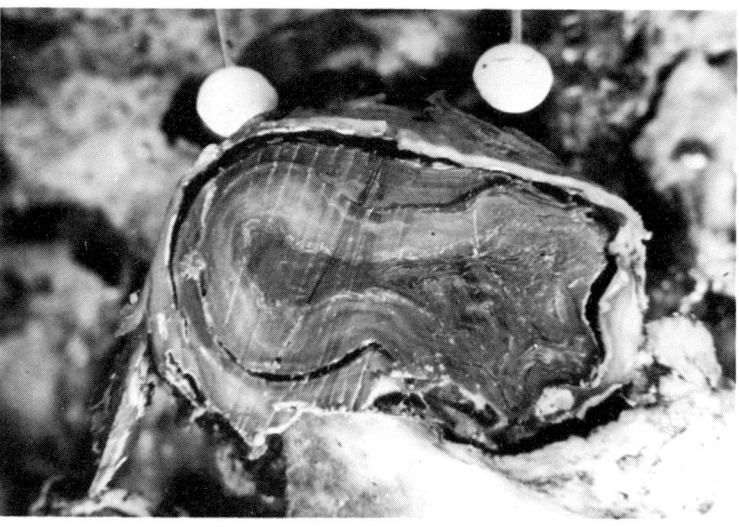

Fig. 7.6. Laminated mycetoma from airway of Nile crocodile. Hyphae and conidiophores of *Paecilomyces lilacinus* observed in outer zones only.

7 FUNGI AND ACTINOMYCETES 201

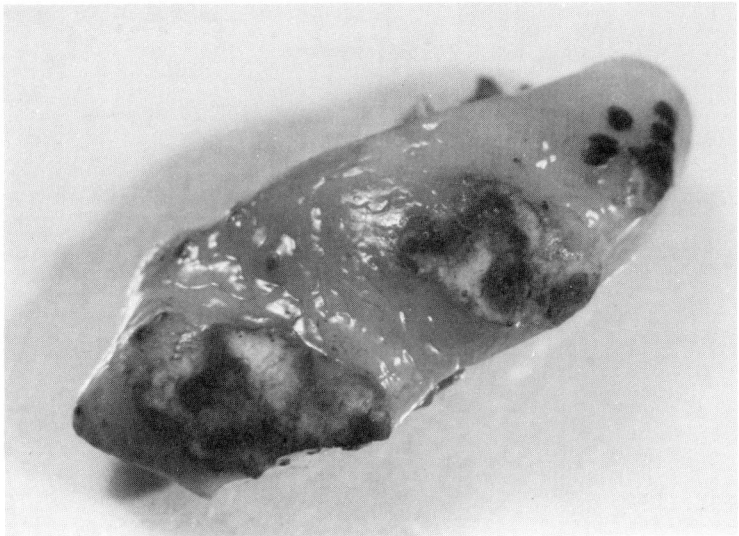

Fig. 7.7. Portion of stomach wall of Nile crocodile with raised greenish ulcers invaded by *Mucor circinelloides*.

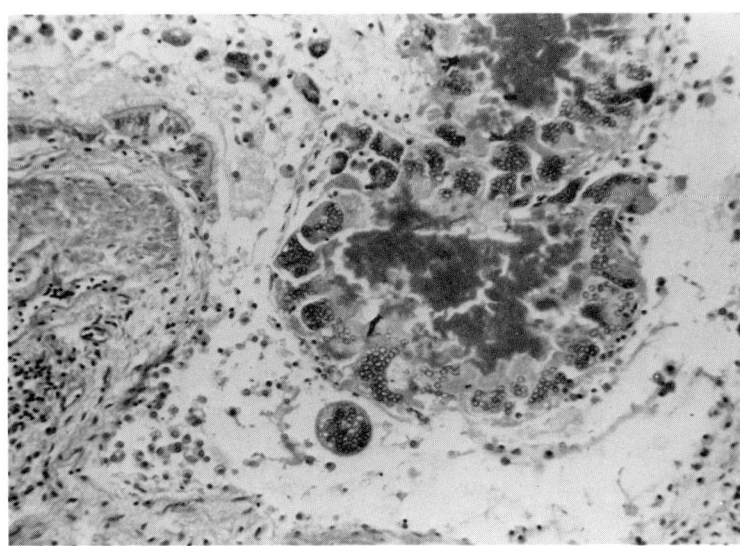

Fig. 7.8. Granuloma from lung of spectacled cayman showing early spindle arrangement of giant cells surrounding caseous centre. *Paecilomyces lilacinus* isolated. (×150)

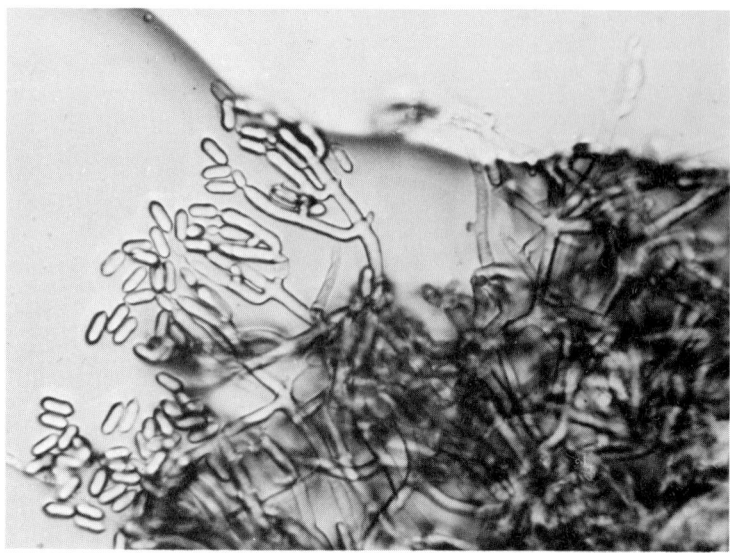

Fig. 7.9. Conidiophores and conidia of *Metarhizium anisopliae* from surface of bullous plaque lesion in lung of Mississippi alligator. (Unstained, ×400)

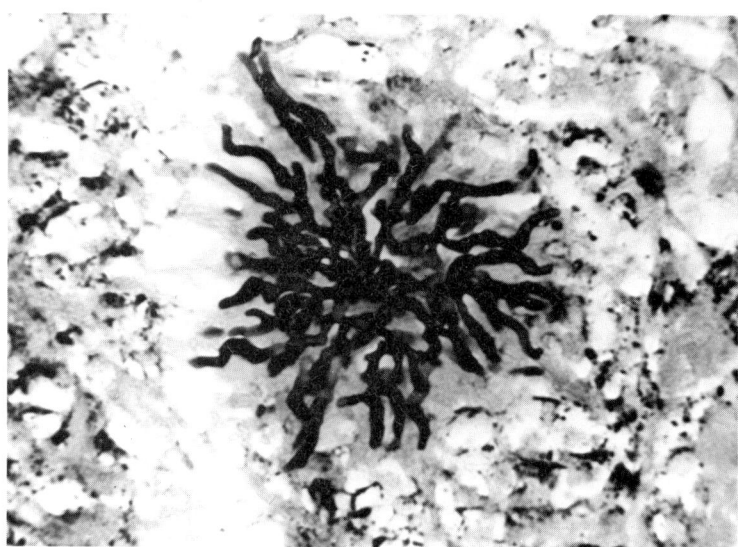

Fig. 7.10. Liver lesion in *Lacerta dugesii* experimentally infected with *Metarhizium anisopliae*, showing contorted hyphae in granuloma (See Fig. 7.6) (Stained Gomori–Grocott, ×400)

D. Egg Infection

Little information exists on fungal infection in reptilian eggs but it is probably a factor influencing hatchability at least in captive animals; only Patterson (1974) and Branch and Patterson (1975) seem to have alluded to the possible role of "moulds" in mortality and abnormal development (see also Chapter 14). Two cases were investigated at the London Zoo; one concerned a batch of incubating Indian python eggs in which *Fusarium oxysporum* was growing over the membranes as a white mycelial felt and invading the embryo and yolk-sac, where it produced a characteristic blue-green colouration. The second involved hatching boipevussu snake eggs from the membrane of which *Chaetomium globosum* was isolated. The pathogenicity of these two fungi to the eggs was not established, but when the hazards of the rotting vegetation of alligator nests is considered it seems likely that certain reptile eggs possess an innate resistance to fungal infection.

IV. Pathogenesis and Pathogenicity

It has not been possible to obtain from the literature analysis a clear idea of the pathogenesis of reptile mycoses and the impressions gained in this important aspect of these diseases have come chiefly from the material examined at the London Zoo. This in itself has been restrictive in that the cases seen were all of long-standing infections and hence it is difficult to envisage the initial processes in the formation of such lesions as the airways mycelial casts. From examination of the miliary lung lesions, it seems that this type may represent the first stages of infection following the inhalation of spores. Many lie free in the lumen of the alveolar sacs and are generally easily separable from the tissue. Each consists of a focus of cellular infiltration surrounding a fungal colony which, as it grows in size, invades the adjacent alveolar or bronchiolar wall. The large granulomata that develop extensively involve the interstitial tissues and probably lead to the formation of the pulmonary nodules seen in a high proportion of infections. Another form of development may result from the colony remaining free from the surrounding tissues and simply enlarging by radial hyphal growth and by accretion, still within the airway, and eventually forming the hard, laminated type of mycetoma seen in a Nile crocodile associated with *P. lilacinus* (Keymer, 1974) (Fig. 7.6). A comparable human pulmonary mycetoma (due to *Aspergillus fumigatus*) might take several years to develop. A second type of mycetoma seen with *M. anisopliae* seems to consist of a number of separate colonies, each within a caseous envelope but embedded in a firm reddish mucilaginous material containing large numbers of heterophil granulocytes (Jones, 1978) (Fig. 7.1d). Plaques are thought to arise from similar colonies which, however, spread concentrically as the fungus grows over the respiratory mucosa. Where there is little physical restriction, this type of lesion seems able to cover the entire internal surface of a lung lobe with sporulating mycelium, e.g. *M. anisopliae* infection, but when contained, perhaps the ultimate development of such lesions is shown by the *Paecilomyces farinosus* infection of the Mississippi alligator in which the coalescing lesions apparently formed the extensive hyphal mat casts, up to 30 mm wide, with extensions into the minor associated airways. It also seems possible that the continued lateral growth of the plaques under the constriction of the airways was responsible for the folding of the mycelial mat and hence the multi-chambered structures with internal sporulation (Fig. 7.5).

The consistent role of certain species of fungi in systemic reptile infection suggests that they have common features of pathogenicity. A property of four of the species is the ability to infect insects, in which they cause epidemic disease (Balfour-Browne, 1960; Bell, 1974; Madelin, 1963). These species are *Beauveria bassiana*, *Metarhizium anisopliae*, *Paecilomyces farinosus* and *P. lilacinus* and because of their importance and the large amount of data now available on them, they are considered here in some detail, whilst other interesting isolates are briefly discussed.

Beauveria bassiana This is the well-known white muscardine fungus of the silkworm which has been used extensively for the biological control of insect pests. It also occurs in soil and has occasionally been isolated from human and animal lungs (Pore *et al*, 1970), but it has not been regarded as a pathogen in this context. Colonies on malt agar are white to pale buff and produce copious conidia 2–3 μm in diameter borne sympodially in acropetal succession. In the lesions from reptile lungs the hyphae are reported up to 7 μm diameter. Fromtling *et al* (1979b), and Georg *et al* (1962) illustrated cephalosporioid conidiophores bearing oval conidia 1·5 × 3–5 μm, which had not been seen previously.

Paecilomyces lilacinus This fungus, along with several others has been taken out of the genus *Penicillium* on account of its tapering phialides and the ovoid conidia. It has also been placed in the genus *Spicaria*, in which the closely related *Paecilomyces fumoso-roseus* was also included.

Cultures on malt agar are characterized by their pale lilac colour. This colour was also seen on the surface of the thin sporulating plaques lining an airway in a Nile crocodile (Keymer, 1974). The main characteristic noted in lesions has been the production of cephalosporioid conidiophores within the caseated tissue. These were seen in 6 out of 7 cases examined and suggest that this is a regular feature as indicated by Thom (1910). Curiously the giant tortoise No. 3 reported by Georg et al (1962) showed identical structures associated with the isolation of *Beauveria bassiana*. The single case (in an African python) which did not show conidia inside the lesions, had copious development of arthrospores on the outside of the tissue, whilst the experimentally infected lizards (see p. 207) showed yeast-like bodies in the lesions. *P. lilacinus* occurs frequently in soil (Gilman and Abbott, 1927).

Paecilomyces farinosus This common insect pathogen is better known as *Isaria farinosa* and is thought by some mycologists to be the imperfect stage of the well-known *Cordyceps militaris*. Although only a single case of this infection has been found, in a Mississippi alligator (Jones, 1978), the nature of the lesions indicates that this fungus may prove to be a potent pathogen of reptiles. Sporulation on the mycelial felts in the airways consisted of phialospores 1·8 to 2 × 0·9 to 1·2 μm but the additional presence of aleuriospores 5 to 7 × 2 to 2·9 μm raises the problem of multiple spore types in these three important species (Brown and Smith, 1957) (Fig. 7.5).

Metarhizium anisopliae This is the green muscardine fungus which is also used as a biological pesticide. It occurs in soil and on plant remains, and its pathogenicity to reptiles has been confirmed by the successful inoculation of a lizard (see p. 207). Colonies are at first bright yellow and floccose but when the columns of conidia develop and coalesce a dark green crust is formed. The appearance and colour of the hyphal mats in the airways of the affected alligator closely resembled those of *Aspergillus fumigatus* as seen in the airsacs in avian aspergillosis. In lesions the hyphae can reach 7 μm diameter and are generally thin-walled and contorted. The characteristic sporulation was seen on one occasion in a tracheal surface plaque (Fig. 7.2).

Aspergillus spp. The aspergilli and especially *Aspergillus fumigatus* do not seem to play a dominant role in reptilian mycoses. The report of Georg et al (1962) of a tumour-like lesion containing the hyphae of *Aspergillus amstelodami* in a giant tortoise is convincing but *Aspergillus niger* recorded from the Mississippi alligator (Jones, 1978) seemed to be a secondary invader of the mycelial felt of *Paecilomyces farinosus* in the airways casts.

Cephalosporium sp. The three cases of respiratory mycosis in caimans described by Trevino (1972) associated with this fungus are of special mycological interest because of both the formation of chlamydospore-like structures in the lesions and the presence, in some areas of the sections, of conidiophores and spores which closely resembled those seen in *Paecilomyces lilacinus* infection.

Chrysosporium spp. Two of the most important fungal pathogens of warm-blooded animals, viz. *Histoplasma capsulatum* and *Blastomyces dermatitidis*, are closely related to species of this genus and the occurrence of *C. keratinophilum* in skin lesions of iguanas (Zwart *et al*, 1968) indicates a pathogenic ability. The isolate from the tumour-like lesions in a corn snake (Elkan, 1974) was probably an undescribed species.

Fusarium spp. The skin infections of reptiles associated with *Fusarium* spp. parallel the situation in mammals, especially the aquatic species, in which reports of dermal, subcutaneous and orbital infection due to *F. oxysporum* and *F. solani* are now quite frequent. These fungi are not systemic pathogens, but they readily colonize damaged skin surfaces and then seem well able to invade the underlying tissues.

Mucor circinelloides The pathogenicity of this species has been demonstrated in amphibia, in which endosporulating spherules are produced in the viscera (Frank, 1976). In the stomach ulcers of the Nile crocodile described by Jones (1978), invasion of the mucosa and sub-mucosa was by wide, sparsely septate hyphae with abundant chlamydospores developing in the outer parts of the lesions (Fig. 7.7). Phycomycosis seems to be rare in reptiles but when reported, has shown a similar range of lesions to that seen in mammals.

V. Experimental Fungal Infection

Very few attempts appear to have been made to reproduce reptile mycoses experimentally, which may well be due to lack of interest and opportunity, but must also be connected with the problem of obtaining suitable reptiles for experiment. Almost all have to be caught in the wild, and hence carry their normal parasitic fauna and bacterial flora. Transfer to the laboratory moreover is not always successful. The following notes outline present knowledge:

Beauveria bassiana A strain isolated by Georg *et al* (1962) from pulmonary mycosis in a giant tortoise, was inoculated into two specimens of *Terrapene carolina*, one of which died in 4 days and showed hyphae in lung abscesses.

Geotrichum candidum Some 7 isolates from plant and animal sources including a lung isolate from a tortoise (Georg *et al*, 1962) were used by Sinclair (1969) to assess the pathogenicity of this species to *Chelydra serpentina* and *Pseudemys elegans*. Some apparent infection occurred and the organism was isolated from the tissues. Low grade granulomata were obtained by Ruiz *et al* (1980) in *Testudo horsfieldii*.

Metarhizium anisopliae Two individuals of *Lacerta dugesii* inoculated subcutaneously with an isolate of this species from the lung of a Nile crocodile (Keymer, 1974) died 12 and 28 days later respectively. Small infectious foci were found in the lungs, liver and kidneys from which the fungus was re-isolated. These small granulomata contained colonies of extensively branching hyphae which were contorted in the manner characteristic for this species when growing in lesions (Fig. 7.10). Intraperitoneal inoculation of a *Pseudemys elegans* also produced extensive visceral lesions (Austwick, unpublished).

Paecilomyces lilacinus An isolate of this species from the lungs of a Nile crocodile and another from those of a broad-fronted crocodile (Keymer; 1974) were inoculated intraperitoneally and subcutaneously respectively into two *Lacerta dugesii*. The fungus was seen in, and recovered from, tissues up to 28 days later and histopathological examination showed microscopic infiltrated foci containing short hyphal fragments and yeast-like cells. One intraperitoneal inoculation of a *Pseudemys elegans* failed to show gross lesions *post mortem* at 19 days, but the fungus was readily isolated from the viscera. Attempts at airborne infection of similar terrapins both with this species and with *M. anisopliae* were unsuccessful (Austwick, unpublished).

VI. Environmental Aspects

A knowledge of the circumstances in which fungal infection becomes established in reptiles is essential to both the study of pathogenicity and to the more practical aspect of the control of these infections in captive animals. The confinement of animals caught in the wild provides the main contributory factor in stress which is manifest in loss of appetite and nutritional deficiency. How much this affects susceptibility to fungal infection is hard to assess but it is notable that in several of the cases involving Crocodilia, severe nutritional disease in the form of degenerative liver lesions was suspected. Another stress factor which has been considered significant in reptile disease is that associated with a sudden drop in temperature. Both Georg *et al* (1962) and Fromtling *et al* (1979b) encountered their cases in animals that had been exposed to thermal shock following brief failure of the heating systems in the reptile house. Intercurrent viral, bacterial and protozoal infection is also a factor in mycoses and several examples are listed in Table 7.2, occurring particularly when the skin has been involved.

Two more general aspects of the relationship of reptiles to insects are also relevant to the epidemiology of reptilian mycoses. One is the curious link between entomophthorous activity and reptilian pathogenicity, in which the acquisition of the fungus could be by eating an infected insect, but in view of the large size and fish diet of the Crocodilia and the herbivorous habit of some of the Testudines affected, it seems more likely that infection could have come from conidia formed on dead insects in the immediate environment. In two attempts to verify this suggestion *Paecilomyces lilacinus* was isolated from the air of the reptile house at the London Zoo, but no other insect pathogens were obtained (Austwick, unpublished). These connections carry an interesting possibility of an evolutionary link between the reptiles and the insects.

The other mycological curiosity of reptile life is the frequent presence of the zygomycetous fungi belonging to the genus *Basidiobolus* as commensals in the gut. These fungi belong to the Entomophthorales which are predominantly insect pathogens, but include two species causing subcutaneous mammalian infection, viz. *Entomophthora (Conidiobolus) coronata* and *Basidiobolus meristosporus*. *Basidiobolus ranarum* (= ? *B. meristosporus*) is a frequent inhabitant of reptile intestines and has been regularly isolated from reptile faeces (Coremans-Pelseneer, 1973; Nickerson and Hutchinson, 1971). It seems it has never been found invading the tissues and the association strengthens the idea of a link between the insects and the reptiles through their normal and pathogenic mycoflora.

VII. Discussion

The presentation of data on reptilian mycoses in the form of extended tables does not allow for adequate discussion of the individual cases, nor for their easy pathological comparison. However there was a serious need for a compilation of the literature on these diseases and for some evaluation of the data in the light of experience gained from the authors' own studies at the London Zoo between 1966 and 1979. A relatively small number of citations found had to be excluded on the grounds of inadequate description, and it has been a surprise to find that 75 cases could be located, albeit often within the reports of zoo pathologists. The addition of hitherto unpublished data from the 25 cases examined at the London Zoo has meant that there is now a fairly comprehensive background to reptilian mycoses for the guidance of pathologists and herpetologists.

This study also highlights the many interesting problems posed by reptile pathology. The pathogenesis of the systemic mycoses is particularly difficult to elucidate in the absence of accounts of early lesions and this allows only speculation on the changes that lead to the chronic lesions. The unique susceptibility to infection by mesophilic (i.e. medium temperature tolerant) fungi which are not normally vertebrate pathogens would indicate some fundamental differences from mammals, not the least of which must be linked with the temperature status of the poikilothermic animal. Part of the seemingly easy, rapid and extensive development of fungal plaques in the airways may be linked to the relatively simple non-rigid bag-like structure with muscular trabeculae demarcating the folds between larger airsacs and alveoli (Bellairs, 1969), but equally, the reptile's apparent deficiency in surfactant (Pattle and Hopkinson, 1963) may contribute to the ability of fungi of low pathogenicity to establish themselves.

The susceptibility of reptile skins to fungal infection clearly does not lie in the direct invasion of the keratinized layers by dermatophytes, for there are as yet no records of these fungi from reptiles. More likely, it seems that the reptile skin is generally resistant to fungal attack unless it is damaged by mechanical trauma or, in the terrestrial species, by prolonged water-soaking. Subcutaneous infection seems to be more important but as yet the known causal fungi show none of the epidemiological relationships which might be expected in such a habitat, as is seen in the systemic fungi. Further records should, in future, enable a better evaluation of fungi isolated from the skin of reptiles.

Table 7.1. Mycosis of the respiratory and alimentary tracts

Host and fungus	Organs affected	Gross lesions	Histopathology	Fungal morphology	Author	Date
Order CHELONIA (TESTUDINES)						
Caretta caretta						
Paecilomyces lilacinus	Lung	Chronic nodular pneumonia with large caseated nodules to 18 mm (Fig. 7.3)	Very wide fibrous capsule, many giant cells, and epithelioid cells	Hyphae septate, spiral, cephalosporioid conidiophores within lesion, conidia 4–6.5 × 1.5–2.5 μm	Keymer Goodwin Elkan and Reichenbach-Klinke	1974 1974 1974 1977
Chelonia-mydas						
Paecilomyces sp. *Sporotrichum* sp. (*Cladosporium* sp.)	Lung	Nodular and acute suppurative pneumonia	Granulomata with central caseation, giant cells, macrophages, and outer fibroblasts; lesions extending into airways	Hyphae septate narrow, sporulating in airways	Jacobson *et al*	1979
Indet.	Lung	Chronic pneumonia with large caseated nodules to 20 mm	Thick capsule, outer vacuolated zone, giant cells absent, little cellular infiltration, satellite lesions	Hyphae, septate, random within caseous material cephalosporioid conidia 4–7.5 × 1.5–2 μm	Keymer Goodwin	1974 1974
Chrysemys d'orbugnyi						
Indet.	Lung	—	—	—	Hill	1956
Hydraspis pilarii						
Aspergillus sp.	Lung	Nodular pneumonia and red hepatization, pleural plaques	Caseating granulomata (mycetomata)	Hyphae extensive in lesions and airways	Hamerton	1934
	Liver, Spleen, Kidney	—	Mycetomata	—		

Host and fungus	Organs affected	Gross lesions	Histopathology	Fungal morphology	Author	Date
Pseudemys ornatus						
Paecilomyces lilacinus	Lung	Caseating pneumonia	Eosinophilic bronchiolar exudate, hyphal felts formed from confluent plaques	Hyphae, narrow, septate with oval $3–6 \times 1\cdot2–1\cdot5\ \mu m$ and limoniform $2\cdot5–3 \times 1\cdot7–2\ \mu m$ conidia	Keymer	1976
Indet.	Rectum Intestine	Proctitis	Diphtheritic membrane	*Pseudomonas aeruginosa* isolated from the lungs and large intestine	Keymer	1978a
	Kidney Liver	Nephrosis nodules	Encapsulated lesions	Hyphae present		
Testudo denticulata						
Paecilomyces lilacinus	Lung	Walls with hyphal layer	—	—	Bemmel et al	1960
Testudo elephantopus						
Aspergillus amstelodami (*Geotrichum candidum*)	Lung	Severe pneumonitis	Exudate with organization, monocytes, granulocytes amorphous material		Georg et al	1962
	Leg	Skin tumours	Bands of uniform monocytes in tumour tissue	Hyphae seen fresh but not in stained sections		
Beauveria bassiana	Lung	Necrotizing pneumonia, thickened pleura	Extensive monocytic infiltration and focal caseation	Hyphae septate, $5\ \mu m$ wide, dense at periphery of lesions, no conidia seen	Georg et al	1962

Table 7.1 (contd.)

Host and fungus	Organs affected	Gross lesions	Histopathology	Fungal morphology	Author	Date
Testudo gigantea elephantina						
Aspergillus sp.	Lung	Greyish exudate, also in nasal and buccal cavities	Inflammation of mucosa with acidophilic infiltration	Hyphae in exudate penetrating lamina propria and cartilage	Andersen et al	1968
Beauveria bassiana	Lung	Necrotizing pneumonitis	Inflammatory exudate of monocytes and few granulocytes, exudate partly organized	Hyphae 4–5 µm wide, septate conidia oval 1·5 × 3·5 µm at aerial surfaces	Georg et al	1962
Paecilomyces fumoso-roseus	Lung	Nodular necrotizing pneumonia	Large and small granulomata with peripheral epithelioid and giant cells, infiltrating monocytes, bronchi and bronchioles filled with mucus	Hyphae 3–4 µm wide, fragmented in central caseation and bronchial lumen, no conidia seen	Georg et al	1962
Indet.	Heart	Chronic fibrotic endocarditis	Generalized mycosis	Not reported	Hamerton	1935
	Plastron } Bone	Infection	—	—		
Testudo nigrita						
Aspergillus sp.	Lung	Consolidation	—	White hyphal felt in airways	Hamerton	1937
Aspergillus sp.	Lung	Cavitation and gangrene	—	Hyphal felt with conidiophores	Hamerton	1939
Penicillium sp.	Lung	Nodular pneumonia	—	Conidiophores on surfaces of air-spaces, hyphae lining stomach wall	Hamerton	1934
	Liver	Nodular lesions	—			
Testudo radiata						
Fusarium solani	Stomach	Ulceration	Not seen	Not seen	Borst et al	1972

Host and fungus	Organs affected	Gross lesions	Histopathology	Fungal morphology	Author	Date
Order SQUAMATA—LACERTILIA (SAURIA)						
Agama agama						
Indet.	Liver	Small foci	Extensive necrosis	Hyphae abundant forming arthrospores	Keymer	1967
Chameleo jacksonii						
Indet.	Intestine Rectum	Enteritis and rectal prolapse	Intussusception of terminal colon with necrosis and infiltration	(a) Hyphae in vascular channels; (b) spherical structures 15–25 μm diam. in intestinal wall and lumen	Shalev et al	1977
Chameleo lateralis						
Paecilomyces viridis	Viscera	Generalized mycosis	?	Yeast form in vivo	Segretain et al	1964
Chameleo vulgaris						
Indet. yeast	Cloaca	None	Cloacal epithelial cells invaded and degenerated	Intracellular yeast cells and filaments in lumen	Wenyon	1921
Crocodilurus lacertinus						
Candida albicans	Oesophagus	Lesions	Oesophageal wall thickened and covered with a superficial film containing yeast cells	Yeast cells	Zwart et al	1968
Iguana iguana						
Chrysosporium keratinophilum	Lung Digestive tract	} Stomach lining	Necrotic zone in stomach thickened to 15 mm	Isolate from lung, stomach, liver, heart and intestine	Zwart et al	1968
Chrysosporium keratinophilum	Lung	Miliary lesions	—	Isolate from lung	Zwart et al	1968
	Gall bladder	Inflammation	Lining inflamed	—		

Table 7.1 (contd.)

Host and fungus	Organs affected	Gross lesions	Histopathology	Fungal morphology	Author	Date
Lacerta viridis						
Indet.	Kidney	—		Septate hyphae	Elkan	1974
Metopoceros cornutus						
Indet.	Trachea	Occlusion	Large mycetoma adherent to part of surface of pericardium and heart	Network of hyphae in necrotic tissue	Hamerton	1941
Tupinambis nigropunctatus						
Aspergillus sp.	Lung	Nodular pneumonia	Generalized mycosis as Hydraspis pilarii above	Hyphae extensive in lesions	Hamerton	1934
Tupinambis tequexii						
Indet.	Lung	Consolidation	—	Mycotic deposits	Hamerton	1935
Order SQUAMATA—SERPENTES (OPHIDIA)						
Bitis arietans						
Aspergillus sp.	Peritoneum, Liver, Spleen	Peritonitis	Multiple granulomata in peritoneum	Hyphal invasion of liver and spleen	Hamerton	1934
Coronella austriaca						
Candida albicans	Liver	Miliary lesions to 1 mm diam.	—	—	Elkan	1962, 1974
	Nose, mouth, throat, eye	Nasal passages blocked, oral mucosa swollen	Pustular lesions with eosinophilic infiltration	Hyphae in foci		
Natrix cyclopion						
Aspergillus sp.	Body cavity	Plaque lesions	Liver necrosis	Hyphae in plaques	Hamerton	1937
Pseustes sulphureus						
Indet., yeast	Lung	—	Abscesses	Yeast cells seen	Jones	1978

Host and fungus	Organs affected	Gross lesions	Histopathology	Fungal morphology	Author	Date
Python sebae						
Paecilomyces lilacinus	Lung	Necrosis	Necrotic focus and extensive haemorrhage and lymphocytic infiltration	Extensive development of septate hyphae to 3 μm diam., arthrospores superficial only, 1·5–5 × 1–2 μm	Keymer	1974
Indet. (S. American water snake)						
Trichosporon sp.	Lung	Abscesses	—	Hyphae and arthrospores	Jones	1978
	Intestine	Small white superficial plaques	Ulceration			
Indet.						
Candida albicans } *Geotrichum candidum*	Viscera	—	—	—	Wallach	1969
Fusarium sp.	Intestine	—	—	—	Grünberg *et al*	1963
Order CROCODILIA						
Alligator mississipiensis						
Aspergillus fumigatus	Lung	Grey pneumonic	Cellular exudate in lesion	Hyphae present in lung and skin	Jasmin *et al*	1968
	Skin	Lesions	—			
Beauveria bassiana	Lungs	(a) Miliary foci with white filamentous lesions to 90 mm diam. pneumonic consolidation and hepatization (three cases)	(a) Thickened alveolar septa with exudate and monocytic infiltration in parenchyma; multifocal granulomata with monocytes, heterophils and giant cells	(a) Hyphae septate, 5–7 μm diam. present in all bronchial and alveolar spaces	Fromtling *et al*	1979 a, b.
	Intestine Liver }	Petechial haemorrhages (b) Nodular lesions	(b) Localized granulomata central necrosis, giant cells, fibroblastic capsule; foci also in spleen	(b) Hyphae present in all granulomata		

Table 7.1 (contd.)

Host and fungus	Organs affected	Gross lesions	Histopathology	Fungal morphology	Author	Date
Metarhizium anisopliae	Lung	Emphysema with (a) miliary nodules in parenchyma; (b) soft hollow bullae lined with dark green fungal mat; (c) mycetomata to 50 mm. diam. in airways; (d) trachea and bronchi with raised yellow firm lesions to 20 mm. diam.; (e) tongue with ulceration (Figs. 7.1, 7.2)	(a) Large and small granulomata with caseation, round cell infiltration heterophils and necrosis of muscle and epithelial tissue, giant cells absent; (b) epithelium destroyed and replaced by sporulating fungal mat, oxalate crystals (?) present; (c) large granulomata to 20 mm diam. centre caseated with vacuolated cells, lymphocytes and peripheral giant cells; (d) lesions to 5 mm thick with extensive invasion of musculature and penetration to cartilage. Round cells and eosinophils and tissue caseated towards surface	(a) Hyphae radiating from centres of granulomata to 4 μm diam. contorted, non-sporulating; (b) hyphae to 6 μm wide and conidia 3–6 × 1·5–3 μm over surface; (c) hyphae to 7 μm wide contorted and radiating when present, non-sporulating; (d) hyphae to 4 μm wide radiating from centre of lesion beneath epithelium, sporulating in lesion; (e) germinating spores (Fig. 7.9)	Jones Goodwin	1978 1978
Paecilomyces farinosus (Aspergillus niger)	Lung	Emphysema with (a) firm bullae lined with white or black fungal mat to 50 mm diam. but elongating into airways giving irregular, spiny casts to 120 mm × 35 mm; (b) white miliary lesions to 2 mm diam.; (c) small plaques on epithelium of airways; (d) mycetomata to 20 mm diam. (Figs. 7.4, 7.5)	(a) Dilated airways lined with single or laminated caseous material with a hyphal felt; epithelium with round cell infiltration, necrosis and loss of basophily; peripheral spindle-shaped giant cells. Occasional mucoid material between laminations (b) } Small granulomata (c) } (d) Centre with many heterophils and round cell nuclei, becoming vacuolate and invaded by bacteria	(a) Hyphae narrow 1·5 μm diam. dense sporulation on inner (aerial surfaces), poorly stained in deeper laminations. Conidia of two types—phialospores 1·8–2·0 × 0·9–1·2 μm limoniform and aleuriospores 5–7 × 2–2·9 μm pyriform: black areas with Aspergillus niger conidiospores (d) Few hyphal fragments seen	Jones Goodwin	1978 1978
Paecilomyces lilacinus	Lung	Miliary, nodular caseating pneumonia with mucoid exudate	Granulomata with central caseation, peripheral spindled-shaped giant cells, monocytic and heterophilic infiltration	Hyphae and cephalosporioid conidia in caseated material but not in all granulomata	Keymer	1974

Host and fungus	Organs affected	Gross lesions	Histopathology	Fungal morphology	Author	Date
Paecilomyces lilacinus	Lung	As above	Large and small granulomata with spindle-shaped giant cells, heterophils and other polymorphonuclear cells	Hyphae with cephalosporioid conidia 5·5–11 × 1·8–2·7 μm within granulomata; external hyphae to 4 μm diam. with limoniform spores 2–3·5 × 2–2·2 μm *Pseudomonas aeruginosa* isolated from lung	Keymer	1976
Penicillium sp.	Lung	No details	—	—	Williamson *et al*	1963
Indet.	Head	Projecting nodule in frontal region	Necrotic foci surrounded by eosinophils and granulation tissue	Hyphae present	Plusiński	1966
Alligator sp.						
Aspergillus fumigatus	Lung Spleen Liver Myocardium Intestine	Miliary pneumonia Nodules Septic degeneration Ulcerated nodules	Nodules with central necrosis and peripheral giant cells	Hyphae within lesions	Pallaske	1957
Caiman crocodilus						
Paecilomyces lilacinus	Lung	Miliary nodular pneumonia with plaques and hollow casts in airways to 10 × 5 mm	Multiple small granulomata with central organised (nucleated) caseous mass surrounded by spindle-shaped giant cells and fibrous capsule (Fig. 7.8)	Hyphae, septate, cephalosporioid cylindrical conidia 5–5·5 μm × 1·5 μm; other hyphae bearing denticles with conidia 2–3 × 1·5–2 μm	Keymer	1976
Caiman sclerops						
Cephalosporium sp.	Lung	Miliary, 1–2 mm diam. grey-white irregular dark-centred nodules	Granulomata surrounded by heterophils and large epithelial cells	(a) Hyphae in lesions tangled, with chlamydospores; (b) hyphae in lumina of vessels with conidiophores bearing elliptical to cigar-shaped conidia 4 × 2 μm	Trevino	1972
	Liver Kidney Muscle	Greyish thick-walled cysts Small white lesions				

217

Table 7.1 (*contd.*)

Host and fungus	Organs affected	Gross lesions	Histopathology	Fungal morphology	Author	Date
Crocodylus niloticus						
Paecilomyces lilacinus *Metarhizium anisopliae* }	Lung	(a) Miliary nodules to 2 mm diam.; (b) plaque-like lesions lining airways, one 80 × 40 mm parchment like, pinkish surface; (c) mycetoma 26 × 16 mm in airway	(a) Granulomata with (i) spindle-shaped giant cells around small caseating foci in mucoid lymphocytic infiltrate (ii) large granulomata with fibrous capsule; (b) plaque seated on relatively unaffected mucosa; (c) firm caseous material, concentrically laminated without nuclei (Fig. 7.6)	(a) Hyphae (i)[a] to 5 ≤m wide diam. contorted, non-sporing (ii)[b] to 2·5 μm straight, cephalosporioid conidia 5–11 × 1–2 μm; (b) hyphae[b] narrow to 1·5 μm abundant penicillate conidiophores and conidia 1·5–2·5 μm diam.; (c) hyphae[b] narrow and conidia on surface, hyphae within caseated mass poorly differentiated	Keymer Goodwin	1974 1974
	Liver	(d) Nodular lesions to 4 mm diam.		(d) Hyphae[a] to 4·5 μm diam. very contorted, non-sporing		
Mucor circinelloides	Stomach	Greenish raised ulcers to 20 mm diam. (Fig. 7.7)	Mucosa mainly necrotic with round cell infiltration	Hyphae to 28 μm diam. thin-walled, sparsely septate, eosinophilic with numerous chlamydospores 9–15 × 7–10 μm	Jones Goodwin	1978 1978
Osteolaemus tetraspis						
Paecilomyces lilacinus *Beauveria bassiana* *Fusarium* sp. }	Lung	(a) Miliary, nodular, 3–4 mm diam. pneumonia; (b) plaque and cavitating lesions	(a) Granulomata with organized centres and staining nuclei; (b) plaques with organised stratification and round cell infiltration	(a) Hyphae 1·5–2 μm diam. septate non-sporing; (b) hyphae to 5 μm diam. septate, extensive, penetrating musculature	Keymer Goodwin	1974 1974
	Kidney	(c) Single large lesion	(c) Complex, old granuloma with necrotic centre	(c) No hyphae seen or fungi isolated		

[a] probably of *Metarhizium anisopliae*
[b] probably of *Paecilomyces lilacinus*

Table 7.2. Mycosis of the skin, orifices and limbs

Host and fungus	Organs affected	Gross lesions	Histopathology	Fungal morphology	Author	Date
Order CHELONIA (TESTUDINES)						
Caretta caretta						
Fusarium solani	Skin, eyes, shell, gastro-intestine	Ulcerative lesions	—	—	Rebell *et al*	1971
Chelonia mydas						
Indet.	Flipper	Generalised *Mycobacterium* sp. infection	Large, deep caseating granulomata with acid-fast bacilli	Hyphae 3 μm to 11 μm, swollen, septate, constricted basophilic	Keymer	1976 1978a
	Buccal cavity	—	—	No hyphae seen		
Chelus fimbriata						
Indet.	Plastron	Mould	Secondary mycetomata	Hyphal felt over plastron	Hamerton	1934
Chelodina longicollis						
Indet.	Plastron	Necrosis	—	Hyphae	Hamerton	1939
Chinemys reevesii						
Indet.	Skin, nose, mouth, eyes	Swelling with Harderian gland affected	—	No information	Elkan	1962
	Intestine	Nodules	Granulomata	Hyphae septate and very contorted		
	Liver	Nodules	Granulomata			

Table 7.2 (*contd.*)

Host and fungus	Organs affected	Gross lesions	Histopathology	Fungal morphology	Author	Date
Pseudemys elegans						
Saprolegnia sp.	Hind-limb skin	Scaling	Little cellular infiltration	Hyphae very wide, non-septate, basophilic, extensive in stratum corneum and lucidum	Keymer	1968a
Indet.	Skin	Ulcers and oedema	Small mycetomata	Hyphae	Hamerton	1932
Sternotherus carinatus						
Mucor sp.	Ventral plastron	—	Not seen	Hyphae	Elkan	1962
Sternotherus odoratus						
Aspergillus sp.	Central digits, metacarpals forefeet	Oedema	Granulomata with infiltration and fibrosis, giant cells, eosinophils	Yeast-like cells in tissue with pseudohyphae	Frye and Dutra	1974
Testudo elephantopus						
Geotrichum candidum	Skin	Ulcers 3 cm diam. on hind legs, neck and head	No tissue reaction	Hyphae and spores in epidermis and dermis	Ruiz *et al*	1980
	Kidney	No lesions seen	Foci of mild inflammation and necrosis	Hyphae present		
Testudo gigantea						
Trichosporon sp.	Mouth	Lesion of commissure	Spinocellular carcinoma macrophages in corium granulosum	Arthrosporic hyphae	Blažek *et al*	1968
Testudo graeca						
Coniothyrium fuckelianum	Shell	Rot on margin	Not seen	Dematiaceous hyphae invading shell	Goodwin	1976

Host and fungus	Organs affected	Gross lesions	Histopathology	Fungal morphology	Author	Date
Testudo radiata						
Candida albicans	Mouth, nose	Ulcers, discharge	Not seen	Not seen	Thoday	1975
Fusarium sp.	Skin scales	—	—	—	Frank	1966
Indet. dematiaceous (Hormodendron ?)	Lower jaw, mouth, lung, spleen, liver, tonsils	Large tumour	Giant cells	Dematiaceous hyphae	Frank	1976
Order SQUAMATA—LACERTILIA (SAURIA)						
Amphibolurus barbatus						
Mucor sp.	Skin	Multiple hyperkeratosis	—	Hyphae in nodules	Frank	1966
Basiliscus americanus						
Indet.	Eye	Tumour of orbit and displacement of eye	Erosion of bony borders of orbit with secondary infection	Fungus seen	Hamerton	1937
Chameleo dilepis						
Fusarium oxysporum	Skin	Chronic lesions	—	—	Poelma	1971
Chameleo melleri						
Indet. yeast	Skin	Lesions on flanks	Secondary pneumonia	Yeast isolated	Hill	1954

Table 7.2 (*contd.*)

Host and fungus	Organs affected	Gross lesions	Histopathology	Fungal morphology	Author	Date
Lacerta viridis						
Fusarium urticearum	Skin	Tumours	Possibly an invaded skin tumour	Hyphae 3 µm diam. and macroconidia in lesion (to 25 × 2·5–4 µm) *Alternaria* spores present	Blanchard	1890
Indet.						
Indet. dematiaceous	Skin	Superficial subcutaneous lesion on right foreleg	Invasion of stratum corneum, corium and subcutaneous muscle	Hyphae dematiaceous at one end of lesion and at other, hyaline, yeast-like, narrow to wide	Rowlatt	1968
Order SQUAMATA—SERPENTES (OPHIDIA)						
Boa constrictor						
Fusarium oxysporum	Eye	Lachrymal sac fluid	—	—	Vroege	1972
Indet. dematiaceous	Skin		—	—	Frank	1970 1976
Crotalus adamanteus						
Indet.	Skin	Dermatitis	—	—	Keymer	1976
Elaphe climacophora						
Aspergillus sp.	Skin	Dermatitis	Inflammatory cell infiltrate	Fungus seen	Mishima *et al*	1975
Elaphe guttata guttata						
Chrysosporium sp.	Subcutaneous	Nodules to 20 mm diam.	Numerous granulomatous foci with giant cells, epithelioid cells and fibrous capsule surrounding central caseation; later stages with marked eosinophilic infiltration and necrosis	Hyphae branching, septate, mainly moniliform 2–8 µm with dense contents	Keymer Elkan	1976 1974

Host and fungus	Organs affected	Gross lesions	Histopathology	Fungal morphology	Author	Date
Prototheca sp.	Skin	Extensive lesion on ventral surface of neck	Encapsulated granulomata, haemorrhages; plasma cells and eosinophils present	Large algal cells in tetrads	Crispens *et al*	1975
Epicrates angulifer						
Indet.	Subcutaneous tissue	Inflammation	Mycetomata	—	Hamerton	1935
Epicrates cenchria maurus						
Fusarium oxysporum	Eye	Bilaterally blind, left eye opaque with white friable mass beneath horny layer	Plug of inflammatory cells with pseudo-eosinophils in horny layer	Hyphae in cheesy mass in horny layer, branching extensively	Zwart *et al*	1973
Eunectes murinus						
Cladosporium sp.	Mouth	Ulcerative stomatitis	Hyperaemic caseous necrosis of mandible with osteomyelitis	Fungus seen	Marcus	1971
Morelia spilotes variegata						
Geotrichum candidum	Skin	Necrosis of wound	—	Fungus seen	McKenzie and Green *et al*	1976
Natrix sipedon						
Geotrichum candidum	Skin	Subcutaneous nodules	(Experimentally inoculated with eastern encephalitis virus)	Fungus isolated	Karstad	1961

Table 7.2 (contd.)

Host and fungus	Organs affected	Gross lesions	Histopathology	Fungal morphology	Author	Date
Python reticulatus						
Indet.	Skin	Subcutaneous mycetomata nodules	Mycetomata	—	Hamerton	1939
Indet. dematiaceous	Skin	Ulcerative lesions on ventral side 2·5–4 mm thick	—	—	Frank	1970 1976
Sistrurus catenatus						
Indet. phycomycete	Skin	Swelling of head	Subcutaneous mass in roof of orbit	Phycomycete hyphae seen	Williams et al	1979
Thamnophis sirtalis						
Aspergillus fumigatus	Skin	Cutaneous ulcers	—	—	Borst et al	1972
Rhizopus arrhizus	Skin	Lesions	—	Hyphae seen in lung	Zwart	1968
Tropidonotus natrix						
Cephalosporium sp.	Trachea	Tumour 35 mm diam. haemorrhagic with yellow foci	Necrosis and leucocytic infiltration	Hyphae seen	Rodhain and Mattlet	1950
Order CROCODILIA						
Crocodylus acutus						
Indet. (Aspergillus, Rhizopus, Mucor)	Skin	Plaques under scales	Necrotic and hyperplastic foci	Erysipelothrix insidiosa infection with hyphae also present	Jasmin et al	1967
Crocodylus sp.						
Indet.	Skin	Vent-slime	—	—	Pooley	1971

Table 7.3. Actinomycosis

Host and actinomycete	Organs affected	Gross lesions	Histopathology	Morphology	Author	Date
Order SQUAMATA—LACERTILIA (SAURIA)						
Amphibolurus barbatus						
Dermatophilus congolensis	Skin	Chronic subcutaneous abscesses on trunk and limbs	—	*Dermatophilus* filaments	Simmons *et al*	1972
Dermatophilus congolensis	Skin	Multiple raised brown lesions on legs, trunk 3–5 mm diam. confluent		Epithelial hyperplasia and hyperkeratosis *Dermatophilus* filaments	Montali *et al*	1975
Calotes mystaceus						
Dermatophilus congolensis	Skin	Hyperkeratinised nodules dorsal and ventral 1–6 mm diam.	Acanthotic epithelium and hyperkeratosis	*Dermatophilus*	Anver *et al*	1976
Indet						
Actinomyces lacertae	—	—	—	—	Terni	1896
Order SQUAMATA—SERPENTES (OPHIDIA)						
Elaphe guttata guttata						
Indet.	Skin	Nodules	Nodules on stratified squamous epithelium with concentric layers of debris	Gram +ve filaments in debris	Beneke *et al*	1966
Elaphe obsoleta quadrivittata						
Indet.	Skin	Nodules	As above	As above	Beneke *et al*	1966

Table 7.3 (*contd.*)

Host and actinomycete	Organs affected	Gross lesions	Histopathology	Morphology	Author	Date
Python sebae						
"*Streptothrix*"	Skin	Subcutaneous suppurating nodules	Granulomata 10–20 mm diam.	Filaments seen	Hamerton	1939
Python spilotes						
"*Streptothrix*"	Skin, pericardium	Subcutaneous nodules	Soft, encapsulated mycetomata in concentric rings	Filaments in tissue	Hamerton	1934
Indet.						
Actinomyces bovis	?		—	—	Meyn	1942

Table 7.4. Fungi and actinomycetes associated with reptilian mycoses

	Viscera	Skin		Viscera	Skin
Deuteromycotina			Zygomycotina		
Aspergillus amstelodami	1	—	*Mucor circinelloides*	1	—
Aspergillus fumigatus	2	1	*Mucor* spp.	—	3
Aspergillus niger	1	—	*Rhizopus arrhizus*	—	1
Aspergillus spp.	8	2	*Rhizopus* sp.	—	1
Beauveria bassiana	4	—	Indeterminate	—	1
Candida albicans	3	1		1	6
Cephalosporium sp.	1	—			
Chrysosporium keratinophilum	2	—	Mastigomycotina		
Chrysosporium sp.	—	1	*Saprolegnia* sp.	—	1
Cladosporium sp.	1	1			
Coniothyrium fuckelianum	—	1	Indeterminate		
Fusarium oxysporum	—	3	Dematiaceous	2	3
Fusarium solani	1	2	Yeasts	—	4
Fusarium urticearum	—	1	Others	10	10
Fusarium spp.	2	1		12	17
Geotrichum candidum	1	3			
Metarhizium anisopliae	2	—	Actinomycetes		
Paecilomyces farinosus	1	—	*Actinomyces bovis*	1	—
Paecilomyces fumoso-roseus	1	—	*Actinomyces lacertae*	—	1
Paecilomyces lilacinus	9	—	*Dermatophilus congolensis*	—	3
Paecilomyces viridis	1	—	Indeterminate	—	4
Penicillium spp.	3	1		1	8
"*Sporotrichum* sp."	1	—			
Trichosporon sp.	1	2	Algae		
	46	19	*Prototheca* sp.	—	1
			Total fungi	59	43
			Total actinomycetes	1	8
				60	51

It is to be hoped that more interest will be shown in the use of reptiles in the development of animal models for the study of chronic fungal infection in man, for the various types of mycetomata seen in reptiles closely mimic those found in such diseases as pulmonary aspergilloma and maduromycosis. Amenable experimental systems are urgently needed for the study of these chronic infections and reptiles could play an important role.

Acknowledgements

The authors would like to thank Dr L. G. Goodwin C.M.G., F.R.S., Director of Science, Zoological Society of London for his kind help and encouragement throughout this work. Acknowledgement is also made to Dr E. Elkan, Mr D. M. Jones, Mr D. Ball and many others who supplied material for examination: to Dr A. H. S. Onions and Mrs M. Tulloch for fungal identifications: to Mr D. Taylor for photography: to Miss Veronica Worth and Mrs Lynne Rolph for technical assistance: to Mrs Sue Bevis for bibliographical help and to Mrs M. Holloman for typing the manuscript.

Grateful acknowledgement is made to the Nuffield Foundation and the Leverhulme Trust for the awards of Senior Research Fellowships to P.K.C.A. for the periods 1970–74 and 1975–76 respectively.

References

Andersen, S. and Eriksen, E. (1968). *In* "Erkrankungen der Zootiere". Verh. Ber. X Int. Symp. Erk. der Zootiere, Salzburg, pp 65–67. Akademie Verlag, Berlin.
Anver, M. R., Park, J. S. and Rush, H. W. (1976). *Lab. Anim. Sci.* **26,** 5, 817–823.
Balfour-Browne, F. L. (1960). *Proc. R. ent. Soc. Lond.* A. **35,** 65–74.
Bell, J. V. (1974). *In* "Insect Diseases". (G. E. Cantwell, ed.), p 300. Marcel Dekker, New York.
Bellairs, A. d'A. (1969). "The Life of Reptiles". Vol. 1, 1–282; Vol. 2, 283–590. Weidenfeld and Nicholson, London.
Bemmel, A. C. V., Peter, J. C. and Zwart, P. (1960). *Tijdschr. Diergeneesk.* **85,** 1203–1213.
Beneke, E. S., Britt, A. L. and Jackson, J. J. (1966). *Mich. St. Univ. Vet.* **26,** 105–106.
Billups, L. H. and Harshbarger, J. C. (1976). *In* "Handbook of Laboratory Animal Science Vol. III". (E. C. Melby and N. H. Altmann, eds.), pp 343–356. C. R. C. Press Inc., Ohio.
Blanchard, R. (1890). *Mém. Soc. zool. Fr.* **3,** 241–255.
Blažek, K., Jaroš, Z., Otčenášek, M. and Konrád, J. (1968). *In* "Erkrankungen der Zootiere". Verh. Ber. X Int. Symp. Erk. der Zootiere, Salzburg, pp 189–192. Akademie Verlag, Berlin.
Borst, G. H. A., Vorge, C., Poelma, F. G., Zwart, P., Strik, W. J. and Peters, J. C. (1972). *Acta. zool. path. antverp.* **56,** 3–19.
Branch, W. R. and Patterson, R. W. (1975). *J. Herpet.* **9**(2), 243–248.
Brown, A. H. S. and Smith, G. (1957). *Trans. Br. mycol. Soc.* **40,** 17–89.
Burtscher, J. (1931). *Zool. Gärten. Leipzig.* (*N.F.*) **4,** 235–243.
Coremans-Pelseneer, J. (1973). *Mycopathol. Mycol. appl.* **49,** 173–176.
Crispens, G. G. Jr. and Marion, K. R. (1975). *Lab. Anim. Sci.* **25,** 788–789.

Elkan, E. (1962). Personal communication with H. Reichenbach-Klinke.
Elkan, E. (1974). Personal communication.
Elkan, E. and Reichenbach-Klinke, H. (1974). "Color Atlas of the Diseases of Fishes, Amphibians and Reptiles." T.F.H. Publications, Reigate, England.
Frank, W. (1966). *Salamandra* **1/2**, 6–12.
Frank, W. (1970). *In* "Erkrankungen der Zootiere". Verh. Ber. XII Int. Symp. Erk. der Zootiere, Budapest, pp 231–235. Akademie Verlag, Berlin.
Frank, W. (1976). *In* "Wildlife Diseases". (L. Page, ed.), pp 73–88. Plenum Press, New York.
Fromtling, R. A., Jensen, J. M., Robinson, B. E. and Bulmer, G. S. (1979a). *Vet. Path.* **16**, 428–431.
Fromtling, R. A., Kosanke, S. D., Jensen, J. M. and Bulmer, G. S. (1979b). *J. Am. vet. med. Ass.* **175**, 934–936.
Frye, F. L. (1973). "Husbandry, Medicine and Surgery in Captive Reptiles." V. M. Publishing Inc., Kansas, U.S.A.
Frye, F. L. and Dutra, F. R. (1974). *VM/SAC*, **69**, 1554–1556.
Georg, L. K., Williamson, W. M., Tilden, E. B. and Getty, R. E. (1962). *Sabouraudia* **2**, 80–86.
Gilman, J. C. and Abbott, E. V. (1927). "A Summary of Soil Fungi." Iowa State College J. Science I, 225–343.
Goodwin, L. G. (1974). *J. Zool. Lond.* **173**, 125–126.
Goodwin, L. G. (1976). *J. Zool. Lond.* **178**, 534.
Goodwin, L. G. (1978). *J. Zool. Lond.* **184**, 379.
Grünberg, W., Kutzer, E. and Otte, E. (1963). *Berl. Münch. Tierärztl. Wschr.* **76**, 90–95.
Hamerton, A. E. (1929–1941). Report on deaths occurring in the Society's Garden for the year

1928	(1929)	*Proc. zool. Soc. Lond.*		49–59
1931	(1932)	ibid.		613–638
1933	(1934)	ibid.		389–422
1934	(1935)	ibid.		443–474
1936	(1937–38)	ibid.	**107A,**	443–474
1938	(1939)	ibid.	**109B,**	281–327
1939–40	(1941–42)	ibid.	**111B,**	151–187

Hill, W. O. (1954). *Proc. zool. Soc. Lond.* **124**, 308.
Hill, W. O. (1956). *Proc. zool. Soc. Lond.* **129**, 438.
Hunt, T. J. (1957). *Herpetologica* **13**, 19–23.
Ippen, R. (1967). *In* "Erkrankungen der Zootiere". Verh. Ber. IX Int. Symp. Erk. der Zootiere, Prague, pp 33–42. Akademie Verlag, Berlin.
Jacobson, E. R., Gaskin, J. M., Shields, R. P. and White, F. H. (1979). *J. Am. vet. med. Ass.* **175**(9), 929–932.
Jasmin, A. F. and Baucom, J. (1967). *Amer. J. Vet. Clin. Path.* **1**, 173–177.
Jasmin, A. M., Carroll, J. M. and Baucom, J. (1968). *Amer. J. Vet. Clin. Path.* **2**, 93–95.
Jones, D. (1978). *J. Zool. Lond.* **184**, 331.

Karstad, L. (1961). Reptiles as possible reservoir hosts for eastern encephalitis virus. Paper presented at the 26th North American Wildlife Conference, Washington, D.C.
Keymer, I. F. (1967). Unpublished data.
Keymer, I. F. (1974). Scientific Report 1971–1973. Zoological Society of London. Report of the Pathologist, 1971 and 1972. *J. Zool. Lond.* **173,** 62, 78.
Keymer, I. F. (1976). *J. Zool. Lond.* **178,** 470–471 and 485.
Keymer, I. F. (1978a). *Vet. Rec.* **103,** 577–582.
Keymer, I. F. (1978b). *Vet. Rec.* **103,** 548–552.
McKenzie, R. A. and & Green, P. E. (1976). *J. Wildl. Dis.* **12,** 405–408.
Madelin, M. F. (1963). *In* "Insect Pathology: an Advanced Treatise." (E. A. Steinhaus, ed.), pp. 233–271. Academic Press, New York and London.
Marcus, L. C. (1971). *J. Am. vet. med. Ass.* **159,** 1626–1631.
Meyn, A. (1942). *Zool. Gärten* NF **14,** 251–253.
Mishima, S., Sawai, Y. and Homma, M. (1975). *Jap. J. Herpetol.* **6,** 9–10.
Montali, R. J., Smith, E. E. and Davenport, M., *et al.* (1975). *J. Am. vet. med. Ass.* **167,** 553–555.
Nickerson, M. A. and Hutchinson, J. A. (1971). *Amer. Midl. Natr.* **86,** 500–502.
Pallaske, G. (1957). *Arch. exp. Vet. Med.* **11,** 30–34.
Patterson, R. W. (1974). *Int. Zoo Yb.* **14,** 81–82.
Pattle, R. E. and Hopkinson, D. A. W. (1963). *Nature,* Lond. **200,** 894.
Plimmer, H. G. (1912). *Proc. zool. Soc. Lond.*, 235–240.
Plusiński, W. (1966). *Medycyna wet.* **22**(7), 398–399.
Poelma, F. G. (1971). Personal communication with Zwart *et al.* (1973).
Pooley, A. C. (1971). *In* "Crocodiles". Vol. 1, pp 104–130. IUCN Publ. New Series Suppl. Paper No. 32. IUCN, Morges, Switzerland.
Pore, R. S., Goodman, N. L. and Larsh, H. W. (1970). *Amer. Rev. resp. Dis.* **101,** 627–628.
Rebell, G., Roth, F. J., Taplin, D. and Wodinsky, J. (1971). *Bacterial Proc.* **71,** 121 (abstract).
Reichenbach-Klincke, H. (1977). "Krankheiten der Reptilien." 2nd edition. G. Fischer Verlag, Stuttgart and New York.
Rodhain, J. and Mattlet, G. (1950). *Ann. Parasitol.* **27,** 77–79.
Rowlatt, U. (1968). Personal communication.
Ruiz, J. M., Arteaga, E., Martinez, J., Rubio, E. M. and Torres, J. M. (1980). *Sabouraudia* **18,** 51–59.
Segretain, G., Fromentin, Huguette, Destombes, P., Brygoo, E.-R. and Dobin, A. (1964) *C. R. Acad. Sci. Paris.* **259**(1), 258–261.
Shalev, M., Murphy, J. C. and Fox, J. G. (1977). *J. Am. vet. med. Ass.* **171,** 872–875.
Simmons, G. C., Sullivan, N. D. and Gree, P. E. (1972). *Aust. vet. J.* **48,** 565–566
Sinclair, J. B. (1969). *Mycologia* **61,** 473–480.
Smith, G. M. and Coates, C. W. (1938). *Zoologica, New York.* **23,** 93–95.

Terni. (1896). *Ufficiale Sanitario*, 160.
Thoday, K. (1975). Personal communication.
Thom. C. (1910). *Bur. Anim. Ind. Bulletin* **118,** 109. (Washington D.C.).
Trevino, G. S. (1972). *J. Wildl. Dis.* **8,** 384–388.
Vroege, C. (1972). Personal communication with Zwart *et al.* (1973).
Wallach, J. D. (1969). *J. Am. vet. med. Ass.* **155,** 1017–1034.
Wenyon, C. M. (1921). *Parasitology* **12,** 350–365.
Williams, L. W., Jacobon, E., Gelatt, K. N., Barrie, K. P. and Shields, R. P. (1979). *VM/SAC* **74,** 1181–1184.
Williamson, W. M., Tilden, E. B. and Getty, R. E. (1963). *Bijdr. Dierk.* **33,** 83–85.
Zwart, P. (1968). *In* "Erkrankungen der Zootiere". Verh. Ber. X Int. Symp. Erk. der Zootiere, Salzburg, pp 45–48. Akademie Verlag, Berlin.
Zwart. P., Poelma, F. G., Strik, W. J., Peters, J. C. and Polder, J. J. W. (1968). *Tijdschr. Diergeneesk.* **93,** 348–365.
Zwart, P., Verver, M. A. J., de Vries, G. A., Hermanides-Nijhof, E. J. and de Vries, H. J. (1973). *J. small Anim. Pract.* **14,** 773–779.

8 Protozoa

I. F. KEYMER

Zoological Society of London, Regent's Park, London, England

Present address: MAFF, Veterinary Investigation Centre, Norwich, Norfolk, England

Owing to the considerable number of species of both reptiles and protozoa which exist and the lack of knowledge concerning reptilian protozoa, it is impossible to deal with these organisms in any depth. Undoubtedly many protozoa await description. Also it is obvious from a study of the earlier literature that some species have been incorrectly identified. Many protozoologists have recognized this fact and attempted to redescribe some species. New names have been created and often changed later by a new generation of protozoologists. This taxonomic activity has unfortunately often led to even more confusion. This is especially so, when not infrequently there is also some doubt about the identity of the host species. Recently, eminent protozoologists such as Drs B. M. Honigberg, N. D. Levine and J. R. Baker have made valiant attempts to reclassify and temporarily stabilize the nomenclature of the Phylum Protozoa. As pointed out by Baker (1973) this is really an impossible task, because classifying any group of living organisms is "trying to impose arbitrary divisions on what is in fact a continuum".

In this chapter the classification is presented in its simplest form and is based mainly upon that of Baker (1973, 1977), but for further information on this complex subject Honigberg *et al* (1964) and Levine (1973) should also be consulted. The Phylum Protozoa is divided by Baker (1973) into four subphyla, each of which is divided into superclasses, classes, subclasses, orders, suborders, genera and species. A few genera are divided in subgenera and a few species into subspecies. From the point of view of pathogenicity, however, it is the identification of protozoa at generic and specific levels that is most important. The other divisions are only given in this chapter in order to clarify the taxonomic position of the organism and to aid the reader in identifying protozoa. Detailed descriptions of morphology and life histories however, are not provided here, being dealt with only sufficiently for a practising veterinarian to diagnose the type of parasite present and enable him to adopt appropriate measures of prevention, control and treatment. For more information on these aspects, text books on protozoology such as those by Wenyon (1926), Kudo (1966), Baker (1973), Levine (1973) and Kreier (1977a, b, c, 1978) should be consulted.

It is probably true to say that in their natural state, all reptiles harbour protozoa of some kind, but there is little evidence that the parasites are pathogenic, except under certain circumstances, in captivity. Indeed even in well-managed collections of reptiles, a relatively high parasite burden may be supported and a normal host–parasite relationship maintained. Factors which may precipitate outbreaks of protozoan diseases in captivity include nutritional disorders and marked alterations in environmental conditions such as excessive fluctuation of temperature, or changes of food. When first acquired from the wild, some species of reptiles may refuse to eat for weeks or even months and this may predispose to parasitic disease. The density of a reptilian population either in captivity or even in the wild obviously influences the spread of protozoan infections. This is particularly facilitated when large numbers of aquatic or semi-aquatic species are involved. Especially under these circumstances a build-up of parasite numbers can occur and lead to an outbreak of disease.

The most important and common protozoa of reptiles dealt with here are represented by all four subphyla, in the Phylum Protozoa. All the genera including protozoan species of veterinary and medical importance occur in reptiles and more besides, so that these animals are a rich source of material for protozoologists. Nevertheless, the study of protozoa of reptiles has been much neglected, mainly because they are of no obvious economic importance and so far as is known reptilian infections include no zoonoses, with the possible exception of *Leishmania* spp. in lizards.

All genera occurring in reptiles are listed and an indication of their host range is given. Owing to problems of nomenclature and the difficulty of analysing the widely scattered publications dealing with protozoa in reptiles, it is, however, impossible to give complete host lists. The classification of reptilian hosts in these lists is based on that given by Matthews *et al* (1970) and outlined in Chapter 2. The class Reptilia is divided into four main orders, namely: (1) Chelonia or Testudines (tortoises, turtles and terrapins); (2) Rhynchocephalia (the tuatara); (3) Squamata (suborder Lacertilia (Sauria), lizards, geckos, chameleons, skinks, slow-worms, etc.), Squamata (suborder

Serpentes (Ophidia), snakes); and (4) Crocodilia (crocodiles, alligators, caimans and gharials). To save space only those orders (and suborders) are given in the lists of hosts when they contain reptile species which have been naturally infected with the protozoan parasite under discussion. Usually only the genera of the parasites and of the hosts are listed. These host lists are based on an analysis of all the references quoted at the end of this chapter and also on unpublished findings by Keymer recorded at the Zoological Society of London. The exact reference for each host record is not given as this would make the lists too cumbersome and difficult to read. Some of the more important references, however, such as those referring to potentially pathogenic or rare organisms, are given. For blood parasites further susceptible species of reptiles are listed in the host list provided by Wenyon (1926), but these include many old records. Care is therefore needed in their interpretation because the names of many parasites and indeed some of the hosts, have now been changed.

I. Subphylum Sarcomastigophora

Locomotion by flagella, pseudopodia or both.

Superclass 1. Mastigophora.

"Flagellates", with locomotion mainly or entirely by flagella. Division symmetrogenic.

Class Zoomastigophorea.

Organisms without chlorophyll.

A. Order Kinetoplastida

Organisms possessing a kinetoplast. All are parasitic.

Genera in reptiles Trypanosoma, Leishmania, Bodo *and* Proteromonas. Potentially the most important are *Trypanosoma* and *Leishmania* spp. *Bodo* spp. are normally free-living and most records in reptiles therefor probably refer to contaminants. There is very little information about *Proteromonas* spp. Records of *Leptomonas* and *Herpetomonas* spp. in reptiles are suspect, because these are exclusively parasites of invertebrates, mainly insects. All species in this Order are seldom if ever likely to be pathogenic to reptiles, although *Trypanosoma* and *Leishmania* are serious pathogens of man and some other mammalian species. However, Wood (1935) observed changes in the blood of geckos (*Tarentola mauritanica*) infected with *T. platydactyli*. He recorded a 20 per cent decrease in eosinophils, 17 per cent increase in basophils, 17 per cent increase in neutrophils and 4 per cent decrease in lymphocytes.

Life-cycles Species of *Trypanosoma* and *Leishmania* require blood-sucking, invertebrate intermediate hosts (see Chapter 10). These are usually insects such as sand flies (*Lutzomyia* and *Sergentomyia* spp.), the latter genus being important for *Leishmania* spp. (Killick-Kendrick, 1979). For trypanosomes of aquatic vertebrates the intermediate hosts include leeches (e.g. *Paecilobdella* and *Placobdella* spp.). Molyneux (1977) gave a host list of all reptilian trypanosomes in which the vectors are known.

(a) *Hosts for* Trypanosoma *spp.*

Many of these blood parasites have been found in reptiles and the majority of those that have been recorded have been given names. They are more common in free-living than in captive reptiles. Numerous *Trypanosoma* spp. were listed by Reichenbach-Klinke and Elkan (1965), Reichenbach-Klinke (1977) and also by Mackerras (1961), Lainson (1977) and Walliker (1965) who gave a list of known reptilian trypanosomes, including old records given by Wenyon (1926).

Order Chelonia

There are records from freshwater chelonians of the genera *Chelodina, Chrysemys, Damonia, Emyda, Emydura, Kinixys, Platemys, Sternothaerus* (= *Pelosios*) and the terrestrial chelonian *Testudo esculenta*.

Order Squamata (Suborder Lacertilia)

Lizards: *Acanthosaura, Agama, Anolis, Gerrhonotus, Plica, Sceloporus, Uranoscodon, Varanus*.

Geckos: *Hemidactylus, Phyllurus, Platydactylus, Psylodactylus, Tarentola, Thecadactylus*.

Chameleons: *Chamaeleo*.

Skinks: *Egernia, Emoia, Lygosoma, Mabuya, Sphenomorphus*.

Order Squamata (Suborder Serpentes)

Snakes: *Bitis, Cyclagras, Demansia, Diemenia, Erythrolamprus, Graya, Helicops, Hypsirhina, Naja, Natrix, Ophis, Philodrias, Psammophis, Python, Thamnophis, Tropidonotus*, and various "South American snakes" (Page, 1966).

Order Crocodilia

Crocodiles: *Crocodylus*.

Caimans: *Caiman*.

(b) *Hosts for* Leishmania *spp.*

Leishmania in reptiles are of particular interest to medical protozoologists because of the possible role of reptiles as reservoirs of human infection in some parts of the world. However, although man has been experimentally infected with *L. adleri* of lizards (Manson-Bahr and Heisch, 1961) there is no evidence of naturally occurring reptilian leishmaniasis in man. The infection in reptiles can normally be diagnosed only by cultural methods using NNN media. Although the organisms can be isolated from various organs and the blood, they can seldom be observed in blood smears. Five important publications dealing with *Leishmania* in reptiles are those by Adler (1964), Belova (1971), Garnham (1971), Mohiuddin (1959) and Wilson and Southgate (1979) and it is from these that the host list below has been compiled.

Order Squamata (Suborder Lacertilia)

Lizards: *Agama, Alsophylax, Anolis, Cnemidophorus, Eremias, Lacerta, Latastia, Phrynocephalus.*

Geckos: *Ceramodactylus, Gymnodactylus, Hemidactylus, Tarentola, Teratoscincus.*

Chameleons: *Chamaeleo.*

Order Squamata (Suborder Serpentes)

"Snakes" are reported to be hosts in the USSR (Garnham, 1971).

(c) *Hosts for* Bodo (= Prowazekella) *spp.*

Most records of these protozoa in reptiles are by Fantham and Porter (1950) and can probably be discounted as either free-living contaminants or parasites of doubtful significance. In the latter category should be included the report of these organisms in the faeces and cloaca of lizards (*Mabuya* and *Lacerta* spp.) by Mohiuddin (1959).

(d) *Hosts for* Proteromonas *spp.*

Kudo (1966) stated that these organisms occur in the intestines of lizards of the genera *Lacerta, Tarentola* and others. According to Reichenbach-Klinke and Elkan (1965) and Reichenbach-Klinke (1977) the parasites are common, but nevertheless there is very little information available concerning the organisms in reptiles.

B. Order Retortamonadida

Organisms with two to four flagella and a cytosome bordered by a fibril. All are parasitic.

Genera in Reptiles (*Retortamonas* and *Chilomastix*.) No evidence of pathogenicity.

Life-cycles Very little is known about these organisms that inhabit the gut, but the life-cycles are probably direct.

(a) *Hosts for* Retortamonas *spp*.

There appears to be only one record of this unimportant genus, species of which occur in the intestine.
Order Chelonia
   Terrestrial tortoises, *Testudo elegans* (Janakidevi 1961, quoted by Reichenbach-Klinke and Elkan, 1965).

(b) *Hosts for* Chilomastix *spp*.

These are also very rare and unimportant intestinal parasites.
Order Squamata (Suborder Lacertilia)
   Geckos *Hemidactylus*.
Order Squamata (Suborder Serpentes)
   Snakes: *Thamnophis*.

C. Order Diplomonadida

Bilaterally symmetrical protozoa with two similar nuclei and four pairs of flagella. Most species are parasitic.

Genera in reptiles *Hexamita* (= *Octomastix*) is pathogenic to chelonians. *Giardia*, an intestinal parasite, is a potential pathogen, although no evidence of pathogenicity has yet been reported. In reptiles, *Hexamita* occurs in the urinary tract and elsewhere (see page 241).

Life-cycles The life-cycles of both *Hexamita* and *Giardia* species are direct. *Giardia* spp. produce cysts that are passed in the excreta. *Hexamita* spp. such as *H. parva* in reptiles probably form cysts because cysts are produced by species of *Spironucleus* which is a recently created synonym for *Hexamita* spp. in other classes of vertebrates, (Kulda and Nohýnková, 1978).

(a) *Hosts for* Hexamita *spp*.

Order Chelonia
   Most records are from this order, both terrestrial and freshwater

species being affected, namely *Clemmys, Cuora, Emys, Geoemyda, Pseudemys, Terrapene* and *Testudo.*
Order Squamata (Suborder Serpentes)
Snakes: *Causus, Naja, Natrix.*

(i) HEXAMITIASIS (*Hexamita parva* INFECTION) OF CHELONIANS

This disease was recently discovered by Zwart and Truyens (1975) and the following account is based almost entirely on their description and also the publication by Zwart *et al* (1976).

Species and Hosts

Although *Hexamita* spp. have been recorded in relatively few reptiles, Zwart and Truyens (1975) reported *H. parva* to be pathogenic in eight different species, including both terrestrial and freshwater aquatic chelonians, of the genera *Testudo, Geochelone, Cuora, Terrapene, Geoemyda* and *Clemmys.*

It is believed that infections with *H. parva* are fairly widespread but that the organisms are only occasionally pathogenic.

Life History

Although there appears to be very little information on the subject, these flagellated protozoa are probably transmitted directly by the voiding of the parasites in the urine. Fresh urine may contaminate food that is eaten by a new host. The urinary system then probably becomes directly infected due to an ascending infection originating from the intestinal tract, with which the ureters have direct connection via the urodaeum. *Hexamita* spp. probably encyst. No sexual reproduction is known. Multiplication is by longitudinal binary fission.

Clinical Signs

The reptiles may show signs of illness for several weeks or months. They fail to thrive, lose weight and become progressively more apathetic.

Diagnosis

The parasites can be found in the excreta of some infected chelonians on microscopical examination. When the flagellates are alive they move fast and in straight lines in the urine, but are able to change direction quickly. In the solid accumulation of faeces, however, they often rotate around their long axes and appear very flexible. In air-dried, stained preparations the organisms are rather pleomorphic, although predominantly egg-shaped. Six flagella are present, two of which are caudal. Zwart and Truyens (1975) found the mean body length to be 8·03 μm and width 4·79 μm.

Differential Diagnosis

On microscopical examination of the excreta, *Hexamita* spp. can be confused with other flagellates that occur in chelonians, i.e. *Trichomonas* an *Retortomonas* spp. However, *Trichomonas* has only one recurrent flagellum and *Retortomonas* has a total of two to four flagella, whereas *Hexamita parva* has six.

Prevention and Treatment

With captive chelonians, strict attention to hygiene to avoid contamination of food by excreta and prevention of over-crowding should control the disease. Zwart *et al* (1976) recommended oral dosage with dimetridazole (40 mg/kg bodyweight) for a period of seven days, but results are variable. The reptile can either be dosed orally by direct methods or the drug can be dissolved in one litre of water and this used as a bath for a fortnight. Repeated treatments are often necessary.

Post Mortem Findings and Pathology

At necropsy the gross findings are non-specific. The kidneys may be enlarged and usually appear pale due to nephritis. Sometimes the renal tubules are obviously dilated. It is impossible, however, to confirm the diagnosis without histological examination of the kidneys. Lesions may also be found in the liver and intestinal tract. In fresh carcasses live *Hexamita* can be found in the excreta. The histopathological appearances of the affected organs were described in detail by Zwart and Truyens (1975). Lesions in the glomeruli were a constant feature. Sometimes the changes were restricted to proliferation of the visceral layer of Bowman's capsule, while in others this layer showed increased cellularity of the mesangium and thickening of the capillary basement membranes. Degenerative changes also occurred in the proximal segments of the renal tubules. In one case hyaline casts were seen. *Hexamita* organisms may be visible in the lumina of tubular distal segments and in collecting ducts. The lesions ranged from acute to chronic inflammatory reactions. In the more chronic cases interstitial round-cell infiltration and some fibrosis were present.

In some cases the parasites were found in the bile. The larger bile-ducts and cystic duct may be macroscopically thickened and have wide lumina. On microscopical examination the hepatic lesions varied in different animals, but included irregularity of the bile-duct epithelium due to proliferation of epithelial cells, inflammatory cell infiltration in the ductal lumina and degenerative or necrotic changes in the epithelial lining of the bile-ducts. *Hexamita* organisms were found in these damaged areas and a periductal fibrosis and proliferation of arteries were also observed. In one *Testudo* (now *Geochelone*) *carbonaria* the duodenum showed focal areas of epithelial destruction associated with the parasites. Colitis was found in four reptiles, this being severe with almost complete loss of the epithelium in *T. carbonaria*.

No specific lesions were found in the heart, lung, spleen, pancreas, adrenals or thyroid.

(b) *Hosts for* Giardia *spp.*

These are rare and unimportant parasites of reptiles, that appear only to have been recorded by Fantham and Porter (1952).
Order Squamata (Suborder Serpentes)
   Snakes: *Causus, Lampropeltis.*

D. Order Trichomonadida

Flagellates with typically four to six flagella, one of which trails and is associated with an undulating membrane. A parabasal body is present. Cysts are typically absent and do not occur in *Trichomonas* spp. infecting reptiles. Probably all genera are parasitic.

Genera in reptiles (*Trichomonas*) Many species are potential pathogens, although there is little evidence of pathogenicity (but see p 243). Little known genera occurring in reptiles include *Hexamastrix, Monocercomonas, Monocercomonoides, Trepomonas* and *Tritrichomonas* spp. They are all parasites of the intestinal tract.

Life-cycles   The life-cycles of *Trichomonas* spp. are direct and cysts are not produced.

(a) *Hosts for* Trichomonas *spp.*

These parasites may not be so common as reports suggest; because veterinarians are familiar with *Trichomonas* spp. in bovine animals and various species of birds, many tend to assume that flagellates found in reptiles must therefore be trichomonads. Numerous other flagellates occur in reptiles and therefore accurate identifications are essential.
Order Chelonia
    Tortoises: *Testudo*, "Galapagos tortoise" (genus not stated—see Fantham and Porter, 1950), *Nicoria* (= *Geoemyda*).
Order Squamata (Suborder Lacertilia)
    Geckos: *Hoplodactylus*.
    Chameleon: Genus unknown.
    Lizards: *Calotes*.
Order Squamata (Suborder Serpentes)
    Snakes: *Ablabes* (= *Liopeltis*), *Agkistrodon*, *Bitis*, *Boa*, *Boaedon*, *Causus*, *Crotaphopeltis*, *Dispholidus*, *Drymarchon*, *Lampropeltis*, *Liopeltis*, *Naja*, *Natrix*, *Pseudaspis*, *Python*, *Thamnophis*, *Vipera*.
Order Crocodilia
    Crocodiles: *Crocodylus*.

(b) *Hosts for* Hexamastrix *spp.*

These parasites were recorded by Reichenbach-Klinke and Elkan (1965) as occurring in the intestine of General Hardwick's lizard (*Uromastix hardwickii*) and the starred tortoise (*Testudo elegans*).

(c) *Hosts for* Monocercomonas (= Eutrichomastix) *spp.*

Records of these organisms in reptiles appear to be almost confined to those of Fantham and Porter (1950) in various genera of snakes. Reichenbach-Klinke and Elkan (1965) and Telford (1971), however, stated that they also occur in the gut of "lizards". Nevertheless, they are not mentioned in reptiles by such an authority as Kudo (1966) and must therefore be regarded as of doubtful validity.

(d) *Hosts for* Monocercomonoides *spp.*

Kudo (1966) made no mention of these parasites in reptiles but Levine (1973) listed them as occurring. The only specific records appear to be those of *M. filamentum* quoted by Murphy (1973) in an Indian starred tortoise (*Testudo elegans*) and *M. lacertae* in the rectum, of the lizard (*Eremias arguta*) by Reichenbach-Klinke and Elkan (1965).

(e) *Hosts for* Trepomonas *spp.*

These organisms occur in chelonians according to Das Gupta (1935), Levine (1973) and Murphy (1973) but they are not listed as parasites of reptiles by Kudo (1966) or Reichenbach-Klinke and Elkan (1965).

(f) *Hosts for* Tritrichomonas *spp.*

Kudo (1966) recorded these organisms in the colon of "lizards" and Murphy (1973) stated that they occur in terrapins (*Lissemys* sp.). Reichenbach-Klinke and Elkan (1965) stated that the parasites inhabit the cloaca of "several lizards".

(i) ENTERITIS OF TERRESTRIAL CHELONIANS AND SNAKES ASSOCIATED WITH FLAGELLATES

Although proof is lacking, a number of workers suspect that flagellates, including *Trichomonas* spp., cause enteritis when present in large numbers or when in association with other parasites or pathogenic bacteria. For example Keymer (1970) stated that it "seemed possible" that these organisms could be pathogenic to snakes. Borst *et al* (1972) found fibrinous, necrotizing enteritis with *Trichomonas* and "*Ascaridea*" spp. of helminths in a Jaboty tortoise (*Testudo denticulata*). Jackson (1976) regarded intestinal flagellates as potential pathogens stating that in snakes they can cause "wet cloacal voidings" and that affected individuals drink excessively. In chelonians he stated that they may cause inappetance, the excreta being "full of flagellate organisms". It is obvious from these brief reports that the role of various species of intestinal flagellates in reptiles needs proper investigation.

For the treatment of intestinal flagellates in reptiles Zwart (1977) recommended dimetridazole at the oral dosage rate of 40 mg/kg bodyweight, for a period of five days. Wallach (1969) provided no evidence of pathogenicity of "trichomonads" and "*Monocercomonas* spp." as common intestinal parasites of lizards and snakes but recommended treatment with sodium sulphadimidine (1 oz/gal of the drinking water for a period of 10 days.) However, perhaps the most promising drug is metronidazole, as recommended by Jackson (1976) who suggested a single administration orally by stomach tube at a dosage rate of 160 mg/kg bodyweight. With large reptiles, however, the dose should not exceed 400 mg.

Superclass 2. Opalinata.
The taxonomy of this group is very confused.

Order Opalinida

Organisms with numerous cilia or short flagella and two to many similar nuclei. All species are parasitic and mainly confined to amphibians, in which they inhabit the large intestine.

Genus in reptiles One genus, *Opalina*, is a rare intestinal protozoon of reptiles. There is no evidence of pathogenicity.

Life-cycle This is probably direct. Cysts are formed and passed in faeces.

(a) *Hosts for* Opalina *spp*.

Order Squamata (Suborder Lacertilia)
According to Reichenbach-Klinke and Elkan (1965) the organisms are occasionally encountered in "saurians".
   Lizard: *Varanus*.

Superclass 3. Sarcodina.
Amoebae with locomotion mainly or entirely by pseudopodia.

Class Rhizopodea.
Subclass Lobosia.

Order Amoebida

"Naked" organisms without a so-called "shell". Many are parasitic, including important pathogens.

Genera in reptiles *Acanthamoeba* (potential pathogen), *Endolimax* (non-pathogenic), *Entamoeba* (one of the most serious of all pathogens, especially to snakes), *Hartmanella* (potential pathogen) and *Naegleria* (non-pathogenic). All these parasites occur in the gut.

According to Frank *et al* (1976a), quoting Bosch and Deichsel (1972), there are several pathogenic amoebae present in reptiles that have only been considered as "types or strains" and which possibly represent true species. They also quoted Frank *et al* (1976a) who showed that immune sera induced in rabbits against the recognized pathogen *Entamoeba invadens* did not react against all pathogenic entamoebae in reptiles. Further investigations are clearly necessary.

Life-cycle The life-cycle of all genera is probably direct and all species infecting reptiles probably produce cysts. The life history of *E. invadens* is described on pages 246–7. The cysts may be carried mechanically by insects such as flies and cockroaches which feed on reptilian excreta, but there is no evidence that arthropods act as true intermediate hosts.

(a) *Hosts for* Entamoeba *spp*.

Herbivorous species of reptiles probably act as healthy carriers for highly susceptible carnivorous species such as snakes.
Order Chelonia
   Tortoises: *Geochelone, Testudo*.
   Freshwater chelonians: *Amboina, Chelodina, Chelydra, Chrysemys, Cuora, Emydura, Emys, Nicoria, Podocnemis, Pseudemys, Trionyx*.
   Marine turtles, accidental infections in captivity only in *Caretta* and *Chelonia*.
Order Rhynchocephalia
   Tuatara (*Sphenodon punctatus*)
Order Squamata (Suborder Lacertilia)
   Lizards: *Agama, Conolophus, Dracaena, Hydrosaurus, Iguana, Lacerta, Physignatus, Tropidurus, Varanus*.
   Skinks: *Chalcides, Eumeces, Tiliqua*.
   Geckos: *Hemidactylus*.
   Slow-worm: *Anguis*.
Order Crocodilia
   Crocodiles: *Crocodylus*.
Order Squamata (Suborder Serpentes)
There is little point in compiling a list of genera containing susceptible

species of snakes, because all carnivorous species of reptiles are unnatural hosts, as described later, and highly susceptible to the pathogen *Entamoeba invadens*.

(i) AMOEBIASIS (*Entamoeba invadens* INFECTION) OF SNAKES

Disease in snakes due to an *Entamoeba* sp. was first recorded by Ratcliffe and Geiman (1934) and there are a considerable number of further reports of the infection, a particularly good description of the disease being that by Steck (1962). The organism has been studied in great detail, especially by medical protozoologists, because of its close relationship to the human pathogen *Entamoeba histolytica*.

Species and Hosts

The organism was originally named *E. invadens* by Rodhain (1934). Judging by the very wide host range of *Entamoeba invadens* it is likely that all species of snakes are susceptible to the infection in captivity. Meerovitch (1958) drew attention to the fact that pathogenic amoebiasis is mainly a disease of carnivorous species, to which the amoebae are ill adapted. He found that encystation (see later) occurs only at 15°C or above and that suitable conditions for commensalism only seem to exist in herbivorous or partially herbivorous chelonians, perhaps due to the presence of a polysaccharide of plant origin that allows the amoebae to accumulate glycogen and encyst without invading the tissues.

Distribution and Incidence

Without doubt *E. invadens* infection is the most serious protozoan disease of snakes, indeed it is probably the most significant of all reptilian infectious diseases. The infection appears to be cosmopolitan and is common in captivity although little is known of the incidence of the parasite in nature.

Life History

The organism has a direct life-cycle. The trophozoites, which are the typical amoebic form of the parasite, normally encyst only in the lumen of the gut, although they often invade the blood and reach the liver via the portal circulation. It is the cyst, however, which is the transmissive stage. The cyst does not develop further in the original host but is passed out in the faeces. Cysts can survive for several days outside the body. McConnachie (1975) found that cysts could survive for at least 14 days at 8°C but for less than 7 days at 37°C. The cysts undergo no development until ingested by another susceptible host. Cysts pass unharmed through the stomach to reach the small intestine where the trophozoites excyst, emerging as quadrinucleate amoebae. Each cyst produces one trophozoite. The nuclei divide, followed by division of the cytoplasm, producing eight small uninucleate amoebae which pass into the colon and mature reaching full size. The trophozoites multiply by binary fission in the colon where encystation occurs and the life-cycle is repeated.

Clinical Signs

Steck (1962) stated that clinical signs are limited to the terminal phase of the disease, when the swollen colon can be palpated in the live snake. The cloacal region may also be swollen and firm on palpation. Food is refused and often the thirst increases. Affected snakes lose weight and become progressively sluggish before dying, sometimes after an illness lasting as long as several weeks. Diarrhoea, often blood-tinged, is a characteristic sign. Fantham and Porter (1952) reported that some snakes become anaemic with haemoglobin indices of 65–70 per cent. It is not known if reptiles ever recover spontaneously or if carriers occur, as in *E. histolytica* infection of man (McConnachie, 1975).

Diagnosis

The disease can only be diagnosed accurately by identification of the parasites in the faeces. Both trophozoites and cysts may be found, although the former can only be recognized in fresh faecal samples. The active amoeboid trophozoites can be seen most easily if fresh excreta are mixed with normal saline and examined microscopically at 37°C. Unlike the trophozoites, the cysts may occur in normal as well as in diarrhoeic faeces. Cysts may be found either by direct microscopical examination (especially in heavy infections) or after concentration. In direct smears the cysts are most readily seen if a drop of faeces is mixed with a 1 per cent aqueous eosin solution. When eosin is used the cysts remain as unstained, white objects against a pink background of eosin solution and red-stained debris. In order to stain the cysts it is necessary to use double-strength Lugol's iodine solution (4 per cent potassium iodide plus 2 per cent iodine in distilled water). When examining the eosin-stained preparation, little detail can be seen in the cysts, except for the chromatoid bodies. In order to help in the identification of the amoebic cysts, it is important at this stage to note the shape of the chromatoid bodies and also the shape and size of the cysts. After this has been done the iodine suspension of faeces should be examined microscopically using the oil-immersion objective in order to study the cysts in more detail. The iodine stains the nuclei of the cysts, when their number and shape should be noted. If vacuoles containing glycogen are present in the cysts these will be conspicuous as they stain a deep golden-brown colour. Further details of the staining and cyst concentration methods, as well as techniques for culturing the organisms *in vitro*, are available in the book by Baker (1973).

It is important, especially when finding cysts in the faeces of healthy snakes, to identify accurately the amoebae because a number of normally non-pathogenic species infect snakes and some other reptiles. These include *Acanthamoeba*, *Hartmanella* and *Naegleria*, although Bosch and Deichsel (1972) and Frank and Bosch (1972) regarded the first two as potential pathogens. In addition to *E. invadens*, Fantham and Porter (1950, 1952) considered *E. serpentis* to be pathogenic. However, Ghosh (1968) after critically examining the type specimen of *E. serpentis* showed that the species "resembles the 'histolytica' type, producing 4-nucleate mature cysts", their measurements falling within the size range occupied by *E. invadens*. As pointed out by Dolensek *et al* (1976) it is generally assumed now that *E. invadens* is the cause of amoebiasis in snakes and other reptiles. Ghosh (1968) tabulated the measurements of both *E. serpentis* and *E. invadens* based on his own specimens and also those of others. For *E. invadens* the body length of the trophozoite in microns, ranges from 9 to 38·6 and the nucleus from 3·5 to 7·3. The cysts vary in diameter from 9 to 24 microns. Not only therefore are *E. serpentis* and *E. invadens* morphologically indistinguishable but they are also morphologically indistinguishable from *E. histolytica* which is the human pathogen (McConnachie, 1975). In fact Geiman and Ratcliffe (1936) were of the opinion that *E. invadens* and *E. histolytica* have identical life-cycles, showing the same details of encystation, excystation and metacystic development. After a more recent detailed study of the two organisms McConnachie (1975) revealed only two significant differences, namely "a difference in the factors controlling their encystation and in their temperature requirements". In other respects they are strikingly similar. Both organisms are adversely affected by free oxygen. Their growth is enhanced by starch and sustained under anaerobic conditions in similar media and in the presence of a mixed bacterial flora or of *Escherichia coli* alone. In their natural environments constant anaerobic conditions occur and the amoebae feed on bacteria and tissue cells.

In addition to the long established methods of diagnosis referred to above and described fully by Baker (1973), *E. invadens* infection can now be diagnosed using the immunofluorescent antibody technique (Frank and Sigmund, 1976). In future it may also be possible to differentiate between *E. invadens* and *E. histolytica* by comparing their electrophoretic isoenzyme patterns, as done for *E. histolytica* and *Entamoeba coli* by Sargeaunt and Williams (1978). However, such tests involve specialized laboratory techniques which are not available to the majority of veterinary clinicians.

Differential Diagnosis

As *Entamoeba invadens* may be the sole truly pathogenic amoeba of snakes (and other reptiles), differential diagnosis is only a problem when trying to trace healthy carriers of *E. invadens*, when as stated above (see Diagnosis) it is essential to distinguish it from other species of amoebae.

Prevention and Treatment

Strict attention to hygiene and avoidance of faecal contamination of food is essential for the prevention of the disease. Cockroaches should also be controlled as they can spread the disease mechanically.

Various treatments have been tried with limited success (see also Chapter 18). Zwart (1977) recommended dimetridazole at the oral dosage rate of 40 mg/kg bodyweight, for a period of 8 days. Gabrisch (1977), however, differentiated between the intestinal and "organ- and liver-invading form". For the intestinal form he recommended dimetridazole at the dosage rate of 20–50 mg/kg bodyweight given *per os* for a period of 10 days by stomach tube. He advocated chloroquine when other viscera are involved, dosing 2–3 times weekly for 3 weeks at the dosage of 1 ml/kg bodyweight. Deakins (1972) suggested a variety of drugs including oxytetracycline in the food at the dosage of 2 mg/g of food. The most promising agent is metronidazole given orally. This is also the drug of choice in human beings for both intestinal and hepatic amoebiasis. Donaldson *et al* (1975) obtained excellent results with several species of snakes using 275 mg/kg in a single dose given by stomach tube. However, Jackson (1976) recommended 160 mg/kg bodyweight given daily for three days.

Post Mortem Findings and Pathology

Good accounts of the pathology of the disease are given by Fantham and Porter (1950), Hill and Neal (1952), Ippen (1959), Steck (1962) and Donaldson *et al* (1975).

As mentioned previously, amoebiasis is mainly a disease of carnivorous species (Meerovitch, 1958). This worker explained this phenomenon by demonstrating that the trophozoites normally derive polysaccharide from food of plant origin. In the intestinal lumen of snakes, however, which are all carnivores, this source of food is not available. The trophozoites therefore resort to feeding on the mucous secretion of the intestinal epithelium which they eventually denude of its protective layer of mucus and thereby gain entry into the deeper tissues. This also assists secondary bacterial invasion and severe lesions result. The primary lesions occur in the colon, but as originally pointed out by Ratcliffe and Geiman (1934) and later by Fantham and Porter (1950, 1952), the posterior part of the small intestine, stomach and liver may later be involved.

The lesions in the colon and lower small intestine are characterized by ulceration and haemorrhages. In the more acute stage the gut epithelium is very congested. In severe and more chronic cases the ulceration leads to granulomatous thickening of the intestinal wall, which may involve the entire colon and lead to occlusion of the lumen. Stomach lesions also consist of congestion of the epithelium, ulceration and haemorrhage, but they are seldom so severe as those affecting the gut. Although the liver is less frequently affected than the intestine, it often becomes swollen and mottled. Multiple, discrete and partly confluent areas of necrosis develop, the size of the lesions varying considerably and depending upon the degree of infection. Sometimes the severe gut lesions cause acute peritonitis, due to perforation of the gut wall through ulceration of the epithelium extending through to the serosal surface.

Page (1966) stated that subcutaneous amoebic cysts have often been seen in newly acquired snakes and he considered that these may have resulted from the bites of "amoeba-infested lice".

Several workers (e.g. Ratcliffe and Geiman, 1934; Ippen, 1959; Steck, 1962 and Donaldson *et al*, 1975) have described the histopathological lesions. Steck (1962) gave a particularly full account with illustrations. Microscopical examination shows that the amoebae produce a circumscribed desquamation of the epithelial lining of the colon and this leads to a necrotic colitis, probably caused by the toxic action of the bacterial flora in the colon (Steck, 1962). Donaldson *et al* (1975) described thickening of the intestinal wall with the formation of multiple, necrotic ulcers extending through the mucosa and submucosa and occasionally deep into the muscularis. Ratcliffe and Geiman (1934) found that leucocytic infiltration was more pronounced in the less advanced lesions.

In the small intestine, the lesions are similar but usually less severe than in the colon.

When the stomach is affected, circumscribed ulcers may occur in all parts of the organ (Ratcliffe and Geiman, 1934) and these are accompanied by an acute inflammatory response. Localized areas of necrosis and ulceration of the mucosa (and occasionally also in the submucosa) occur.

In the liver, Ratcliffe and Geiman (1934) found multiple and usually circumscribed abscesses, these being largest in the cephalic half of the organ. The more advanced areas of degeneration and necrosis occur in the region of the central veins. These lesions vary in size and necrotic areas are often surrounded by areas of fatty degeneration leading to destruction of the parenchymal cells with only the stroma remaining (Donaldson *et al*, 1975).

In association with the above lesions, non-specific lesions are often found in other organs, particularly the kidneys.

(ii) AMOEBIASIS (*Entamoeba* sp. INFECTION) OF TORTOISES AND TERRAPINS

Four species of *Entamoeba* have been recorded from chelonians (Donaldson *et al*, 1975), namely *E. invadens*, *E. testudinis*, *E. barreti* and *E. terrapinae*. All species including *E. invadens* are normally commensals and these reptiles are therefore dangerous sources of *E. invadens* in mixed reptilian collections. However, although *E. invadens* is a natural commensal in chelonians (Barker, 1965; Kramer, 1972; Donaldson *et al*, 1975) there are a few records of the organism being pathogenic to captive chelonians. Gabrisch (1976) diagnosed amoebiasis in 1 per cent of tortoises and Ippen (1971) in 2·9 per cent of 170 chelonians in captivity. As long ago as 1952, Hill and Neal strongly suspected the disease in a Greek tortoise (*Testudo graeca*) that died during an outbreak of amoebiasis in snakes at London Zoo. The lesions resembled those of amoebiasis but they were unable to find the amoebae. Nevertheless there are few convincing records of amoebiasis in chelonians and this is not surprising if the opinion of Meerovitch (1958) concerning the mechanism of commensalism in these reptiles is correct (see earlier).

(iii) AMOEBIASIS (PROBABLE *Entamoeba invadens* INFECTION) OF TURTLES

The only record of the disease in marine chelonians, i.e. true turtles, appears to be that by Frank *et al* (1976a). Two species, namely green turtles (*Chelonia mydas*) and a loggerhead turtle (*Caretta caretta*) became infected. A healthy Amboina box tortoise or terrapin (*Cuora* (= *Cyclemys*) *amboinensis*) which was acting as a carrier, was probably the source of the infection. The young infected green turtles had been kept in fresh water together with terrapins.

At necropsy the green turtles showed extensive abscess formation in the liver and typical intestinal lesions associated with an *Entamoeba* sp.

As *Entamoeba invadens* cannot survive in sea water, there is little likelihood of turtles becoming infected, except accidentally as in this report.

(iv) AMOEBIASIS (*Entamoeba* spp. INFECTION) OF LIZARDS

The disease is often said to occur in "lizards", but there are only a few reports in specific species. These include the iguana (*Iguana iguana*) by Hill and Neal (1952), the Komodo dragon (*Varanus komodoensis*) by Gray *et al* (1966), the blue-tongued skink (*Tiliqua scincoides*) and Thailand water dragon (*Physignathus cochinchinus*) by Donaldson *et al* (1975).

Clinical Signs

Those in the Komodo dragon consisted of inappetance and "evidence of abdominal pain by frequent colonic spasms".

Life History

The life history of the parasite and pathogenesis in lizards appear to be essentially the same as those described in snakes.

Prevention and Treatment

This is the same as that given for snakes, although Gray *et al* (1966) had success treating a Komodo dragon using the human amoebicides diiodohydroxyquin and emetine hydrochloride. They used 650 mg of the former in 150 ml of 0·9 per cent saline given daily as a retention enema for 14 days. However, this drug is only effective against the enteric form of the disease and as the liver is often affected in reptiles it is necessary to supplement the treatment with the systemic amoebicide, emetine hydrochloride. This was given intramuscularly into the tail at a dosage rate of 65 mg for a 40 lb *Varanus* lizard. However, as Donaldson *et al* (1975) pointed out, this form of therapy is impracticable in many cases because of the excessive handling required. The use of metronidazole, as recommended for snakes, has obvious advantages over this method.

(v) AMOEBIASIS (*Entamoeba* sp. INFECTION) OF THE TUATARA

Frank *et al* (1976b) recorded amoebiasis due to an *Entamoeba* sp. in a tuatara (*Sphenodon punctatus*) that had been kept in captivity for eight years. They stated that the reptile showed typical lesions of the disease with inflammation and thickening of the posterior part of the gut. No clinical signs or other *post mortem* findings were described.

(vi) AMOEBIASIS (*Entamoeba* sp. INFECTION) OF CROCODILES

Ippen (1965) stated that he found the disease once in a crocodile and this appears to be the only record. The lesions were similar to those occurring in snakes.

(b) *Hosts for* Endolimax *spp.*

Freshwater terrapin: *Pseudemys*.

(c) *Hosts for* Hartmanella *spp.*

Order Chelonia
   The genus is found in "turtles" (presumably freshwater terrapins) according to Telford (1971).

Order Squamata (Suborders Lacertilia and Serpentes)
"Lizards" and "snakes" were reported to be infected by Telford (1971).

(d) *Hosts for* Naegleria *spp*.

Although these organisms were recorded in reptiles by Frank and Bosch (1972) and Will (1975), they were not mentioned in reptiles by Kudo (1966) and are therefore probably spurious parasites.

(e) *Hosts for* Acanthamoeba *spp*.

Order Chelonia
The genus is found in "turtles" (presumably freshwater terrapins) according to Telford (1971).
Order Squamata (Suborders Lacertilia and Serpentes)
"Lizards" and "snakes" are infected according to Telford (1971) and Levine (1973).

II. Subphylum Sporozoa

Protozoa that typically produce simple, resistant spores or which have a stage in the cycle that is derived from one and contains one or more sporozoites. No cilia or flagella are present except on the male gametes of some species. All are parasitic. Many are serious pathogens.

Class Telosporea

All species have sexual reproduction. Spores are present in most and sporozoites in all.
   Subclass Coccidia   The mature trophozoites are small and intracellular.

Order Eucoccida

Schizogony occurs with asexual and sexual phases of multiplication.

(1) SUBORDER ADELEINA

Spores present in some genera. Syzygy—male and female gametocytes develop in association. One or two hosts are required.

Genera in reptiles Haemogregarina and *Hepatozoon* spp. are common blood-borne parasites but only rarely pathogenic. *Karyolysus* and *Klossiella* are potential pathogens but not known to be pathogenic. *Karyolysus*, unlike *Klossiella*, is blood-borne, whereas *Klossiella* occurs in the kidneys.

Life-cycles Intermediate hosts of *Hepatozoon* spp. include ticks and mosquitoes although other invertebrates also transmit haemogregarines (see below). For example, the leech (*Placobdella catenigera*) is the vector of the haemogregarines (*Haemogregarina stepanowi*) of the European pond terrapin (*Emys orbicularis*) according to Noble and Noble (1976) and leeches are vectors of haemogregarines of other aquatic vertebrates (Paterson and Dresser, 1976) (see Chapter 10).

Sexual reproduction of *Karyolysus* takes place in mites, which therefore act as intermediate hosts. In the case of *K. lacertae* of the wall lizard (*Lacerta muralis*), the mite involved is *Neoliponyssus saurarum* (Reichenbach-Klinke and Elkan, 1965). However, according to Svahn (1975), four species of *Karyolysus* occurring in the sand lizard (*L. agilis*) and the viviparous lizard (*L. vivipara*) develop in the mite *Sauronyssus saurarum*.

The life-cycle of *Klossiella* in reptiles appears to be unknown, although oocysts are passed in the urine.

(a) *Hosts for* Haemogregarines

Hosts for confirmed *Hepatozoon* spp. are given separately below this section. Many parasites classed as *Haemogregarina* may belong to the genus *Hepatozoon* because the parasites can only be separated on the basis of their endogenous schizogony or type of development in a given vector (Ball, 1967). Often this is unknown. All are blood-borne parasites.

Order Chelonia

There appear to be no records of this parasite in marine turtles and the parasites are relatively uncommon in tortoises.

Freshwater terrapins: *Chelodina, Chelydra, Chrysemys, Cinosternum* (= *Kinosternon*), *Elseya, Emydoidea* (= *Emys*), *Emydura, Emys, Graptemys, Kinosternon, Nicoria, Pelusios, Pseudemys, Terrapene, Trionyx*.

Tortoises: *Geomyda, Testudo*.

Order Rhynchocephalia

Tuatara (*Sphenodon punctatus*)

Order Squamata (Suborder Lacertilia)

Examples are given below. Many others are listed by Wenyon (1926) and most are probably valid.

Lizards: *Agama, Ameiva, Physignathus, Sphenomorphus, Tiliqua, Tropidurus, Varanus*.

Geckos: *Gecko, Gehyra, Gymnodactylus, Hemidactylus, Heteronota, Hoplodactylus, Lepidodactylus, Phyllodactylus, Phyllurus, Platydactylus, Tarentola*.

Wood (1935) observed changes in the blood of geckos (*Tarentola mauritanica*) infected with haemogregarines, but with the exception of snakes this appears to be the only indication that the parasites may be pathogenic.

Chameleons: *Chamaeleo*.
Skinks: *Egernia, Emoia, Lygosoma* (? = *Leiolopisma*), *Mabuya, Sphenomorphus*.
Order Squamata (Suborder Serpentes)
There are hundreds of records of haemogregarines in a considerable variety of snakes from all over the world. It is likely therefore that all snakes are susceptible.
Order Crocodilia
Crocodiles: *Crocodylus*.
Alligators: *Alligator*.
Caimans: *Caiman*.
Gharials: *Gavialis*.

(i) HAEMOGREGARINIASIS (HAEMOGREGARINE INFECTIONS) OF SNAKES

As heavy infections of haemogregarines are common in captive reptiles of many species, especially snakes, it is surprising that there is so little evidence of pathogenicity.

Species and Hosts

An indication of the wide host range of haemogregarine infections has already been given. Reports of pathogenic infections to date appear to be confined to snakes. Those which have been mentioned specifically include the Californian king snake (*Lampropeltis getulus californiae*) by Keymer (1976).

Distribution and Incidence

Haemogregarine infections in snakes are world wide. The incidence of the disease, unlike the infection, is apparently very low, although most reptiles with heavy infections are potentially at risk. In the opinion of Hilgenfeld (1968), when more than one third of the erythrocytes are infected with haemogregarines, clinical signs can be expected. In the opinion of Zwart (1973) such heavy infections are certain to be fatal but in the experience of Keymer (unpublished) snakes with much heavier infections apparently die from other causes.

Life History

The life-cycles of the vast majority of haemogregarines which infect reptiles are unknown. Therefore, as stated previously, most haemogregarines in reptiles cannot be allocated to a specific genus, because accurate identification of these protozoa depends upon the structure of the stages in the vectors. Nevertheless all species of haemogregarines are transmitted by invertebrates and in reptiles these include ticks (*Hyalomma* sp.), mites (*Liponyssus* sp.), bugs (*Triatoma* sp.), mosquitoes (*Culex* sp.), tsetse flies (*Glossina* sp.) and leeches (*Haementeria*, *Ozobranchus* and *Placobdella* spp.). Although there appears to be no proof it would be surprising if the common snake mite (*Ophionyssus natricis*) did not transmit some of the haemogregarines which infect snakes (see Chapter 10).

The life-cycle is basically similar to that of *Plasmodium* (see page 273). Sexual reproduction occurs in the invertebrate and asexual multiplication (schizogony) in the reptilian host. The parasites (sporozoites) may either be transmitted when the invertebrate sucks the blood of its host, as occurs for example in those species with leeches as vectors, or the host may become infected by eating the vector, for example certain mites.

In the snake, schizonts occur in a variety of organs including liver, spleen, pancreas and lung.

Clinical Signs

Heavy infections can lead to anaemia by dehaemoglobinization, as noted by Hoare (1932) and Fantham and Porter (1950, 1952). This is because the intra-erythrocytic parasites are capable of causing distortion of the red blood cells and displacement of the host cell nucleus leading to destruction of the erythrocytes.

Diagnosis

During life, diagnosis is made by microscopical examination of the blood and finding large numbers of the intra-erythrocytic, sausage-shaped gametocytes associated with anaemia. Histological examination is also necessary at necropsy in order to detect lesions associated with the exo-erythrocytic schizonts.

Differential Diagnosis

Unlike most of the malaria parasites the intra-erythrocytic gametocytes of haemogregarines do not contain refractile pigment granules.

Prevention and Treatment

Destruction and control of all ectoparasites and possible invertebrate vectors.

No chemotherapeutic drug appears to have been tried against haemogregarine infections.

Post Mortem Findings and Pathology

Keymer (1976) recorded the presence of multiple, minute, whitish foci in the liver of a Californian king snake. On histological examination the lesions were found to be due to focal necrosis and partly organized blood clots apparently caused by the presence of numerous schizonts. Similar lesions were found in the spleen and pancreas. The lung was very congested and also contained schizonts. In the opinion of Hilgenfeld (1968) the schizonts in the lung capillaries expand these vessels as they enlarge leading to extension of the vascular congestion as well as perivascular and interstitial oedema. At necropsy affected snakes may also appear thin and anaemic.

(b) *Hosts for* Hepatozoon *spp.*

Many parasites termed "haemogregarines" probably belong to this genus. These are all blood-borne parasites with schizonts occurring in the liver, spleen and other organs and gametocytes in the blood.
Order Chelonia
   Tortoises: *Testudo*.
   "Turtles", the genus was not given by Telford (1971); presumably he referred to freshwater terrapins.
Order Squamata (Suborder Lacertilia)
   Lizards: *Sceloporus, Tupinambis*.
   Geckos: *Gecko*.
   Chameleons: *Chamaeleo*.
Order Squamata (Suborder Serpentes)

Snakes: *Bothrops, Drymarchon.* It is likely that many more genera of snakes harbour *Hepatozoon,* that at present are still referred to as haemogragarines.
Order Crocodilia
Crocodiles: *Crocodylus.*
Caimans: *Caiman.*

(c) *Hosts for* Karyolysus *spp.*

There appear to be no reports from chelonians. Lizards are the main hosts of this relatively rare blood parasite.
Order Squamata (Suborder Lacertilia)
Lizards: *Lacerta, Psammodromus.*
Order Squamata (Suborder Serpentes)
Snakes: It is possible that the haemogregarine found in an African "green tree snake" by Hoare (1920) may have been a *Karyolysus* sp.

(d) *Hosts for* Klossiella *spp.*

This appears to be a very rare parasite; it was not recorded in reptiles by Pellérdy (1974).
Order Squamata (Suborder Lacertilia)
Lizard: *Varanus* (Colley and Else, 1975).
Order Squamata (Suborder Serpentes)
Snake: *Boa* (Zwart, 1964).

(2) SUBORDER EIMERINA

Spores present in some genera. There is no syzygy and zygotes are non-motile. One or two hosts required.

Genera in reptiles *Eimeria* and *Isospora* are both potential and occasional pathogens. Parasites of both genera occur mainly in the gut epithelium but also infect the bile-duct epithelium of some snakes, e.g. *Bitis, Cerastes, Natrix, Ptyas* and *Thamnophis* spp. and also chelonians—*Emyda* and *Lissemys* spp. *Globidium** spp. have been recorded in a few reptiles but these are now regarded as synonyms of *Eimeria* spp. *Cyclospora* can also be pathogenic. *Tyzzeria, Wenyonella, Dorisiella, Pythonella, Hoarella, Caryospora, Cryptosporidium, Mantonella* and *Octo-*

---

* This name has also been used for *Besnoitia.*

sporella are all probably non-pathogenic and occur in the gut epithelium. *Schellackia* (= *Lankesterella* = *Atoxoplasma*) spp. are potentially pathogenic. Schizonts occur in the gut and sporozoites in the blood. *Toxoplasma* and *Besnoitia* spp. are potential pathogens, and likewise *Sarcocystis* spp., two of which are a known pathogen (see page 271–2).

Life-cycles   Most of the above genera have a direct life-cycle but there are exceptions. Sporozoites of *Schellackia* spp. in the blood are apparently transmitted by small mites such as *Geckobia* spp. (Bonorris and Ball, 1955) or *Geckobiella texana* in the case of the fence lizard (*Sceloporus undulatus*), according to Pellérdy (1974). The life-cycle of *Toxoplasma*, represented by the one species (*T. gondii*), is still imperfectly understood in most species. However, there is now evidence that it is divided into two separate cycles, namely an entero–epithelial one and an extra-intestinal (tissue) cycle. The typical coccidian-type entero–epithelial cycle with the production of oocysts passed in the faeces appears to be confined to the cats (Felidae). The extra-intestinal cycle occurs in both feline and non-feline hosts, but it is the only cycle in non-felids. In the latter (i.e. mammals) infection occurs either from the ingestion of sporulated oocysts of feline origin or the ingestion of tissue cysts. However, transplacental infection of the foetus from an infected dam can also occur. The mode of transmission in birds and reptiles remains unknown but may be similar to mammals.

Much less is known about the life-cycles of *Sarcocystis* and *Besnoitia* but they are believed to be similar to that of *T. gondii*.

Hosts for Eimeria, Isospora, Tyzzeria, Cyclospora, Wenyonella, Dorisiella, Pythonella, Hoarella, Caryospora, Cryptosporidium, Mantonella, Octosporella *and* Schellackia

Complete host lists together with descriptions are given for all these genera by Pellérdy (1963, 1969, 1974) on which the therefore abbreviated list of susceptible hosts given below is based. However, more recent records by other workers are included.

(a)   *Hosts for* Eimeria *spp.*

Eimeria spp. are the most common and widespread coccidians.
Order Chelonia
There are relatively few records from tortoises and terrapins. There appear to be no reports of *Eimeria* in marine turtles.

Order Squamata (Suborder Lacertilia)
There are numerous records from lizards of many species, including geckos, skinks and chameleons.
Order Squamata (Suborder Serpentes)
Many reports in numerous species of snakes.
Order Crocodilia
There are few records, although *Eimeria* has been recorded from crocodiles, alligators, caimans and gharials.

(i) COCCIDIAL CHOLECYSTITIS (*Eimeria bitis* and *E. cascabeli* INFECTION) OF SNAKES

Species and Hosts

Eimeria bitis, which was originally described by Fantham (1932), was reported by Fantham and Porter (1950) to be pathogenic to the puff adder (*Bitis arietans* = *lachesis*). Fantham and Porter (1952) recorded disease due to *E. bitis* in the garter snakes (*Thamnophis sirtalis* and *T. sauritus*) and also in the smooth green snake (*Liopeltis vernalis*). Vetterling and Widmer (1968) described a new and pathogenic species, *E. cascabeli* in the rattlesnake (*Crotalus viridis*).

Distribution and Incidence

Like intestinal coccidiosis caused by *Isospora naiae* (see page 264), these cases were also encountered at London Zoo by Fantham and Porter (1950, 1952) and the same remarks concerning intestinal coccidiosis in snakes apply to this infection.

Life History

The complete life histories of *Eimeria bitis* and *E. cascabeli* have not been described. However, the life-cycles of *Eimeria* and *Isospora* species are very similar and therefore the direct cycle described for *Isospora* spp. is likely to be applicable, except that the schizonts of *E. bitis* and *E. cascabeli* attack the epithelium of the bile-ducts and gall bladder instead of the intestine. The parasites do not penetrate the liver tissue. The sporozoites released from ingested oocysts in the gut probably make their way up the bile-duct and into the gall bladder.

Clinical Signs

None has been described.

Diagnosis

The oocysts of both parasites are passed in the excreta. However, as other *Eimeria* spp. occur in snakes, diagnosis on the basis of finding oocysts of *Eimeria* in the excreta is not sufficient to make a definite diagnosis. It is necessary therefore, after the oocysts have been sporulated, not only to confirm that they are *Eimeria* by the presence of four sporocysts each containing two sporozoites, but for the oocysts to be accurately measured. The measurements given by Fantham (1932) for *E. bitis* were $30 \times 20 \mu m$ for young oocysts occurring in the bile and $28–36 \times 18–24 \mu m$ for mature oocysts in the intestinal lumen where sporulation commences. Pellérdy (1974) gave further measurements for other stages. Vetterling and Widmer (1968) described various stages of *E. cascabeli* in detail. They stated that sporulated oocysts measure $34–40 \times 14–20 \mu m$.

Differential Diagnosis

The disease must be differentiated at necropsy from intestinal coccidiosis due to both *Eimeria* and *Isospora* infections.

Prevention and Treatment

See *Isospora naiae* infection (page 264).

Post Mortem Findings and Pathology

In *Bitis arietans*, Fantham and Porter (1950) reported that although the liver tissue was not invaded by *E. bitis*, the organ was congested and the bile bright green in colour and very viscid. The mucosa of the gall bladder, however, was very ragged and denuded in many areas. On histological examination carried out immediately after death, some of the infected epithelial cells were found to protrude beyond the general level of the epithelium and were ultimately shed into the lumen of the gall bladder. A similar appearance was seen in the epithelium of the bile-ducts. Both the gall bladder and the bile-ducts were hardened by the formation of fibrous tissue. Inflammatory exudate occurred in the submucosa of the worst denuded areas. The lesions led to hypersecretion of mucus and some of the bile had the consistency of jelly. Similar lesions were encountered by Fantham and Porter (1952) in the other species of snakes.

In *E. cascabeli* infections, Vetterling and Widmer (1968) described hypertrophy of the connective tissue around bile ducts and erosion of the epithelial layer. The livers and gall bladders were slightly enlarged.

(ii) COCCIDIOSIS (*Eimeria* and *Isospora* INFECTIONS) OF CHAMELEONS AND LIZARDS

Pellérdy (1974) listed *Eimeria* and *Isospora* species infecting the cholecystic and intestinal epithelium of various species of chameleons and lizards, but did not mention any evidence of pathogenicity. Zwart (1973) stated that coccidiosis of the gall bladder occurs in *Anolis* spp. of lizards and he also referred to "coccidiosis in the intestine" of chameleons stating that sometimes intestinal invagination occurs. These appear to be the only records. Obviously these infections need further investigation.

(iii) INTESTINAL COCCIDIOSIS (*Eimeria* sp. INFECTION) OF SNAKES

The only report of this disease appears to be that by Lehmann (1972) on which the present brief account is based.

Species and Hosts

The species of *Eimeria* was not identified by Lehmann (1972). He found the parasite to be pathogenic to reticulated pythons (*Python reticulatus*) and golden tree snakes (*Chrysopelea ornata*).

Distribution and Incidence

Lehmann's snakes had been recently imported into Germany from Bangkok and Thailand. Lehmann did not consider intestinal coccidiosis to be a common disease of snakes, an observation endorsed by Keymer (unpublished).

Life History

See the discussion for *Eimeria bitis* and *Isospora naiae*.

Clinical Signs

Diarrhoea leading to death.

Diagnosis

Use of the same methods as described for *Eimeria bitis* and *Isospora naiae* infections.

Differential Diagnosis

Although of only academic interest to the clinician, it is not possible to differentiate this disease with certainty from *Eimeria bitis* infection of the gall bladder without carrying out a necropsy, because there is no accurate description of the sporulated oocysts for comparison with *E. bitis*.

Prevention and Treatment

As recommended for *Isospora naiae* infection.

Post Mortem Findings and Pathology

Lehmann (1972) recorded an intensive catarrhal and diphtheroid inflammation involving the small and proximal part of the large intestine.

(b) *Hosts for* Isospora *spp.*

These coccidia are also fairly widespread, although not common. There appear to be no records from chelonians.
Order Squamata (Suborders Lacertilia and Serpentes)
 Lizards and snakes seem to be equally susceptible. There are a few records only from geckos, skinks and chameleons.
Order Crocodilia
 There are single records from a crocodile and a caiman (Pellérdy, 1974).

(iv) INTESTINAL COCCIDIOSIS (*Isospora naiae* INFECTION) OF SNAKES

Intestinal coccidiosis due to *Isospora naiae* has apparently only been described by Fantham (1932), Fantham and Porter (1950, 1952), and these publications form the basis of this account.

Species and Hosts

Isospora naiae was reported to be pathogenic in the cape cobra (*Naja nive*) by Fantham (1932) and North American banded rattlesnake (*Crotalus horridus*) by Fantham and Porter (1950, 1952).

Distribution and Incidence

The cases reported by Fantham and Porter (1950, 1952) were in snakes that died at London Zoo, but obviously coccidiosis due to *I. naiae* may occur in almost any zoological collection where carrier and/or susceptible snakes are kept. Nevertheless, the parasite was not identified and no cases of intestinal coccidiosis were encountered over a 10-year period by Keymer (unpublished) whilst Pathologist at London Zoo. During this time numerous snakes were necropsied, so the disease would appear to be rare.

Life History

The life-cycle is presumably direct, as for other *Isospora* spp. that inhabit the intestinal tract of vertebrates.

Snakes become infected by ingesting oocysts, which on reaching the intestine release sporozoites that invade the epithelial lining. Once inside a tissue cell, the sporozoite becomes a trophozoite, and this gradually develops into a mature schizont containing numerous merozoites. When the schizont ruptures, motile merozoites are released and these then penetrate other epithelial cells to become trophozoites and form a second generation of schizonts. This process of sexual reproduction may be repeated several times before some of the merozoites that are released penetrate other epithelial cells and develop into either microgametocytes or macrogametocytes. The microgametocyte undergoes multiple division to produce a large number of motile microgametes (males), whereas the macrogametocyte enlarges and eventually develops into a single macrogamete (female). Fertilization takes place when a microgamete penetrates a macrogamete, producing a zygote. The zygote then secretes a cyst wall around itself and becomes an oocyst. This encysted and relatively resistant stage is passed out in the faeces and matures on the ground to form sporocysts, still within the confines of the cyst wall. Within the sporocysts, sporozoites are produced which invade the epithelial cells of the intestine when the oocyst is ingested by a suitable host.

Clinical Signs

Loss of weight and poor condition.

Diagnosis

During life the infection may be diagnosed by microscopical examination of the excreta. Fantham and Porter (1952) drew attention to the importance of saline enemata when collecting excreta samples from snakes. They pointed out that food may be retained in the alimentary tract for long periods and when passed it is often very hard. Saline enemata help to soften the faeces and facilitate microscopical examination. Excreta are examined on a slide beneath a cover slip, when oocysts are clearly seen if present in sufficiently large numbers to be of any pathological significance. The oocysts are visible as oval, distinct, thin-walled objects. The oocyst wall can be seen to have a double contour if the objective of the microscope is focused up and down. In all *Isospora* spp. the oocysts after sporulation contain two sporocysts, both of which contain four sporozoites. The oocysts of *I. naiae* measure 14–20 × 8–14 μm. Free sporocysts and free sporozoites were detected in scrapings of the anterior part of the intestinal mucosa by Fantham (1932) which may mean that autoinfection can occur. Measurements of all stages were given by Pellérdy (1974).

Differential Diagnosis

The infection should not be confused with intestinal coccidiosis due to *Eimeria* sp. although the treatment for both diseases is the same.

Prevention and Treatment

Strict attention should be paid to hygiene to minimize the spread of infection by faecal contamination of food.

Although Fantham and Porter (1950, 1952) gave no specific treatment for *I. naiae* infection, treatments for intestinal coccidiosis in reptiles have been recommended by other workers. These include Lehmann (1972) and Gabrisch (1976) who both advocated sulphamethoxydiazone (2-sulphanilamido-5-methoxypyrimidine) using a dosage level of 80 mg/kg for the initial dose and 40 mg/kg daily from the second to the fifth day. The drug is given by subcutaneous or intramuscular injection using a 20 per cent solution. Gabrisch (1976) stated that intraperitoneal injection of sulphamethoxydiazine is an alternative method of administration, but the drug has to be diluted in physiological saline. Wallach (1969) suggested the administration of sodium sulphadimidine in the drinking water at a dosage rate of 1 oz/gal for ten days.

Post Mortem Findings and Pathology

Fantham and Porter (1950) reported that most of the small intestine was heavily parasitized in *Naja nivea*. The intensity of the infection diminished from the duodenum to the beginning of the large intestine. Haemorrhagic areas occurred throughout and on histological examination the mucosa and submucosa of the villi were the chief seats of infection. In some areas long shreds of mucous membrane were present in the lumen of the gut, the villi being stripped of mucosa. In places the parasites had not only destroyed the mucosa, but had also penetrated deep into the submucosa.

(c) *Hosts for* Tyzzeria *spp.*

Order Squamata (Serpentes)
    A single record from a snake by Pellérdy (1974) appears to be the only report in any reptile.

(d) *Hosts for* Cyclospora *spp.*

There are a few records from reptiles in the Order Squamata only.
Order Squamata (Suborder Lacertilia)
    Reported in lizards and geckos.
Order Squamata (Suborder Serpentes)
    There are a few records in snakes of various genera.

(v) CYCLOSPORIOSIS IN SNAKES

According to Pellérdy (1974) *C. niniae* can be pathogenic to the snake *Ninia sebae sebae*, massive invasion of the intestinal epithelium provoking "an inflammatory cellular reaction resulting in detachment of the intestinal epithelium". Nothing more appears to have been recorded about this infection.

(e) *Hosts for* Wenyonella *spp.*

Order Squamata (Suborder Serpentes)
The brown house snake (*Boaedon lineatus*) appears to be the only known reptilian host (Pellérdy, 1974).

(f) *Hosts for* Dorisiella *spp.*

Order Squamata (Suborder Serpentes)
Pellérdy's (1974) report in a snake appears to be the only record in a reptile.

(g) *Hosts for* Pythonella *spp.*

This is another rare parasite.
Order Squamata (Suborder Lacertilia)
There is a single record in a *Sceloporus* spp. of lizard.
Order Squamata (Suborder Serpentes)
The parasite was first recorded in a *Python* sp. and there appear to be no further reports.

(h) *Hosts for* Hoarella *sp.*

Order Squamata (Suborder Lacertilia)
The original record of *H. garnhami* in a lizard (*Cnemidophorus* sp.) remains as the only report of this parasite.

(i) *Hosts for* Caryospora *spp.*

These uncommon parasites appear to be confined to the order Squamata.
Order Squamata (Suborder Lacertilia)
Pellérdy (1974) recorded the parasite in a gecko and a lizard.
Order Squamata (Suborder Serpentes)
There are a few reports from snakes.

(j) *Hosts for* Cryptosporidium *spp.*

These parasites appear to be even more uncommon than *Caryospora* spp. and apparently confined to the Squamata.
Order Squamata (Suborder Lacertilia)
Only reports are from a lizard and a gecko.

Order Squamata (Suborder Serpentes)
There is one record from a snake.

(k) *Hosts for* Mantonella *sp.*

Order Chelonia
This parasite appears to be confined to terrapins and was not recorded in reptiles by Pellérdy (1974). Wacha and Christiansen (1976) reported *M. hammondi* from *Chrysemys, Graptemys, Kinosternon* and *Trionyx*.

(l) *Hosts for* Octosporella *spp.*

Order Squamata (Suborder Lacertilia)
This is a very rare parasite recorded in a skink and in agama lizards.

(m) *Hosts for* Schellackia *spp.*

Order Squamata (Suborder Lacertilia)
This rare parasite seems to be confined to lizards.

(n) *Hosts for* Sarcocystis *spp.*

Order Chelonia
  Tortoises: *Testudo*. One report only (Keymer, 1978).
  Terrapins: *Kinosternon*. Single record of *S. kinosterni* by Lainson and Shaw (1971, 1972).
Order Squamata (Suborder Lacertilia)
The list below is based mainly on that given by Lainson and Shaw (1971).
  Lizards: *Eremias, Lacerta, Sceloporus, Uta*.
  Geckos: *Tarentola* (= *Platydactylus*).
  Chameleons: *Chamaeleo*.
  Skinks: *Chalcides* (= *Gongylus*).
Order Squamata (Serpentes)
  Snakes: *Atractaspis, Morelia* (= *Python*). The parasite recorded in *Atractaspis* by Parenzan (1947) was regarded as of doubtful authenticity by Lainson and Shaw (1971).

(vi) SARCOSPORIDIOSIS (*Sarcocystis kinosterni* INFECTION) OF AQUATIC CHELONIANS

Sarcocystis infections of skeletal and cardiac muscle occur in a wide range of hosts, including man and other mammals, birds, reptiles and fish, but they are seldom pathogenic. In reptiles the parasite is also rare. The following account of the disease is based mainly on the report of Lainson and Shaw (1971).

Species and Hosts

Sarcocystis kinosterni is a replacement name given by Lainson and Shaw (1972) to *S. gracilis*, which they originally described (Lainson and Shaw, 1971) from its only known host, the Brazilian "tortoise" or scorpion mud terrapin (*Kinosternon scorpioides*). The only other record in a chelonian of an organism that was almost certainly *Sarcocystis* was that by Keymer (1978) in a terrestrial chelonian—a Jaboty tortoise (*T. denticulata*). The latter parasite, however, showed no evidence of pathogenicity.

Distribution and Incidence

Lainson and Shaw (1971) found the parasite in 18 *K. scorpioides* out of a total of 206 that they examined. All the reptiles came from the Island of Marajó, northern Brazil. The parasite therefore is obviously rare.

Life History

The life-cycle of this particular *Sarcocystis* species is completely unknown. Lainson and Shaw (1971), however, discussed various hypotheses including its possible relationship with *Isospora* coccidia and *Toxoplasma*.

Clinical Signs

None described.

Diagnosis

Sarcocystis infections can only be diagnosed with certainty at necropsy or from biopsy specimens of muscle tissue by finding the typical intramuscular cysts. Occasionally the zoites are accidentally liberated from the cysts when infected animals are bled, so that the zoites contaminate blood smears and are found on microscopical examination. It was in this way that the infection was diagnosed by Lainson and Shaw (1971). These authors described the parasite in detail.

Cysts were found only in skeletal muscle. They were cylindrical in shape with pointed ends and measured up to 8 mm long and approximately 230 μm in diameter when measured in fresh preparations. Fresh and unstained zoites were long, slender and curved, measuring 18·4 × 1·4 μm.

Differential Diagnosis

On histological examination of intramuscular cysts great care is necessary to differentiate the parasite from *Toxoplasma* and *Besnoitia* spp. This involves detailed studies of the morphology of the parasite by a skilled protozoologist. However, if the intramuscular cysts are visible to the naked eye they are most likely to be those of *Sarcocystis*. It should also be remembered that *Toxoplasma* is an exceedingly rare parasite of reptiles, probably the only authentic case being that found in a lizard by Elkan (1976) and recorded by Reichenbach-Klinke (1977). *Besnoitia* appears also to have been found only in lizards.

Prevention and Treatment

No information available.

Post Mortem Findings and Pathology

Some of the infected chelonians examined by Lainson and Shaw (1971) showed severe muscular lesions, these usually being associated with cysts that had ruptured and released zoites into surrounding muscle. Remnants of the cysts were visible in the centre of intense round-cell infiltration. Eventually the cellular infiltration appeared to replace the zoites. The affected musculature was seen to be pale, soft and pulpy. Most of the sarcocysts were visible to the naked eye as white streaks. Reptiles which were very heavily infected died in captivity.

(vii) SARCOSPORIDIOSIS (*Sarcocystis chamaeleonis* INFECTION) OF CHAMELEONS

This account is based on the description given by Frank (1966).

Species and Host

Frank (1966) described *Sarcocystis chamaeleonis* in its only known host,

Fischer's chameleon (*Chamaeleo fischeri multituberculatus*). Although *Sarcocystis* species have been recorded in a few other saurians this appears to be the only record in the family Chamaeleonidae.

Distribution and Incidence

Unknown.

Life History

Like virtually all *Sarcocystis* spp. this is unknown.

Clinical Signs

Frank (1966) described swelling of all the legs and the "chewing muscles". The reptile had great difficulty in drinking and refused to eat.

Prevention and Treatment

No information available.

Post Mortem Findings and Pathology

All affected muscles were whitish-grey in colour and appeared anaemic. In the worst affected areas the muscles formed an almost gruel-like mass. Mainly the masseter and occipital muscles and those of the tail and extremities showed the typical "Miescher's tubes", but the dorsal and intercostal muscles were also infected.

(o) *Hosts for* Besnoitia *spp.*

The only records so far are from lizards. Schneider (1965, 1967) and Garnham (1966a) should be consulted for more information on these rare parasites.
Order Squamata (Suborder Lacertilia)
   Lizards: *Ameiva, Basiliscus*.

(p) *Hosts for* Toxoplasma gondii

In spite of the fact that Levine (1973) stated that *Toxoplasma* occurs in "turtles, lizards, geckos, chameleons and skinks", most protozoolo-

gists doubt the existence of the parasite in reptiles. However, the recent report by Elkan (1976) seems convincing.
Order Squamata (Suborder Lacertilia)
  Lizard: *T. gondii* was recorded in *Lacerta muralis* by Elkan (1976) and briefly described in the book by Reichenbach-Klinke (1977).

(3) SUBORDER HAEMOSPORINA

No syzygy and no spores formed. Zygote is motile. Two hosts are required, with asexual development in a vertebrate and sexual reproduction in a dipterous insect. These are all blood parasites.

Genera in reptiles Plasmodium (potential and occasional pathogen), *Simondia, Haemocystidium* (= *Haemoproteus*), *Garnia, Fallisia* and *Saurocytozoon* (all potential pathogens, but pathogenicity unproven).

Garnham (1966b) created three new subgenera of *Plasmodium*, namely *Sauramoeba* for those parasites with large schizonts, *Carinamoeba* for those with small schizonts and *Ophidiella* to accommodate the species described in snakes. Many of the old records of *Plasmodium* are incorrect, the genus having been confused with *Haemocystidium* (= *Haemoproteus*) and even haemogregarines. There are no true *Plasmodium* spp. in chelonians.

Life cycle of Plasmodium *spp.*   The intermediate hosts for virtually all species in reptiles are unknown. The sand fly (*Lutzomyia*) transmits *P.* (*Sauramoeba*) *floridense* (see page 275) and *Culex* species of mosquitoes or gnats may be involved in some species of *Plasmodium* and possibly also mites (*Hirstiella* sp.), (Garnham 1966b). The life history of *P. (S.) floridense* is probably similar to other *Plasmodium* spp. in reptiles, except that the vector will undoubtedly be found to be different in most cases.

(a) *Hosts for* Plasmodium (Sauramoeba) *spp. and* P. (Carinamoeba) *spp.*

Garnham (1966b) gave a list of *Plasmodium* spp. and indicated the type of host. This list was updated by Ayala (1978) who provided a checklist, host index and annotated bibliography of all *Plasmodium* spp. in reptiles. However, he included *Garnia, Fallisia* and *Saurocytozoon* spp. in his checklist as he did not recognize these genera only using the terms in a descriptive rather than a taxonomic sense.

No attempt is made here to list the genera of reptiles in which *Plasmodium* spp. have been found. Up until 1975, Ayala (1978) stated that the world literature on *Plasmodium* of squamate reptiles included 54 valid species and subspecies. The majority of *Plasmodium* spp. in squamate reptiles infect lizards, but they also occur in skinks, chameleons and geckos. All parasites previously named as *Plasmodium* spp. in chelonians are now regarded as *Simondia* spp. (see later).

(b) *Hosts for* Plasmodium (Ophidiella) *spp.*

Order Squamata (Suborder Serpentes)

Snake: *Thamnodynastes pallidus*. This South American snake is the only known host of *P. (O.) wenyoni* and indeed according to Garnham (1966b), it was probably the only true *Plasmodium* reported in snakes up until that time. Nevertheless there were other records of *Plasmodium* spp. in snakes (*Bitis, Causus, Naja* and *Python*) by Fantham and Porter (1950) and the colubrine snakes, *Clelia, Leptophis, Oxybelis* and *Pseustes* spp. by Gorgas (1964) quoted by Garnham (1966b). Ayala (1978) listed additional snake hosts for *Plasmodium* spp. (unnamed), namely *Chironius, Corallus, Lachesis* and *Spilotes* spp. He also listed another named species *P. (O.) tomodoni* from the snake *Tomodon dorsatus*.

(i) MALARIA (*Plasmodium* spp. INFECTIONS) OF LIZARDS

Although malaria is an important disease of man and to a lesser extent, certain species of birds, it is a rare disease of reptiles.

Species and Hosts

Plasmodium species occur mainly in lizards, skinks and chameleons (Garnham, 1966b) but are not common, especially in captive reptiles. *Plasmodium (Sauramoeba) floridense, P. (S.) zonuriae* and *P. (S.) mexicanum* are the only species which appear to be pathogenic (excluding experimental infections). The former infects North American spiny lizards (*Sceloporus undulatus* and *S. formosus*), and the so-called American "chameleon" (*Anolis carolinensis*). *P. (S.) zonuriae* is found in the girdled lizard (*Cordylus* (= *Zonurus*) *vittifer*) of South Africa. It may also occur in the robust plated lizard (*Gerrhosaurus vallidus*) according to Garnham (1966b). *P. (S.) mexicanum* is widespread in the North American western fence lizard (*Sceloporus occidentalis*).

Distribution and Incidence

The infection is likely to be confined to the areas where the natural hosts occur. It might also be encountered in other areas in recently imported lizards.

Life History

As with all *Plasmodium* spp. the vertebrate host originally becomes infected with sporozoites. These stages of the parasite are injected into the blood stream usually via the saliva of an infected female mosquito whilst it is taking a blood meal. In the case of *P. (S.) floridense* infections in *Sceloporus occidentalis*, the vector has been found to be the sand fly (*Lutzomyia*) according to Noble and Noble (1976). *P. (S.) zonuriae*, however, may possibly be transmitted by the prostigmatic mite (*Zonurobia circularis*), but *P. (S.) mexicanum* is also transmitted by species of *Lutzomyia* (Ayala, 1970). The sporozoites penetrate fixed tissue cells, which in lizards are "the early haemopoietic cells and wandering or fixed mesodermal elements" (Garnham, 1966b), and give rise to schizonts. In some reptiles, merozoites produced by these primary exo-erythrocytic schizonts invade lymphoid–macrophage cells to give rise to secondary exoerythrocytic schizonts. Some of the merozoites produced by these secondary schizonts may also invade other lymphoid–macrophage cells, while others infect red blood cells to initiate erythrocytic schizogony. Merozoites produced by the erythrocytic schizonts are capable of invading other erythrocytes or lymphoid–macrophage cells, where in the latter they develop as secondary exo-erythrocytic schizonts. Some of the merozoites that invade erythrocytes develop into gametocytes. These are of two types, females or macrogametocytes and males or microgametocytes. When a suitable mosquito feeds on the blood of the infected vertebrate host, the gametocytes continue their development in the insect's stomach, where they develop into gametes. The microgametes swim actively to find and fertilize the macrogametes. The resultant zygote or ookinete penetrates the stomach wall of the mosquito and forms an oocyst. The nucleus of the oocyst divides to produce sporozoites which break out of the oocysts into the body cavity from where they migrate to the salivary glands. The cycle is repeated when the infected vector feeds. For more precise information on the life-cycle of *Plasmodium* spp. in reptiles and for *P. (S.) floridense*, the reader should consult the classic work by Garnham (1966b).

Clinical Signs

Very little information is available, although in *P. (S.) floridense* infections, anaemia may develop and lizards die after unusually high parasitaemias (Garnham, 1966b; Huff and Marchbank, 1953). Garnham (1966b) also reported marked asthenia and anaemia in heavy infections with *P. (S.) zonuriae*. Some lizards overcome this infection and pass into a state of premunition. *P. (S.) mexicanum* can produce massive infections in young *S. occidentalis* lizards producing "greatly distorted" blood pictures and death (Ayala, 1970).

Diagnosis

This is based on finding intra-erythrocytic schizonts and/or gametocytes in large numbers on microscopical examination of the blood. Like all true *Plasmodium* spp. (except *Garnia*, see pages 277–8) the parasites contain pigment granules derived from the breakdown products of infected erythrocytes. *P. (S.) floridense*, *P. (S.) zonuriae* and *P. (S.) mexicanum* in blood smears stained by Giemsa's method have all been illustrated in colour by Garnham (1966b).

Differential Diagnosis

If no intra-erythrocytic schizonts can be found in blood smears, then *Plasmodium* infections cannot with certainty be differentiated from those caused by *Haemoproteus*, reptilian species of which are now called *Haemocystidium*. Even on histological examination of exo-erythrocytic stages in tissues, combined with a critical examination of the erythrocytic gametocytes it is exceedingly difficult to diagnose *Plasmodium*. However, *Haemocystidium* (= *Haemoproteus*) spp. have not yet been recorded in iguanid lizards or *Cordylus* spp., although they are known to occur in geckos.

Prevention and Treatment

No information available; however, susceptible reptiles should be protected from possible vectors.

Post Mortem Findings and Pathology

In experimental infections with *P. (S.) floridense*, according to Garnham (1966b), phagocytosis becomes intense in the course of the disease and "malaria pigment" accumulates in the liver and spleen.

Disintegrating parasites may also be observed in the blood after the crisis of parasitaemia.

(c) *Hosts for* Simondia

Garnham (1966b) created this genus for all protozoa of chelonians previously classified as *Plasmodium* spp. He described them as "large bladder-like pigmented sexual parasites found in the blood" and provided a host list. The genus includes some organisms previously named *Haemoproteus* and *Haemocystidium* in chelonians. At present it contains the single species *S. metchnikowi*.
Order Chelonia
  Tortoises: *Testudo*.
  Terrapins: *Chelodina, Chitra, Chrysemys, Cinixys, Clemmys, Elseya, Emydura, Emys, Graptemys, Pseudemys, Staurotypus, Trionyx*.

(i) MALARIA (*Simondia* previously *Plasmodium* INFECTION) OF CHELONIANS

Mention of the disease in chelonians is based entirely on the brief report by Murphy (1973) who quoted Hunsaker (1966). "A mosquito" is stated to transmit *Plasmodium* (= *Simondia*) to "turtles". As this is an American report it is probable that "turtles" refers to fresh water terrapins. The disease is stated to have been associated with parasites in the erythrocytes and manifested by general emaciation and lesions in the liver, gut and spleen. The parasite is reputed to have caused death. Obviously much more detailed information is required before malaria can be confirmed as a cause of death in chelonians.

(d) *Hosts for* Haemocystidium (= Haemoproteus) *spp.*

This genus includes the pigmented haemoproteid parasites of erythrocytes of reptiles. The blood stages are confined to gametocytes. Erythrocytic schizogony has not been observed (Mackerras, 1961).
Order Squamata (Suborder Lacertilia)
  Geckos: *Gehyra, Hemidactylus, Heteronota, Oedura, Phyllurus, Tarentola*.
  Lizards: *Agama*.
  Skink: *Sphenomorphus*.

(e) *Hosts for* Garnia *spp.*

Some of these parasites were previously reported as *Plasmodium* spp.

prior to the creation of the genus *Garnia* by Lainson *et al* (1971) for these pigmentless intra-erythrocytic malaria parasites. The vectors and sporogonic stages are unknown.
Order Squamata (Suborder Lacertilia)
 Lizards: *Ameiva, Plica, Uranoscodon.*
 Skinks: *Mabuya.*

(f) *Hosts for* Fallisia *sp.*

This genus was created by Lainson *et al* (1974) for malaria parasites inhabiting leucocytes and thrombocytes of reptiles, both schizogony and gametogony occurring in these cells.
Order Squamata (Suborder Lacertilia)
 Lizards: *Plica, Uranoscodon.* (See Lainson *et al*, 1974, 1975.)

(g) *Hosts for* Saurocytozoon *spp.*

This genus was created by Lainson and Shaw (1969) for an intra-leucocytic parasite of reptiles with round gametocytes which morphologically resembles *Leucocytozoon*, a parasite of birds. It is pigmentless and the asexual stages are still unknown. The life cycle is unknown. *Aedes* spp. of mosquitoes may be vectors.
Order Squamata (Suborder Lacertilia)
 Lizards: *Crocodilurus, Tupinambis.*
 'Skinks: *Mabuya.*

Class Piroplasmea

(See page 254 for description of subphylum Sporozoa.) No spores formed. Small, non-pigmented parasites of erythrocytes and sometimes other cells of vertebrates. They have an invertebrate host (usually a species of tick) and reproduce by schizogony or binary fission. Presence of sexual process is uncertain.

Order Piroplasmida

Genera in reptiles *Dactylosoma* (see Kudo, 1966), possibly *Babesia* and various piroplasma-like parasites have been recorded under the following generic names—*Nuttallia, Sauroplasma* and *Tunetella* (= *Aegyptianella*). The identity and pathogenicity are uncertain in the majority of cases and parasites such as the latter two genera are probably not protozoa but Rickettsiales. All are blood-borne parasites.

(*a*) *Hosts for piroplasms*

Owing to the considerable confusion and uncertainty concerning the identification of many piroplasms, it is not possible to compile any sort of host list in the present state of our knowledge. These organisms, however, have been recorded or suspected in chelonians, geckos, lizards (Reichenbach-Klinke and Elkan, 1965), chameleons (Keymer, 1972) and in snakes (Fantham and Porter, 1952; Keymer, 1970).

III. Subphylum Cnidospora

Organisms having spores with one or more polar filaments. All are parasitic and have a single host.

Class Myxosporidea

All species in this class have multicellular spores.

Order Myxosporida

All are parasitic in cold-blooded vertebrates. Each spore contains one or two sporoplasms and usually two polar capsules containing a coiled polar filament. The organisms attack various organs including the gut and gall bladder.

Genera in reptiles (*Myxidium* and *Henneguya*) Myxosporidians are important pathogens of fish and therefore potential pathogens of aquatic reptiles, although very little is known about myxosporidian infections of the Reptilia. A good account of this complex group is given by Mitchell (1977).

Life-cycle Vertebrates become infected by ingesting spores. Although the life-cycle is imperfectly known, it is believed that the sporoplasm then emerges from the spore as a small amoeba. This penetrates the gut wall and eventually reaches other internal organs, where it encysts. Spores develop in the cyst. Although it is not yet clear how the cysts infect other individuals, it is likely that in some cases, at least, the spores are liberated from the cysts when these are ingested.

(a) *Hosts for* Myxidium *spp*.

The parasite has only been recorded in freshwater chelonians.
Order Chelonia
  Will (1975) stated that "tropical aquatic chelonians are affected". Reichenbach-Klinke and Elkan (1965) and Reichenbach-Klinke (1977) mentioned terrapins of the genera *Emys* and *Trionyx*.

(b) *Hosts for* Henneguya *spp*.

Very little is known about this parasite in reptiles.
Order Chelonia
  The only record appears to be that by Will (1975) in "tropical aquatic" species.

(i) MYXOSPORIDIOSIS (*Myxidium* and *Henneguya* INFECTIONS) OF AQUATIC CHELONIANS

Apparently the only indication that myxosporidian parasites can produce disease in reptiles is the report by Will (1975). He stated that tropical aquatic chelonians are frequently affected by myxosporidian infections of the gall bladder. The parasites responsible were said to be mostly of the genera *Myxidium* and *Henneguya*. Unfortunately he provided no further information. Reichenbach-Klinke (1977) quoting Kudo (1919) also listed three species of aquatic chelonians as hosts of *Myxidium*.

Class Microsporidea

Organisms with unicellular spores, one polar filament and one sporoplasm. All have invertebrate or vertebrate hosts.

Order Microsporida

Suborder Monocnidina   Organisms with single independent spores.

Genera in reptiles   *Glugea* and *Pleistophora* (= *Plistophora*) spp. are important pathogens of fish but, with the exception of *Pleistophora* in the tuatara, there is little evidence of pathogenicity to reptiles. A good account of the Microsporida was given by Canning (1977). These parasites attack various organs including the gut.

Life-cycle This is described below in the description of the disease in the tuatara.

(a) *Hosts for* Glugea *and* Pleistophora *spp.*

In a review of microsporidians in reptiles and amphibians, Canning *et al* (1964) concluded that a record of *Glugea* in "turtles" by Danilewsky (1891) probably referred to a *Pleistophora* sp. Similarly the record of *Glugea danilewskyi* in grass snakes (species not given) by Guyénot and Naville (1920, 1922), they assigned to a *Pleistophora* sp. Canning *et al* (1964), however, accepted the record of *Glugea danilewskyi* in the grass snake (*Tropidonotus natrix*) by Debaisieux (1919). *Pleistophora* sp. infection has also been described in the tuatara (see below).

(i) MICROSPORIDIOSIS (*Pleistophora* sp. INFECTION) OF THE TUATARA

Microsporidiosis is primarily a disease of arthropods, fish and, more rarely amphibians, a number of genera (e.g. *Nosema* and *Thelohania*) being involved.

Species and Host

In reptiles the only pathogenic microsporidian infection recognized to date appears to be that caused by a *Pleistophora* (= *Plistophora*) sp. in the primitive and rare New Zealand tuatara (*Sphenodon punctatus*) described by Liu and King (1971).

Distribution and Incidence

Nothing is known since the infection described in tuataras occurred after the reptiles had been in captivity for several months.

Life History

Microsporidians produce infective spores. When a spore is swallowed by a susceptible host, a polar filament from within the spore is extruded into the lumen of the host's gut and a sporoplasm migrates along this hollow filament to emerge as a small amoeba. Eventually this stage of the parasite reaches its chosen location in the body, where it enters a cell, grows and divides repeatedly, becoming an aggregation of unicellular sporonts, which although often referred to as a "cyst" is really a pseudocyst. Each sporont gives rise to one or more spores (according to the genus of Microsporida); 16 or more being produced by *Pleistophora*. When pseudocysts occur in deep tissues such as muscle as in the tuatara, the release of spores is presumably dependent upon the host's death. The infective spores then require to be ingested by another susceptible host in order to repeat the life-cycle.

Clinical Signs

Infected tuataras became increasingly lethargic, lost weight and showed anorexia for 8 to 12 weeks prior to death.

Diagnosis

In tuataras diagnosis was made on the basis of the *post mortem* findings and the presence of *Pleistophora* "cysts" in the muscle fibres of the tongue and skeletal muscles.

Prevention and Treatment

There is very little information available about prevention or treatment of microsporidiosis in any species of animal, although Baker (1973) stated that the antibiotic Fumagillin is used to control *Nosema apis* infection of bees.

Post Mortem Findings and Pathology

Both infected tuataras were reported as having "white and fragile" tongues and skeletal muscles. On histological examination numerous parasitic "cysts" were found containing up to 100 or more spores within the degenerated muscle fibres. There was no membrane surrounding the groups of spores or pseudocysts that they probably represented. Around disintegrated cysts, mineralization and eosinophilic and monocytic infiltration had occurred. Liu and King (1971) illustrated the lesions and parasites in their account of the disease.

IV. Subphylum Ciliophora

Protozoa having cilia present at some or all stages of the life-cycle. Nuclei are of two dissimilar types. Binary fission occurs and sexual reproduction is usually by conjugation.

Class Ciliatea

Subclass Holotrichia. The body ciliature is simple and uniform in most orders. Special buccal cilia are absent or inconspicuous.

Order Trichostomatida

A cystosome is present at the base of the vestibule. Some species are parasitic.

Genus in reptiles (*Balantidium*) Potential pathogen especially in chelonians. The parasites occur in the intestine, especially the colon.

The life-cycle of all *Balantidium* spp. is direct, resistant cysts being excreted by the host.

(a) *Hosts for* Balantidium *spp.*

The parasite appears to be most common in tortoises.
Order Chelonia
    Tortoises: *Testudo*.
    Terrapins: "Herbivorous turtles" (Telford, 1971).
Order Squamata (Suborder Lacertilia)
Telford (1971) stated that *Balantidium* occurs in lizards, but this appears to be the only evidence.
Order Squamata (Suborder Serpentes)
    Snakes: *Ablabophis, Boaedon, Trimerorhinus*.

(i) COLITIS AND ENTERITIS OF TERRESTRIAL CHELONIANS AND SNAKES ASSOCIATED WITH CILIATE INFECTIONS

The role of *Balantidium* and other related enteric protozoa in the cause of inflammatory lesions of the gut is not clear. There is evidence that such protozoa may be pathogenic when they are present in very large numbers or found in association with other parasites or pathogenic bacteria. For example, Keymer (1978) suspected that ciliates (probably *Balantidium* sp.) were at least partly responsible for a severe colitis in a Horsfield's tortoise (*T. horsfieldi*) and Fantham and Porter (1950) believed *Balantidium* to be responsible for pin-head ulcers in the intestine of the South African snake *Boaedon lineatus*.

Subclass Spirotrichia   The body ciliature is usually sparse and the oral ciliature conspicuous, winding in a clockwise fashion.

Order Heterotrichida

Body ciliature is usually present and uniform.

Genus in reptiles   *Nyctotherus*. No evidence of pathogenicity.

Life-cycle   The life-cycle is direct, with the formation of cysts which are passed in the faeces.

(a) *Hosts for* Nyctotherus *spp.*

Except where stated otherwise, all these records are those of Fantham and Porter (1950, 1952). Kudo (1966) recorded these parasites in amphibians but not in reptiles.
Order Chelonia
   Tortoises: *Testudo*.
   Terrapins: "Herbivorous turtles" recorded by Telford (1971).
Order Squamata (Suborder Lacertilia)
   Lizards: *Iguana, Trachydosaurus*.
   Geckos: *Tarentola*.
Order Squamata (Suborder Serpentes)
   Snakes: *Ablabophis, Agkistrodon, Boaedon, Leimadophis, Liophis, Opheodrys, Ophis, Pseudoboa, Trimerorhinus*.

V. Protozoa of Doubtful Taxonomic Position and Pathological Significance

The organisms listed below have all been recorded in reptiles but there is no evidence that any are pathogenic. The identity of some must remain in doubt especially those in early records and those not listed in reptiles by Kudo (1966).
   (a) *Alexeifella* in terrapins (*Lissemys* sp.) was listed by Murphy (1973) but not mentioned by Kudo (1966).
   (b) *Chilodon* (= *Chilodonella*) in the intestine of snakes (*Ablabophis*,

Boaedon, Naja and *Trimerorhinus*) was recorded by Fantham and Porter, (1950). The organism was not mentioned as a reptilian parasite by Kudo (1966).

(c) *Protoopalina* in the monitor lizard *Varanus niloticus* was reported by Lavier (1927) and quoted by Reichenbach-Klinke and Elkan (1965). Kudo (1966), however, only listed this organism as a parasite of axolotls and marine fish.

(d) *Sauroplasma* in chameleons (*Chamaeleo* spp.) and a girdled lizard (*Zonosaurus madagascariensis*) was recorded by Mackerras (1961) and in the sand lizard (*Lacerta agilis*) by Svahn (1976).

(e) *Trichocercomitus* (= *Trimitus*; = ? *Alexeifella*). There is little doubt that some of these organisms are flagellates belonging to the subphylum Sarcomastigophora, superclass Mastigophora, but others are of doubtful taxonomic position. Reichenbach-Klinke and Elkan (1965) referred to *Trichocercomitus* spp. in snakes and chelonians.

(f) *Tricercomonas* (= *Enteromonas*) was recorded in the intestines of snakes (*Causus* and *Dispholidus* spp.) by Fantham and Porter (1950) but was only recorded as a parasite of mammals by Kudo (1966).

(g) *Vahlkampfia* was recorded in the intestine of lizards (*Lacerta* and *Sceloporus* spp.) by Reichenbach-Klinke and Elkan (1965). Kudo (1966) did not list it as a parasite of reptiles.

(h) Miscellaneous genera. In addition to the genera listed above, Ball (1965) gave a useful summary of obscure protozoa and other bodies of uncertain nature found in the blood of reptiles and amphibians. These included the following "genera" which have not been mentioned previously in this chapter, namely: *Babesiosoma, Bertarellia, Besnomoitia, Cingula, Cytamoeba, Dactylosoma, Sauromella, Serpentoplasma, Toddia* and structures known as "Todd bodies".

Ball (1965) pointed out that many of these forms have been observed only in a single host or in very few hosts. Some may even be artefacts or viral in nature as recently shown (Stehbens and Johnston, 1966) for *Pirhemocyton* which was one of the organisms listed by Ball (1965).

Acknowledgements

The author is grateful for the invaluable help that was received from Dr J. R. Baker, Professor D. H. Molyneux and Dr R. Killick-Kendrick. The former helped to solve some of the difficult, protozoological, taxonomic problems of nomenclature and all lent reprints and drew the author's attention to many publications that might otherwise have been overlooked. Dr E. Elkan helped to translate most of the German papers quoted in the text and help was also obtained in this respect from Dr M. Böttcher.

References

Adler, S. (1964). *In* "Advances in Parasitology." (B. Dawes, ed.) Vol. 2, pp 35–96. Academic Press, London and New York.
Ayala, S. C. (1970). *J. Parasit.* **56,** 417–425.
Ayala, S. C. (1977). *In* "Parasitic Protozoa." (J. P. Kreier, ed.) Vol. III, pp 267–309. Academic Press, London and New York.
Ayala, S. C. (1978). *J. Protozool.* **25,** 87–100.
Baker, J. R. (1973). "Parasitic Protozoa." Hutchinson University Library, London.
Baker, J. R. (1977). *In* "Parasitic Protozoa." (J. P. Kreier, ed.) Vol. 1, pp 35–56. Academic Press, London and New York.
Ball, G. H. (1965). *In* "Progress in Protozoology." pp 127–128. Abstracts of papers presented at the second International Conference, London.
Ball, G. H. (1967). *J. Protozool.* **14,** 198–210.
Barker, D. C. (1965). *In* "Progress in Protozoology.", p 105. Abstract of papers read at the Second International Conference, London.
Belova, E. M. (1971). *Bull. Org. mond. Santé Bull. Wld. Hlth. Org.* **44,** 553–560.
Bonorris, J. S. and Ball, G. H. (1955). *J. Protozool.* **2,** 31–34.
Borst, G. H. A., Vroege, C., Poelma, F. G., Zwart, P., Strik, W. J. and Peters, J. C. (1972). *Acta zool. path. antverp.* **56,** 3–19.
Bosch, I. and Deichsel, G. (1972). *Z. ParasitKde.* **40,** 107–129.
Canning, E. J. (1977). *In* "Parasitic Protozoa." (J. P. Kreier, ed.) Vol. IV, pp 155–196. Academic Press, London and New York.
Canning, E. J., Elkan, E. and Trigg, P. I. (1964). *J. Protozool* **11,** 157–166.
Colley, F. C. and Else, J. G. (1975). *Annls Parasit. hum. comp.* **50,** 669–673.
Danilewsky, B. (1891). *Zentbl. Bakt. ParasitKde* I. **9,** 9–10.
Das Gupta, B. M. (1935). *J. Parasit.* **21,** 125–126.
Deakins, D. E. (1972). *Annual Proc. Am. Ass. Zoo Veterinarians*, 37–48, Washington D.C.
Debaisieux, P. (1919). *La Cellule* **30,** 153–183.
Dolensek, E. P., Bihn, J. P. and Napolitano, R. L. (1976). *J. Protozool.* **23,**(2) 19A.
Donaldson, M., Heyneman, D., Dempster, R. and Garcia, L. (1975). *Am. J. vet. Res.* **36,** 807–817.
Elkan, E. (1976). *In* "Krankheiten der Reptilien." (H. H. Reichenbach-Klinke, ed.) p 59. G. Fischer, Stuttgart and New York.
Fantham, H. B. (1932). *S. Afr. J. Sci.* **29,** 627–640.
Fantham, H. B. and Porter, A. (1950). *Proc. zool. Soc. Lond.* **120,** 599–647.
Fantham, H. B. and Porter, A. (1952). *Proc. zool. Soc. Lond.* **123,** 867–898.
Frank, W. (1966). *Z. ParasitKde.* **27,** 317–335.
Frank, W. and Bosch, I. (1972). *Z. ParasitKde.* **40,** 139–150.

Frank, W., Sachsse, W. and Winkelsträter, K. H. (1976a). *Salamandra* **12,** 120–126.
Frank, W., Bachmann, U. and Braun, R. (1976b). *Salamandra* **12,** 94–102.
Frank, W. and Sigmund, U. (1976). *Kleintier-Praxis* **21,** 196–205.
Gabrisch, K. (1976). *Praktische Tierarzt.* **57,** 37–40.
Gabrisch, K. (1977). *Veterinary Medical Review* **1,** 98–101.
Garnham, P. C. C. (1966a). *Parasitology* **56,** 329–334.
Garnham, P. C. C. (1966b). "Malaria Parasites and Other Haemosporidia". Blackwell Scientific Publications, Oxford.
Garnham, P. C. C. (1971). *Bull. Org. mond. Santé Bull. Wld. Hlth. Org.* **44,** 477–489.
Geiman, Q. M. and Ratcliffe, H. L. (1936). *Parasitology* **28,** 208–228.
Ghosh, T. N. (1968). *J. Protozool.* **15,** 164–166.
Gorgas, ——. (1964). 35th Ann. Report U.S. Govt. Printing Office, Washington, D.C. Quoted by Garnham, P. C. C. (1966) *In* "Malaria Parasites and Other Haemosporidia." p 820. Blackwell Scientific Publications, Oxford.
Gray, C. W., Marcus, L. C., McCarten, W. C. and Sappington, T. (1966). *Int. Zoo Yb.* **6,** 279–283.
Guyénot, E. and Naville, A. (1920). *C. r. Séanc. Soc. Biol.* **83,** 965–966.
Guyénot, E. and Naville, A. (1922). *Revue suisse Zool.* **30,** 1–62.
Hilgenfeld, M. (1968). *In* "Erkrankungen der Zootiere." Verh. Ber. X Int. Symp. Erk. der Zootiere, Salzburg, pp 67–72. Akademie Verlag, Berlin.
Hill, W. C. O. and Neal, R. A. (1952). *Proc. zool. Soc. Lond.* **123,** 731–737.
Hoare, C. A. (1920). *Parasitology* **12,** 315–327.
Hoare, C. A. (1932). *Parasitology* **24,** 210–224.
Honigberg, B. M., Balamuth, W., Bovee, E. C., Corliss, J. O., Gojdics, M., Hall, R. P., Kudo, R. R., Levine, N. D., Loeblich, A. R., Weiser, J. and Wenrich, D. H. (1964). *J. Protozool.* **11,** 7–20.
Huff, C. G. and Marchbank, D. F. (1953). *Nav. med. Res. Inst. Res. Rep.* **11,** 509–516.
Hunsaker, D. (1966). *Int. Turtle Tortoise Soc. J.* **1,** 6–7, 23, 37, 46.
Ippen, R. (1959). *Kleintier-Praxis* **4,** 131–137.
Ippen, R. (1965). *Zbl. allg. Path.* **107,** 520–529.
Ippen, R. (1971). *In* "Erkrankungen der Zootiere." Verh. Ber. XIII Int. Symp. Erk. der Zootiere, Helsinki, pp 173–187. Akademie Verlag, Berlin.
Jackson, O. F. (1976). *In* "A Manual of the Care and Treatment of Children's and Exotic Pets." (A. F. Cowie, ed.) pp 24, 26. British Veterinary Association, London.
Janakidevi, K. (1961). *Parasitology* **52,** 165–168.
Keymer, I. F. (1970). *In* "Scientific Report 1967–69." pp 15–16. Zoological Society of London, London.
Keymer, I. F. (1972). *J. Zool. Lond.* **166,** 538.
Keymer, I. F. (1976). *J. Zool. Lond.* **178,** 471.
Keymer, I. F. (1978). *Vet. Rec.* **103,** 548–552.
Keymer, I. F. (1978). *Vet. Rec.* **103,** 577–582.

Killick-Kendrick, R. (1979). *In* "Biology of the Kinetoplastida." (W. H. R. Lumsden and D. A. Evans, eds) Vol. 2, pp 395–460. Academic Press, London and New York.
Kramer, M. (1972). *Lacerta* **30,** 87–96.
Kreier, J. P. (1977a). "Parasitic Protozoa." Vol. I. Academic Press, London and New York.
Kreier, J. P. (1977b). "Parasitic Protozoa." Vol. III. Academic Press, London and New York.
Kreier, J. P. (1977c). "Parasitic Protozoa." Vol. IV. Academic Press, London and New York.
Kreier, J. P. (1978). "Parasitic Protozoa." Vol. II. Academic Press, London and New York.
Kudo, R. (1919). *Illinois biol. Monogr.* **5,** 3–4.
Kudo, R. H. (1966). "Protozoology." 5th edition. Charles C. Thomas, Illinois.
Kulda, J. and Nohýnková, E. (1978). *In* "Parasitic Protozoa." (J. P. Kreier, ed.) Vol. II., pp 1–138. Academic Press, London and New York.
Lainson, R. (1977). *In* "Protozoology." Vol. III, pp 87–93. London School of Hygiene and Tropical Medicine, London.
Lainson, R., Landau, I. and Shaw, J. J. (1971). *Int. J. Parasit.* **1,** 241–250.
Lainson, R., Landau, I. and Shaw, J. J. (1974). *Parasitology* **68,** 117–125.
Lainson, R. and Shaw, J. J. (1969). *Parasitology* **59,** 159–162.
Lainson, R. and Shaw, J. J. (1971). *J. Protozool.* **18,** 365–372.
Lainson, R. and Shaw, J. J. (1972). *J. Protozool.* **19,** 212.
Lainson, R., Shaw, J. J. and Landau, I. (1975). *Parasitology* **70,** 119–141.
Landau, I., Chabaud, A. G., Michell, J. C. and Brygoo, E. (1970). *J. Protozool.* **17,** (Suppl.), 36.
Lavier, G. (1927). *C. R. Soc. Biol. Paris* **97,** 1709–1710.
Lehmann, H. D. (1972). *Salamandra* **8,** 48–49.
Levine, N. D. (1973). "Protozoan Parasites of Domestic Animals and Man." 2nd edition. Burgess Publishing Company, Minnesota.
Liu, S.-K. and King, F. W. (1971). *J. Am. vet. med. Ass.* **159,** 1578–1582.
McConnachie, E. W. (1954). *Parasitology* **44,** 342–348.
McConnachie, E. W. (1975). *Parasitology* **45,** 452–481.
Mackerras, M. J. (1961). *Aust. J. Zool.* **9,** 61–122.
Maier-Rittermann, P. F. (1973). *Zool. Gart., Lpz.* **43,** 144–147.
Manson-Bahr, P. E. C. and Heisch, R. B. (1961). *Ann. trop. Med. Parasit.* **55,** 381–382.
Matthews, L. H., Carrington, R., Boorer, M. and Oates, J. F. (1970). "The Living World of Animals." Classification of Reptiles, pp 392–395. Reader's Digest Association, in conjunction with World Wildlife Fund, London.
Meerovitch, E. (1958). *Can. J. Zool.* **36,** 513–523.
Mitchell, L. G. (1977). *In* "Parasitic Protozoa." (J. P. Kreier, ed.) Vol. IV, pp 115–154. Academic Press, London and New York.
Mohiuddin, A. (1959). *E. Afr. med. J.* **36,** 171–176.
Molyneux, D. H. (1977). *In* "Advances in Parasitology." (B. Dawes, ed.)

Vol. 15, pp 11–14. Academic Press, London and New York.
Murphy, J. B. (1973). *Hiss News-Journal* **1,** 123–128.
Noble, E. R. and Noble, G. A. (1976). "Parasitology. The Biology of Animal Parasites". Lea and Febiger, Philadelphia.
Page, L. A. (1966). *Bull. Wildl. Dis. Assoc.* **2,** 111–126.
Parenzan, P. (1947). *Boll. Soc. Nat. Napoli* **55,** 117–119.
Paterson, W. B. and Dresser, S. S. (1976). *J. Protozool.* **33,** 294–301.
Pellérdy, L. P. (1963). "Catalogue of Eimeriidea (Protozoa, Sporozoa). Class Reptilia" 109–112. Akadémiai Kiadó, Budapest.
Pellérdy, L. P. (1969). "Catalogue of Eimeriidea (Protozoa, Sporozoa) Supplementum 1. Class Reptilia." pp 58–59. Akadémiai Kiadó, Budapest.
Pellérdy, L. P. (1974). "Coccidia and Coccidiosis." 2nd edition. Verlag Paul Parey, Berlin and Hamburg.
Ratcliffe, H. L. and Geiman, Q. M. (1934). *Science, N. Y.* **79,** 324–325.
Reichenbach-Klinke, H. and Elkan, E. (1965). "The Principal Diseases of Lower Vertebrates. Book III; Diseases of Reptiles". T. F. H. Publications, New Jersey.
Reichenbach-Klinke, H. H. (1977). "Krankheiten der Reptilien". 2nd edition. G. Fischer Verlag, Stuttgart and New York.
Rodhain, J. (1934). *C. R. Soc. Biol. Paris.* **117,** 1195–1199.
Sargeaunt, P. G. and Williams, J. E. (1978). *Trans. R. Soc. trop. Med.* **72,** 164–166.
Schneider, C. R. (1965). *J. Parasit.* **51,** 340–344.
Schneider, C. R. (1967). *J. Protozool.* **14,** 674–678.
Steck, F. (1961). *Abt. I. Originale Zentbl. Bakt. ParasitKde I* **181,** 551–553.
Steck, F. (1962). *Acta trop.* **19,** 318–354.
Stehbens, W. E. and Johnston, M. R. L. (1966). *J. Ultrastruct. Res.* **15,** 543–554.
Svahn, K. (1975). *Norw. J. Zool.* **23,** 277–295.
Svahn, K. (1976). *Norw. J. Zool.* **24,** 1–6.
Telford, S. R. (1971). *J. Am. vet. med. Ass.* **159,** 1644–1652.
Tiegs, O. W. (1931). *Parasitology* **23,** 412–414.
Vetterling, J. M. and Widmer, E. A. (1968). *J. Parasit.* **54,** 569–576.
Wacha, R. S. and Christiansen, J. L. (1976). *J. Protozool.* **23,** 57–63.
Wallach, J. M. (1969). *J. Am. vet. med. Ass.* **155,** 1017–1034.
Walliker, D. (1965). *Parasitology* **55,** 601–606.
Weber, A. (1910). *Arch. Anat. Micr.* **11,** 167–178.
Wenyon, C. M. (1926). "Protozoology." Vols. 1 and 2. Baillière, Tindall and Cox, London.
Will, R. (1975). *Zbl. Vet. Med. B.* **22,** 626–634.
Wilson, V. C. L. C. and Southgate, B. A. (1979). *In* "Biology of the Kinetoplastida." (W. H. R. Lumsden and D. A. Evans, eds) Vol. 2, pp 241–268. Academic Press, London and New York.
Wood, S. F. (1935). *Zoology* **41,** 9–22. University of California Publications.
Zwart, P. (1964). *J. Protozool.* **11,** 261–263.
Zwart, P. (1973). *Lacerta* **31,** 116–120.

Zwart, P. (1977). *In* "Proceedings 6th World Congress, World Small Animal Veterinary Association, Voorjaarsdagen 1977." The Netherlands Small Animal Veterinary Association, Post Academisch Onderwijs Publikatie No. 8, 40–42.

Zwart, P., Borst, G. H. A. and Truyens, E. H. A. (1976). *In* "Erkrankungen der Zootiere." Verh. Ber. XVII Int. Symp. Erk. der Zootiere, Tunis pp 317–319. Akademic Verlag, Berlin.

Zwart, P. and Truyens, E. H. A. (1975). *Vet. Parasit.* **1,** 175–183.

9 Endoparasites

W. FRANK*

Universität Hohenheim, Abteilung Parasitologie, D7000 Stuttgart 70, Emil-Wolff Strasse 34, West Germany

I. Introduction

The reptiles are suitable intermediate, paratenic and definitive hosts for many endoparasites, including the protozoa (see Chapter 8).

The noxious effect of parasites is accentuated when reptiles are kept in captivity where reinfection with reproductive stages can lead to heavy parasitism and death of the host; common examples include ascarid worms in pythons and oxyurid worms in iguanids.

Even in natural surroundings parasites can multiply excessively. Kutzer and Grünberg (1965a) reported that an *Eunectes murinus* was infested with 1547 specimens of the tapeworm *Crepidobothrium gerrardii* and Frank and Loos-Frank (1977) found over 1000 cestodes of the genus *Bothridium* in a *Python reticulatus*. In both these cases the parasites were considered to be the cause of death.

Various papers on reptilian disease have emphasized the importance of endoparasites. For example, Ippen (1971) carried out 1100 dissections of reptiles and reported a 40 per cent mortality rate due to parasites. Martin (1972) searched for helminths in 287 turtles belonging to seven American species and found 80·8 per cent to be parasitized; the 125 *Pseudemys scripta* examined in this series were all found to harbour worm parasites. Extensive reviews of parasites affecting reptiles have been published by Reichenbach-Klinke (1977), Reichenbach-Klinke and Elkan (1965), Page (1966), Marcus (1968), Wallach (1969), Telford (1970), Frye (1973), Zwart (1972, 1973, 1974), Frank (1976b), Frank and Loos-Frank (1977) and Cooper (1974).

* Dedicated to the author's most esteemed teacher, Prof Dr O. Pflugfelder, on the occasion of his 75th birthday (15.2.79).

Many animals have an obligatory or facultative relationship with others. Optimally this is a symbiotic relationship with mutual benefit or a type of commensalism where the smaller and less well organized partner utilizes food which is of no value for the host. The borderline between symbiosis, commensalism and parasitism is ill-defined; parasites are dependent on their hosts, but it is frequently not easy to decide whether they are detrimental. In some instances the relationship may be well balanced and neither party appears to suffer. In other instances the parasite is pathogenic and the host shows clinical signs of disease or may die from the infection.

Laboratory techniques for the demonstration of parasites are discussed in Chapter 4. However, brief mention should be made of helminth eggs and larvae.

Eggs of helminths (and pentastomids) living in the lung are usually shed in the faeces, as are those of species parasitizing the intestinal tract, the bile-ducts and the gall bladder. Eggs of trematodes and a few nematodes inhabiting the ureter or the tubules of the kidney are found in the urates. Eggs of pentastomids and certain nematodes may also be observed in the oral mucus and in a few cases—for example members of the order Rhabditida—larvae may also be seen in this site.

Helminth eggs can be demonstrated using standard techniques but it is often difficult to identify them. No comprehensive illustrated keys exist and reference must be made to publications such as Frank and Reichel (1977).

The term "pseudoparasite" is sometimes used. This refers to organisms which are normally parasites of earthworms, insects, snails and other prey items of reptiles. Most are eggs of helminths and of mites but whole mites and eggs of pentastomids may pass through the intestinal tract and be found in the faeces of reptiles.

In captive reptiles fed on mice and rats the developmental stages of *Demodex* species (mites) may be found since these mites are common in laboratory rodents. Mice and rats from particularly unhygienic breeding colonies may also harbour other mites, such as *Myobia*, *Sarcoptes* and *Notoedres* spp. while spoiled dry food given to chelonians or iguanas may contain mites of the family Tyroglyphidae.

Nematode and cestode eggs may also originate from rodents or birds supplied as food. Examples of rodent parasites are the nematode *Syphacia* and the cestode *Hymenolepis*.

Examination of the faeces of snakes of the genus *Thamnophis* frequently yields primary and secondary cysts of gregarines (*Monocystis agilis*) which live in the seminal vesicles of earthworms, a common food of these reptiles.

II. Main Sites for Parasites in Reptiles

(This table should be read in conjunction with Chapters 8 and 10.)

Skin (external surface):   Ectoparasites (mites and ticks)

Skin (internal surface):   Dracunculoidea. Plerocercoids of pseudophyllidean cestodes. *Capillaria recurva* eggs in *Crocodylus acutus*.

Intestinal tract

Oral cavity: Trematodes, nematodes (*Rhabdias*) in crypts and in dental abscesses. Rarely Pentastomida.

Oesophagus: Nematodes (*Kalicephalus*), Trematodes (rarely).

Stomach: Nematodes (Ascaridida, Spirurida). Nematode larvae in the gastric wall.

Mid-gut: Nematodes (*Kalicephalus*, *Capillaria* and others). Cestodes (*Bothridium*, *Ophiotaenia* and others). Acanthocephala (very rarely).
Flagellates (trichomonads in cases of bacterial enteritis). *Entamoeba invadens* (rare). Coccidial oocysts.
Sarcocystis oocysts and/or sporocysts (rare).

Colon: Nematodes (oxyurids and others).
Flagellates (*Leptomonas*, Bodonidae, Trichomonadidae, Opalinidae (rare)). *Entamoeba invadens* and other amoebae. Ciliatea.

Mesentery and serous membranes of the intestinal tract: Trematode larvae (metacercariae). Larvae of acanthocephalan plerocercoids, tetrathyrids. Larvae of Trypanorhynchidae (in sea snakes and sea turtles only). Nematode larvae. Dracunculoidea, Filarioidea.
Pentastomid larvae (very rare).

Abdominal cavity: Dracunculoidea (rare), Filarioidea.

Muscular system: Plerocercoids, nematode larvae. Larvae of Acanthocephala. Dracunculoidea, Filarioidea (rare). Spiruroid larvae (Gnathostomatidae) (very rare). "Miescher's tubes" (*Sarcocystis* stages), *Besnoitia* cysts.

Serous membranes: Dracunculoidea. Filarioidea.

Fat body:	Metacercariae. Vegetative stages of "haemogregarines".
Heart:	Filarioidea (lumen). Nematode larvae around the heart (rare). "Miescher's tubes" in the muscle.
Blood vessels:	Spirochidae, especially in turtles (rare). Filarioidea.
Blood, circulating:	Trypanosomes and microfilariae in plasma. In the cells: malaria parasites, "*Babesia*" (both rare). Gametocytes of haemogregarines (very common). Gametocytes of *Saurocytozoon* (very rare), gametocytes of Haemoproteidae (very rare).
Lungs:	Vegetative stages of "haemogregarines" and species of *Saurocytozoon* and *Plasmodium*. *Entamoeba invadens*. Larvae of Ascaridida (rare).
Gall bladder:	Flagellates (trichomonads), Coccidia, Trematodes.
Bile-ducts in the liver:	(Coccidia). Trematodes.
Pancreas:	Vegetative stages of "haemogregarines". Trematodes.
Spleen:	Vegetative stages of "haemogregarines" and species of *Plasmodium*.
Kidney:	Trematodes. Vegetative stages of "haemogregarines" and other Adeleidea (*Klossiella*). Coccidia.
Oviduct:	Nematodes (extremely rare).
Brain:	Vegetative stages of "haemogregarines". *Besnoitia*.
Cloaca and nostrils:	Fly larvae (myiasis in tortoises—rare). Mites (rare).

III. Zoonoses

With a few exceptions mature reptilian parasites are species specific and pose no threat to humans.

The importance of reptiles as reservoir hosts for arboviruses is discussed in Chapters 5 and 10.

Where mammals function as intermediate hosts of parasites man may occasionally be drawn into the cycle—for example, in some species of Pentastomida and certain spirurid worms (Daengsvang, 1949; Mazaud *et al*, 1973).

In Asia, open wounds are sometimes treated by the application of reptilian meat and this may facilitate the introduction of plerocercoids of Diphyllobothriidae.

IV–V. GROUPS OF ENDOPARASITES

IV. Phylum Parenchymia
A. Subphylum Platyhelminthes (Flatworms)

The subphylum is divided into three classes, the Turbellaria, the Trematoda (flukes) and the Cestoda (tapeworms). The turbellarians are mainly free-living; only members of the order Neorhabdocoela live as commensals or parasites on invertebrates and vertebrates (turtles). All the trematodes and the cestodes, on the other hand, are vertebrate parasites as adults. Their immature stages are commonly found in invertebrate hosts but various vertebrates can also serve as intermediate hosts for certain cestodes.

Trematodes have a varying number of intermediate hosts. Only the Monogenea have a direct life-cycle while the Digenea may require one or several intermediate hosts to complete their life-cycle.

(1) Class Trematoda (Flukes)

This class is divided into three subclasses, the Monogenea, the Aspidogastrea and the Digenea. The last group consists of those trematodes which are of most importance to man and vertebrates. Monogeneans are mainly found on the skin, the gills and in the mouth cavity of fish; they are less commonly seen in amphibians and rarely in reptiles, with the exception of chelonians where they may inhabit the urinary bladder and the naso-pharyngeal area. Only about 40 species are known of the less important Aspidogastrea but their distribution is world-wide. They are found in invertebrates (for example crustaceans) and occasionally in lower vertebrates.

Subclass Monogenea

Few of these flukes exceed 3 mm in length. They have a direct life-cycle, with no intermediate host.

Monogenetic trematodes occur mainly on fish. A few are known from amphibians and only about 20 species from reptiles. The latter are all in the family Polystomatidae (Bychowsky, 1962; Yamaguti, 1963a).

These parasites inhabit the urinary bladder of turtles (*Polystomoidella* spp.), the nostrils and the urinary bladder (*Neopolystoma* spp.), or the urinary bladder, the nasal passages, the oropharynx and the oesophagus (*Polystomoides* spp.). The report of *Neopolystoma orbiculare* in a chelonian lung (Reichenbach-Klinke, 1977) may have been due to *post mortem* migration.

The main hosts of these parasites are freshwater chelonians of the genera *Amyda* (syn. *Trionyx*), *Chelodina*, *Chrysemys*, *Clemmys*, *Emys*, *Geoemyda*, *Graptemys*, *Kachuga*, *Kinosternon*, *Malaclemys*, *Pseudemys*, *Sternotherus* (*Trionyx*). It is doubtful whether the genus *Terrapene*, which is mainly terrestrial, should be included in the list.

Clinical signs None reported.
Pathology Not reported.
Diagnosis Characteristic eggs, often with filaments, are found in the appropriate part of the body.

Subclass Aspidogastrea (Aspidocotylea)

These flatworms live deeply embedded in their hosts and have a large ventral holdfast organ with a chambered sucking disc. Rohde (1972), when discussing these parasites, pointed out that they seem to combine features of both the Monogenea and the Digenea. He stated that they "are most closely related to the Digenea but a number of reasons can be given for placing the Aspidogastrea in a group of their own." All the species known up to 1958 were discussed by Dollfus (1958a) and subsequently listed by Yamaguti (1963a).

The invertebrate hosts of these parasites are freshwater snails of the families Ampullariidae, Viviparidae and Bythiniidae.

Aspidogastrea occur in both sea and freshwater vertebrates. About 40 species are known but representatives of only four genera (*Lophotoaspis*, *Cotylaspis*, *Multicotyle* and *Lyssemysai*) parasitize chelonians.

Clinical signs None reported.
Pathology Not reported.

Subclass Digenea (Flukes)

Digenetic trematodes parasitize a number of organs in vertebrates but the digestive system, bile-ducts and gall bladder are mainly affected.

There are numerous publications which deal with their taxonomy, for example Yamaguti (1958, 1971) and Skrjabin (1947–1964). Studies on their life-cycle, on the other hand, are rare (Yamaguti, 1975) and there are few publications dealing with their pathology in reptiles.

The subclass Digenea embraces two orders of which only one, the Prostomatida, are parasites of reptiles.

The biology of digenetic trematodes

(a) *Adults*

Although only a few life-cycles are known it can be assumed that most follow a similar pattern. The eggs are shed with the faeces, urine or oral mucus. In the case of the Spirorchidae, which live in blood vessels, this necessitates traversing tissue barriers. In many species free-swimming miracidia emerge from the eggs and these are capable of penetrating a first intermediate host, commonly an aquatic snail, where further development (sporocyst, redia and daughter generations) occur up to the cercarial stage. In a number of species however, free-swimming miracidia are not known; the eggs must be ingested by suitable snails in whose digestive tract the miracidia emerge. The specificity for molluscs is very strict and in many cases only closely related species of snails are acceptable as hosts.

One miracidium can produce innumerable cercariae, the larvae of the next generation. These larvae leave the snail host and live free in the environment. They must either locate a suitable second intermediate host or penetrate the skin of a definitive host. The complicated life-cycle of these trematodes inhibits the spread of infection from one reptile to another in captivity.

(b) *Larvae*

Reptiles may occasionally serve as second intermediate hosts for trematode species of other reptiles, birds or mammals. These metacercariae are frequently found in the mesenteries and the fat body. For example, Odening (1960, 1961) reported metacercariae of *Neodiplostomulum* spp. in snakes (*Natrix natrix* and *Vipera berus*) in Europe; as adults these trematodes parasitize birds. It is not known as yet whether reptiles may play any part in the life-cycles of trematodes injurious to man.

Clinical signs Not characteristic; anorexia has been reported in infections with adult *Styphlodora* spp.

Pathology Although trematodes are commonly seen in reptiles little has been published on their pathology. Perhaps the best documented cases are where the kidneys are infested with *Styphlodora* spp. (Grünberg and Kutzer, 1964; Tury and Kobulej, 1973a,b; Kazacos and Fisher, 1977.) Reichenbach-Klinke quoted Elkan who found 37 specimens of *Styphlodora horrida* in a *Boa constrictor*. The author examined a young *Python reticulatus* which harboured several hundred specimens of the same genus in its ureters and a water snake (*Erpeton tentaculatum*) where the gall bladder was affected by trematodes (Frank, 1966a).

Styphlodora spp. bear spines which may damage the renal tubules. The widely dilated ureters can usually be detected with the naked eye and if the worms are very numerous the colour of the ureter changes to white or yellow or its lumen may be filled with pale yellow material. The latter consists of mucus and cellular debris which contains the brown-coloured trematodes. The kidneys in such cases may show white lesions, these being tubules filled with urates. Nephritis and visceral gout may result.

The histology of such cases was described by Grünberg and Kutzer (1964) who found three different species of *Styphlodora* in 8 boids (*Python* spp. and *Boa constrictor*). Tury and Kobulej (1973a,b) recorded *S. condita* in a *Boa constrictor* and Kazacos and Fisher (1977) found *S. horrida* in the same species. According to Tury and Kobulej (1973a) the narrower the tubules the more severe the pathological changes. Grünberg and Kutzer (1964) reported severe damage to the tubular epithelium while Kazacos and Fisher described "tubular epithelial hyperplasia". Tury and Kobulej (1973a) noted that the epithelium in some areas was replaced by giant cells.

The severity of the damage depends on the number of worms and the consequent deposition of urates. The bulk of the ureteric debris consists of urates mixed with small amounts of salts of calcium and mucopolysaccharides, the latter being derived from disintegrated parasites. It may, however, take several years—30 months according to Grünberg and Kutzer (1964)—before the affected animal dies.

Infestation of the gall bladder of several *Erpeton tentaculatum* snakes with *Gogatea serpentium* was described by Frank (1966a). Blockage of the main bile duct caused concentration of the bile, back pressure and the accumulation of material containing trematodes and thousands of eggs. In view of the disparity between the number of worms and the number of eggs a long standing condition was suspected and this was supported by the thickness of the walls of the bile-duct and the gall

9 ENDOPARASITES 299

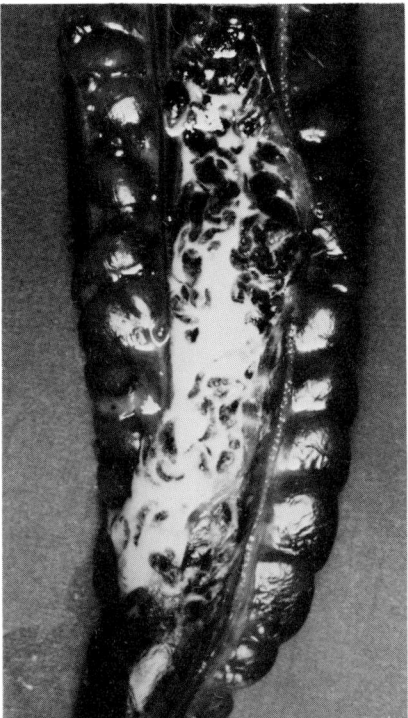

Fig. 9.1. Ureter of python (*Python reticulatus*) opened to show dilatation caused by trematodes of the genus *Styphlodora*. Between the numerous flukes the white deposits of uric acid can be seen.

bladder. The outcome was severe jaundice which eventually killed the snake.

Sections of kidneys, livers and bile-ducts of reptiles frequently show portions of undetermined trematodes without any concomitant pathological changes. These trematodes are often too small to be detected at *post mortem* examination. They do not seem to endanger the reptile's health.

Trematode infections are diagnosed on the appearance of the eggs, which are usually operculated. The eggs may contain a number of blastomeres or a miracidium. (See Fig. 9.10.)

(2) Class Cestoidea (Tapeworms)

The Class Cestoidea is divided into two subclasses, the Cestodaria

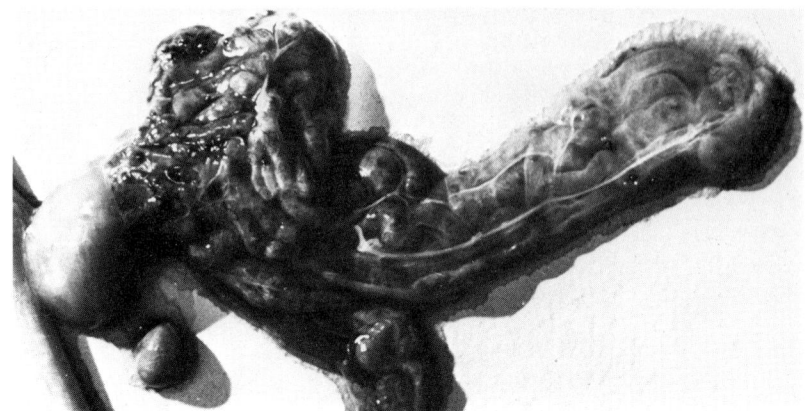

Fig. 9.2. Numerous trematodes of the genus *Infidum* have caused diverticula in the wall of the gall bladder of a colubrid snake.

(unsegmented tapeworms) and the Eucestodea (segmented or true tapeworms), the latter being generally known as cestodes.

Detailed descriptions of the biology of cestodes may be found in Wardle and McLeod (1968), Freeman (1973), Šlais (1973), Voge (1967, 1973) and Wardle *et al* (1974).

More than a thousand cestode species have been described. The mature worms parasitize the intestinal tract of all classes of vertebrates. In rare cases they may be found in ducts, such as those of the pancreas and gall bladder, which are in direct communication with the gut. Shoop and Janovy (1978) recorded mature cestodes (*Oochoristica bivitellobata*) in the coelomic cavity of a lizard (*Cnemidophorus sexlineatus*) but this may have been due to contamination at some stage.

In general the development of the cestodes is less complicated than that of the trematodes. The multiplication of larvae in a first intermediate host is absent in most cestodes. Only the larvae of some genera are capable of vegetative budding and in reptiles this appears to be restricted to second stage of larvae (tetrathyridia) of the genus *Mesocestoides* (Specht and Voge, 1965).

Accounts of the ontogeny and the larval development of cestodes may be found in Freeman (1973), Šlais (1973) and Voge (1967, 1973).

Reptiles may serve as definitive hosts of mature tapeworms but appear less often infested than other vertebrates.

In addition to the comprehensive systematic treatment by Yamaguti (1959) attention must be drawn to the publications by Spasskii

(1951) and Freze (1965) and other texts which limit themselves to certain geographical regions, for example Brazil (Rego, 1973).

In addition to functioning as definitive hosts, reptiles may also serve as intermediate hosts for cestodes whose definitive hosts are other vertebrates. They may be first intermediate, second intermediate or, occasionally, paratenic hosts.

Several authors have emphasized that cestode infestation is relatively uncommon in reptiles. Ippen (1965), for example, found only 30 such cases in 500 *post mortem* examinations of captive reptiles; 73 reptiles from the same series were infested with nematodes.

Subclass Cestodaria (Unsegmented tapeworms)

The Cestodaria mainly parasitize the gut and the coelomic cavity of various primitive fish but are occasionally found in chelonians. They display characters of both the trematodes and the true tapeworms.

The absence of a gut and the embryonic development indicate their relationship to the cestodes (Price, 1967).

Classification and biology

Only one species, *Austramphilina elongata*, belonging to the order Amphilinidea, has been found in chelonians. It parasitizes the body cavity of the freshwater terrapin *Chelodina longicollis* in Australia. The exact biology of this species is not yet known. It is probably similar to that in fish, starting with a procercoid in small crustaceans (amphipods) and progressing to a plerocercoid-like stage which develops either in the amphipod or in a second intermediate host.

Neither clinical signs nor pathological lesions have been reported.

Subclass Cestoda (True tapeworms)

Of all the metazoan parasites the tapeworms are among the most highly specialized. At the distal end of the strobila, the chain of proglottides, gravid segments filled with eggs are constantly discarded and passed out whole with the faeces (apolytic forms), or the eggs escape from the uterine pore into the host's intestinal lumen (anapolytic forms). In the latter case single eggs, egg-clusters or egg-capsules are found in the faeces while the emptied proglottides are digested.

The proximal end of a tapeworm bears a special holdfast organ, the scolex, which is equipped with sucking structures and often, in addition, with hooks.

All true tapeworms start life as a first-stage larva (the oncosphere or hexacanth larva) which is enveloped in several membranes or sheaths. With a few exceptions all cestodes require at least one, sometimes two or more, intermediate hosts. Adult tapeworms vary in size from 1 mm to 30 metres; even species parasitizing reptiles may reach a length of 1 metre. A large number of adult worms may be found inhabiting the same host; Kutzer and Grünberg (1965a) reported 1547 specimens of *Crepidobothrium* in an anaconda (*Eunectes murinus*). Under such circumstances the presence of many cestodes in one host may prevent all of them from reaching maturity, a fact which suggests a reciprocal crowding effect (Frank, 1976b; Frank and Loos-Frank, 1977). The latter authors found more than 1000 specimens of *Bothridium pithonis* in a *Python reticulatus* which has been in captivity for several months. *B. pithonis* is a fast-growing species of tapeworm and needs only a few weeks to reach maturity. However, in spite of this all the parasites were immature.

A summary of the pathogenicity of tapeworms was published by Rees in 1967. Adult tapeworms do not generally appear to injure their hosts and Rees could not quote one example of reptiles being injured by tapeworms. Cooper (1973) mentioned that "proglottides are commonly passed per cloacam by freshly caught snakes but these parasites do not seem to be pathogenic". However, Jackson and Muller (1976) reported clinical signs of weight loss and fatality associated with tapeworms, and other evidence of pathogenicity is discussed later.

Classification

Adult tapeworms found in reptiles belong to the orders Proteocephalidea, Pseudophyllidea and Cyclophyllidea. Some members of other orders use reptiles as intermediate and paratenic hosts or may infest them accidentally. For example, larval stages of trypanorhynchid cestodes are often found in sea snakes (*Laticauda* spp.) (Frank, unpublished) and, rarely, in sea turtles and crocodiles.

Present understanding of cestode biology has been summarized by Wardle and McLeod (1968), Freeman (1973) Šlais (1973), Voge (1967, 1973) and Wardle *et al* (1974).

ORDER PROTEOCEPHALIDEA

(a) *Adults*

The mature worms of this order are small and inhabit the small intestine of various reptiles, mainly snakes and varanid lizards. The development cycle includes an oncosphere, a procercoid in small crustaceans and a plerocercoid either in invertebrates or in vertebrates serving as paratenic (or intermediate) hosts. A second intermediate host does not seem to be obligatory. Proteocephalan cestodes are mainly found in evolutionary ancient hosts and are generally regarded as primitive forms.

The order represents more than half of all the tapeworms found in reptiles. Most of them (about 50) belong to the genus *Ophiotaenia* and another 25, according to Yamaguti (1959), to the genera *Proteocephalus*, *Acanthotaenia* and *Crepidobothrium*.

Proteocephalus	Mainly in varanid lizards
Acanthotaenia	Mainly in varanids, rarely in snakes
Crepidobothrium	In snakes
Ophiotaenia	Mainly in snakes, rarely in saurians or in aquatic chelonians

Biology

Only the life-cycles of a few species found in reptiles are fully known. It can probably be assumed, however, that those of the Proteocephalidea are similar.

The eggs, excreted with the faeces, are usually free and not within a proglottis. They are distinguished by their thin-walled "embryophore" which contains one or several oncospheres. These eggs are taken up by small crustaceans (Copepoda) and in the haemocoel of the latter they subsequently develop into a procercoid. If infested copepods are ingested by a suitable definitive host the procercoids invade the intestinal wall, the liver or the muscles and develop into the next stage, the plerocercoid. Having reached this stage the larvae return to the intestinal canal, evert their scolex and mature.

Since they are resistant to digestive juices of vertebrates plerocercoid larvae can use tadpoles, frogs, fish and possibly also reptiles as paratenic hosts. True second intermediate hosts do not seem to be obligatory. Experimental studies have been carried out on several species of the genus *Ophiotaenia* but not as yet for species belonging to the other genera.

Proteocephalus niloticus probably requires three hosts: a crustacean (as yet unidentified) for the development of the procercoid, an amphibian (frog) for the plerocercoid and monitor lizards (*Varanus niloticus*) for the adult stage (Rees, 1963). *Ophiotaenia perspicua* occurs in *Natrix rhombifer*, *N. sipedon* and *Thamnophis sirtalis*. Intermediate hosts are *Cyclops viridis*, *C. vulgaris*, *Mesocyclops obsoletus* and *Microcyclops varicans*. Paratenic hosts are tadpoles and frogs of *Rana clamitans*, *R. pipiens* and *Umbra lima* (Thomas, 1934, 1941; Herde, 1938). *Ophiotaenia racemosa* occurs in *Liophis merremi*, *Coluber* spp. and *Natrix natrix*. Larvae have been found in *Cyclops* spp. in a fish (*Salmo irideus*) (Joyeux and Baer, 1933, 1936). *Ophiotaenia testudo* occurs in *Amyda* (syn. *Trionyx*) *spinifera*. The life-cycle was studied by Magath (1929). *Ophiotaenia japonensis* occurs in *Natrix tigrina* and *Elaphe quadrivirgata*. Plerocercoids found in *Rana nigromaculata* are possibly the larval stages of this species (Yamaguti, 1935, 1959).

Clinical signs None documented but anorexia may occur in cases of heavy infestation.

Pathology Kutzer and Grünberg (1965a) gave a detailed account of a severe infestation of an anaconda (*Eunectes murinus*), the parasites being *Crepidobothrium gerrardii*. The snake had been in captivity for six years and *post mortem* examination yielded 1547 tapeworms. Although the snake had fed regularly it appeared emaciated when it died.

Kutzer and Grünberg found the majority of the cestodes in the proximal section of the mid-gut, suggesting that the cestodes preferred to settle in the locality where most of the nutritional absorption takes place, and where the mucosa, deeply corrugated with villi and crypts, offers the greatest chance for a solid attachment of the holdfast organs. The columnar epithelium at the site of attachment showed pressure atrophy and abrasion. The suckers were filled with desquamated epithelium. Superficial necrotic patches were seen close to the scolices and there were frequent mitotic figures in the regions of the damaged epithelium. The reticular network of the tunica muscularis mucosae contained many granular eosinophils and lymphoid cells, the capillaries supplying the villi were hyperaemic and in part thrombosed. The lymphatic spaces of the villi were dilated.

Cases of severe tapeworm infestation have also been reported in other species. Elkan (1974) reported a *Thamnophis sirtalis* whose gut "was filled with *Ophiotaenia perspicua*". There was a firm constriction of the gut in the upper third of the cestode mass and resultant intestinal obstruction.

Diagnosis Typical eggs are seen in the faeces. (See Fig. 9.10.)

(b) *Larvae*

There are no definite records of larval stages (plerocercoids) of Proteocephalidea from reptiles, but such stages probably occur.

ORDER PSEUDOPHYLLIDEA

(a) *Adults*

Adult pseudophyllidean cestodes live mainly in the small intestine of fish but also occur in reptiles and mammals. Their holdfast organs are the most primitive type known in cestodes. *Duthiersia*, for example, has a scolex shaped like a flower, and with a very poor adhesive power. This structure represents a simplified remnant of the bothria. In the genus *Bothridium* the two bothria are joined forming two tubular organs with anterior and posterior apertures along each side of the very prominent scolex. These organs can firmly adhere to the intestinal mucosa and may even cause haemorrhage (Wiesenhütter, 1964). (See Fig. 9.3.)

The life-cycle of the Pseudophyllidea starts with a coracidium and proceeds to a procercoid stage in small crustaceans (mainly copepods) and then to a plerocercoid in vertebrate second intermediate or in secondary paratenic hosts. Only members of one family, the Diphyllobothriidae, parasitize reptiles. Yamaguti (1959) divided them into four genera with about a dozen species. The species which infest reptiles are of moderate length from 10 cm to 80 cm and up to 8 mm wide. The numerous proglottides are broader than they are long. The genera are:

Duthiersia	Occurs exclusively in varanid lizards. Scolex compressed, broadly fan-shaped, triangular or circular.
Bothridium	Occurs mainly in boid snakes. Scolex up to 4 mm long with 2 tube-like bothria which have apertures at each end.
Scyphocephalus	Occurs only in varanid lizards. The scolex has only one pair of rudimentary bothria. The whole structure resembles a deep cup.
Spirometra	One species, *S. serpentis*, occurs in the Taiwan cobra *Naja naja atra*. The worms are only 115 mm long and 4 mm wide; the scolex measures about 1 mm and is equipped with two well developed bothria which are very mobile.

Biology

Few reports of the life-cycles of those Pseudophyllidea parasitizing reptiles have been published.

They do not seem to differ from those species which live in fish, amphibia, birds or mammals. The eggs are liberated from the uterine pore of the proglottis in the gut of the host. The empty proglottides are digested (anapolytic species). Since eggs of trematodes and the Diphyllobothriidae both have an operculum differentiation is not always easy. To assure further development the larva (coracidium) must be ingested by a suitable host, usually a copepod crustacean, in which the procercoid develops.

If such infested copepods are ingested by a second obligatory intermediate host the larvae develop into long, slender plerocercoids. Many vertebrates seem to be suitable as second intermediate hosts. Plerocercoids which gain access to unsuitable hosts survive in the muscular system of these "collecting" or paratenic hosts. Such plerocercoids are also known as "spargana".

Some of the plerocercoids are large larvae, several centimetres long. Usually they are found coiled up, surrounded by a thin membrane, in the muscles of the host. If such a host is in turn devoured by a suitable host the spargana develop into mature cestodes.

Only one species infesting reptiles has been fully investigated experimentally, this being *Bothridium pithonis*. This tapeworm occurs in various boid snakes (Pythoninae) in Africa, India, Sri Lanka, the Philippines and Australia. The first intermediate host is *Cyclops viridis*, the second the carnivorous mammal *Paradoxurus philippinensis* (Solomon, 1932). It is interesting to note that European *Cyclops* are equally suitable for development of this parasite (Frank, unpublished).

Clinical signs Snakes heavily infested with such worms sometimes regurgitate part of the strobila, particularly when they are suffering from gastroenteritis and are voiding half-digested prey items. General debility and emaciation often accompany severe cestode infestation (Frank, unpublished).

Pathology Heavy infestations with pseudophyllidean cestodes are not rare (Allroggen and Allroggen, 1959; Wiesenhütter, 1964; Frank and Loos-Frank, 1977). However, there are few descriptions of the pathology of these cases.

Wiesenhütter (1964) examined a *Python reticulatus* which was heavily infested with *Bothridium pithonis*. The proximal 1·5 m of the mid-gut was full of tapeworms. The mucosa in this area was severely oedematous and there was haemorrhage at the points where the large scolices were attached. The first 20 cm of the mid-gut showed superficial ulcerations and the whole intestinal wall was friable. Sections showed an inflammatory reaction at the site of attachment of the large scolices. Individual cells could hardly be identified and there was widespread pyknosis. Many lymphoid cells and cells rich in cytoplasm and eosinophilic granules were distributed in the mucosa. The tubular bothria of the scolices had penetrated deeply among the mucosal villi. Capillaries in such areas were hyperaemic and showed diapedesis; cells filled with eosinophilic granules were numerous. Cells inside the bothria showed pyknosis. Even where the damage caused by tapeworms is limited, it provides a portal of entry for bacteria. In such cases, however, it is not easy to ascertain whether death is due directly or only indirectly to the cestodes.

Diagnosis Characteristically shaped eggs are seen in the excreta. The eggs resemble those of trematodes in that they have an operculum. Differentiation is possible by cultivating the eggs in shallow water;

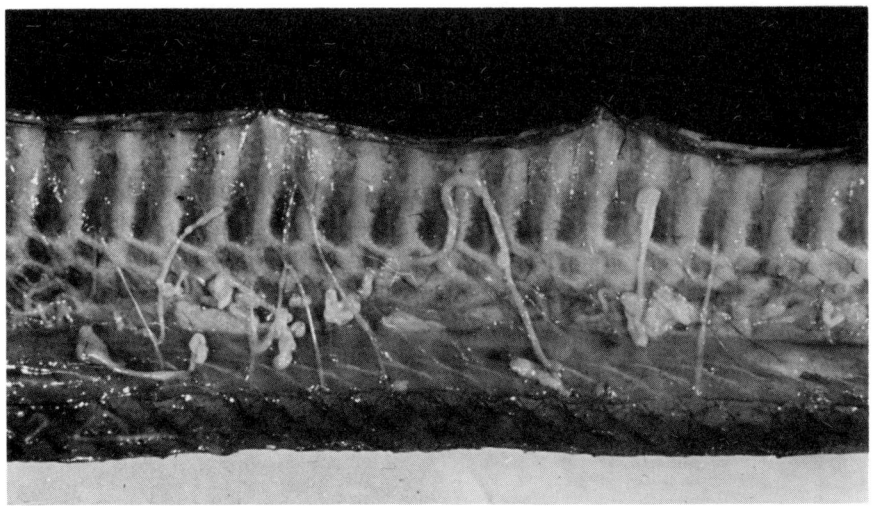

Fig. 9.3. Pleroceroids of the genus *Spirometra* under the skin of a colubrid snake.

after a few days the pseudophyllidean eggs clearly show the oncosphere or the coracidium whereas trematode eggs develop into miracidia. (See Fig. 9.10.)

(b) *Larvae*

Plerocercoids or spargana are frequently found in reptiles. In a *Morelia* of 1·5–2 metres' length hundreds of such spargana occurred (Frank, unpublished). Most of them were subcutaneous, sometimes visible externally as soft swellings, but others were deeply embedded in the intercostal muscles, peritoneal cavity or the serous membranes. Such spargana lie coiled up and are either free in the muscles or are surrounded by a thin membrane. Their length, depending upon species, ranges from a few centimetres to over 30 cm. Alongside the living larvae, others, noticeable by their yellowish colouration, may be in various stages of degeneration.

Snakes from E. Asia and Australia and some S. American species appear particularly prone to these infestations, while African, European and North American reptiles are rarely affected. Useful references are those of Odening and Bockhardt (1976), Hubbard (1933) and Mueller (1937).

The final hosts of the reptilian sparganids are usually carnivores but may, rarely, be other reptiles and birds. The cestode can be reared by feeding sparganids to their final hosts but this method does not seem to be very widely used. Plerocercoids from Australian snakes develop in the domestic cat within 6–7 days into fully mature tapeworms. Within 7 or 8 days typical eggs appear in the cat faeces (Frank, 1966b).

It is impossible to identify plerocercoids with any certainty because their features are too similar. Nor can definite conclusions be drawn from the hosts in which they are found, since plerocercoids may develop in a variety of species. Mueller (1974), for example, considered American species of *Natrix* to be the most important second intermediate hosts of *Spirometra mansonoides* although the same spargana may also be found in frogs and rodents.

Definitive diagnosis and identification are only possible by feeding experiments, but even so difficulties may arise, as pointed out by Wardle and McLeod (1968). It appears on the basis of our present (incomplete) knowledge that the plerocercoids (sparganа) found in reptiles belong to the genus *Spirometra* and the definitive hosts of these are usually Felidae, exceptionally Canidae.

In some regions of the world human sparganosis is a fairly common disease. Seo and Cho (1972) reviewed 45 cases of human sparganosis from Korea which appeared in the literature between 1924 and 1971. In the New World cases appear to be less common and there are relatively few reports—examples are those by Mueller (1974) and Rolón (1976). The latter was probably only the seventh case reported from the South American continent. The author discussed the mode of infection, reporting that "in the republic of Paraguay *Diphyllobothrium* has been observed in cats, which reveals the existence of intermediaries (rats, water snakes, birds, etc.) as sources of human infection."

Human infections with pseudophyllidean sparganids follow the ingestion of raw snake meat. Cho *et al* (1973) referred to "the traditional belief that snake meat is useful in the treatment of such conditions as tuberculosis, arthritis and impotence."

Plerocercoids are also important in the aetiology of so-called "ocular sparganosis" of humans in areas of Eastern Asia. In these regions the uncooked flesh of amphibians and reptiles is applied to inflammatory lesions of various kinds. Plerocercoids can rapidly penetrate into the eye which they may destroy completely. But sparganosis is not limited to the ocular region: it can appear in any part of the body. Reports of such cases have come from Japan, China and elsewhere.

Spirometra mansonoides
The true final host is probably *Lynx rufus* but this worm is also found in domestic cats in New York State where 3 per cent are infested (Mueller, 1974). Cats can be experimentally infected with spargana from snakes (*Natrix*) or spargana reared in mice fed on procercoid-bearing *Cyclops*. Mueller's (1974) two human cases of sparganosis in the United States were possibly due to this species.

Spirometra decipiens
The final hosts of *S. decipiens* are feline mammals. Procercoids develop experimentally in several species of *Cyclops*. Frogs and snakes are second intermediate hosts. The parasite is found in the Far East and, possibly, South America.

Spirometra mansoni
The final host of this species is the dog while plerocercoids, according to Wardle and McLeod (1968) occur "in a wide range of Indo-Chinese animals". Olsen and Haas (1976) reported this species from dogs and cats in Hawaii and suggested that reptiles may form part of the spectrum of intermediate or paratenic hosts. Spargana are

occasionally seen in man. If the species *"Spargana mansoni"* is the larval stage of *Spirometra mansoni*, as suggested by Cho and Seo (1972) and Cho *et al* (1973), reptiles, particularly snakes, may also serve as second intermediate or paratenic hosts.

Spirometra okumurai

Sparganids of *S. okumurai* are found in Japanese frogs and snakes (species not mentioned). Adults develop in dogs which are fed plerocercoids.

Spirometra ranarum

Sparganids of this species are found in Italian frogs (*Rana esculenta?*) and in Burmese frogs (*R. tigrina*); they have been transmitted experimentally to *R. esculenta* and *Natrix natrix*. Adult tapeworms develop in dogs or cats. It is doubtful, however, whether sparganids found in Europe and E. Asia are the same species (Wardle and McLeod, 1968).

Spirometra reptans

Sparganids are found in Burmese boid snakes (*Python* spp?) while adults develop readily in dogs and, possibly, in cats.

Clinical signs

When reptiles with relatively thin skins, such as snakes and geckos, are infested with pseudophyllidean plerocercoids, a diagnosis can often be made clinically. Soft swellings are seen, often close together, and usually in a dorsal or dorso-lateral position. In snakes such lesions are often in the caudal region of the body. A predilection for this part of the body is not only a feature of plerocercoids but also of tetrathyridia of cyclophyllidean cestodes and, particularly, acanthocephalan larvae. This suggests that all these parasitic stages need a stimulus before they penetrate the intestinal wall and it is probable that they obtain this from the bile.

Plerocercoid lesions rarely rupture spontaneously, but they may do so if secondarily infected by bacteria. Heavily infested animals in captivity may become anorectic and lose weight. Surgical removal under local anaesthesia poses no problems. Plerocercoids in reptiles may remain viable for years and even if fully developed may change their locality. Frank and Loos-Frank (1977) reported on a specimen of *Agkistrodon rhodostoma* which had been kept in a collection for six years and then suddenly developed an oedematous lesion behind the head.

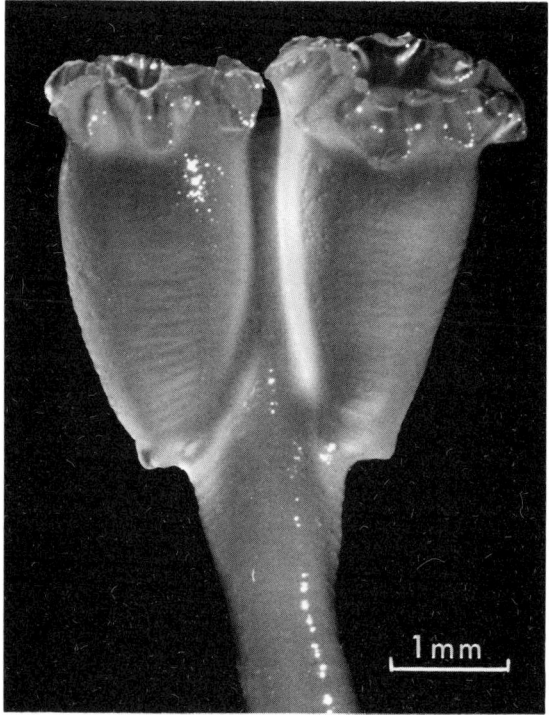

Fig. 9.4. Scolex of the tapeworm *Bothridium pithonis* from *Python reticulatus*.

Incision yielded blood-stained fluid and a plerocercoid, which was 10 cm long.

Pathology Plerocercoids in muscles are frequently associated with oedema and haemorrhage.

If the number of plerocercoids is very large even the myocardium may be damaged (Frank and Loos-Frank, 1977).

In other cases, however, there may be no reaction in the muscles.

Spargana may remain viable in reptiles for years and dead or degenerate larvae are usually few in numbers. The latter may be distinguished from the chalk-white living parasites by virtue of their yellow tint.

Diagnosis This is usually based on clinical lesions and the finding of larvae.

ORDER CYCLOPHYLLIDEA

Adult cyclophyllidean cestodes vary in size from a few millimetres to many metres. They are found mainly in reptiles, birds and mammals. In reptiles there are about 60 species belonging to only three families and few genera. One of these, the Oochoristica (Anoplocephalidae) contains over 40 species. Relatively little is known of the development of Cyclophyllidea in reptiles.

Family Nematotaeniidae
These parasites are small, have a holdfast without a rostellum, a cylindrical body and proglottides in the distal part only. Egg capsules contain one or more embryonated eggs enclosed in a parauterine organ. Only a few species from this family are known from reptiles.

Nematotaenia tarentolae	Occurs in the lizards *Tarentola mauritanica* and *Platydactylus guttata*. It may be identical with the "forma minor" of *N. dispar* known from various amphibians in Europe (Dollfus, 1957).
Nematotaenia lopezenyrai	Parasite in *Tarentola mauritanica*. It was described by Soler in 1945.
Nematotaenia mabuiae	Occurs in the lizard *Mabuia carinata* in India (Shinde, 1968).
Baerietta gerrhonoti	Found in *Gerrhonotus multicarinatus*. It was described by Telford (1965c) from one southern North American host only; it is the only representative of this genus occurring in reptiles.

Biology No studies on the life-cycle of species from this family have been published.

Family Anoplocephalidae
Members of this family are medium to large with a small globular scolex and four prominent suckers but no rostellum.

The eggs have a pyriform capsule which encloses the oncosphere. The typical larva is the cysticercoid. All known life-cycles include arthropods as intermediate hosts. Within the one genus *Oochoristica* the host specificity may vary greatly (Telford, 1970).

These cestodes were discussed by Spasskii (1951). Yamaguti (1959) divided the species occurring in reptiles into four genera, the majority belonging to the *Oochoristica*.

Biology

Relatively little is known of the life-cycles of the *Oochoristica* occurring in reptiles, but it can be assumed that their first intermediate hosts are arthropods such as *Tribolium*, *Attagenus* and *Anthrenus* (Dupouy and Kechemir, 1973). According to Telford (1970) *O. scelopori* has been successfully reared in laboratory arthropods.

Lizards and chelonians become infected with *Oochoristica* by ingestion of first intermediate hosts infested with cysticercoids, but it is difficult to imagine a similar situation in snakes. Accidental ingestion of infected intermediate hosts would hardly be sufficient to maintain the population of the parasite in these reptiles.

Several species of lizard and snake are quoted as final hosts and it remains to be seen whether some species may infect themselves by more than one method. For example, the cysticercoid may survive in a host that is unsuitable for final development and remain there until the animal is eaten by a suitable final host. Alternatively, a further optional larval stage (tetrathyridium) may be involved. Research on this subject is required.

Clinical signs and pathology None reported.

Diagnosis Based on the identification of eggs, or whole proglottides with uterine capsules containing single eggs, in the faeces.

Family Dilepididae

Small to medium-sized tapeworms. Scolex with four suckers which may or may not be armed with hooks and with a retractable rostellum. They are mainly parasites of birds and mammals.

According to Meggitt (1927), most of the cyclophyllidean larvae found in reptiles belong to the family Dilepididae, particularly species of the genus *Dipylidium* and *Diplopylidium*. The same author stated that cysticercoids found in reptiles also belong to this genus. Witenberg (1932), however, asserted that *Dipylidium* "requires a bloodsucking insect as intermediate host". No complete life-cycle has yet been established for a species affecting reptiles.

The unsatisfactory classification of this group was discussed by Yamaguti (1959), Wardle and McLeod (1968) and Wardle *et al* (1974).

Diplopylidium spp. The larvae (cysticercoids) are found in the liver and peritoneum of snakes and small lizards. Final hosts are birds and carnivores. Cysticercoids belonging to species of this genus have been found in *Coluber viridiflavus* and in *Gymnodactylus caspus*.

Observations by Dupouy and Kechemir (1973), however, suggested other definitive hosts. These authors found cysticercoids of *Joyeuxiella* in the mesenteries and in the intestinal wall of *Cerastes cerastes* in North Africa. These, according to Grenot and Vernon (1973), can only develop in hedgehogs (*Paraechinus ethiopicus*) and not in carnivores.

Family Mesocestoididae

Mesocestoides spp. The typical infective larva is the tetrathyridium which develops in vertebrates following ingestion of first intermediate hosts harbouring cysticercoids. The latter develop in invertebrates, probably in mites; Soldatova (1944) demonstrated larvae in several species of oribatid mites. Possible first intermediate hosts are mites of the genera *Trichoribates*, *Scheloribates* and *Punctoribates*. However, so far no mesocestoid life-cycle has been completely determined.

Tetrathyridia have frequently been found in reptiles (Voge, 1953; Dollfus, 1958b; Telford, 1964 and 1970; Frank, unpublished) but the identity of larvae and adults has only rarely been confirmed (Joyeux and Baer, 1932; Joyeux *et al*, 1933; Witenberg, 1934; Webster, 1949; Specht and Voge, 1965; Eckert *et al*, 1969). Such confirmation is complicated by the fact that tetrathyridia are able to leave the intestinal canal of unsuitable hosts and, still as tetrathyridia, to settle elsewhere.

The tetrathyridia from reptiles may also be responsible for occasional human infections with *Mesocestoides*. Kumada *et al* (1972) suggested that dietary habits could contribute to this; in their case the patient had consumed the raw liver, heart and fat of the Pallas's pit viper (*Agkistrodon halys*) as a tonic about five times a year for more than twenty years. This hypothesis was supported by the finding of many tetrathyridia in snakes caught in the vicinity of the patient's home.

The following reptiles are described as second intermediate hosts for larvae of *Mesocestoides*:

Elaphe scalaris, Coluber hippocrepis	*M. ambiguus*
Elaphe scalaris, Tropidonotus platyceps,	*M. lineatus**
Coluber hippocrepis, Agama stellio	
(and various mammals)	
Agkistrodon halys	*M. lineatus**
	(in man in Japan)
Sceloporus occidentalis biseriatus	*M. corti*

* Recent investigations by Loos-Frank (1980) indicate that this name probably applies to several species.

The final hosts of these parasites are mainly carnivorous mammals. The differentiation of the mature cestodes is difficult; not all the species listed by Yamaguti (1959) are accepted as valid.

Pathology Tetrathyridia may be numerous; for example, in an *Agama bibroni* the liver was so riddled with tetrathyridia that it appeared dotted with white spots (Frank, unpublished, quoted by Will, 1975b).

Although severe infestation with cyclophyllidean cestode larvae must certainly damage the host, the author knows of only a few publications describing pathological changes. Telford (1970, 1971) reported that tetrathyridia were common in some species of lizards in the Western USA and considered them to be of considerable significance. He stated that massive infections "must greatly reduce the functional capacity of the liver due to the extensive invasion of hepatic tissue that can occur". Singh and Pande (1972) reported "destruction of the liver parenchyma occupied by the cysticercoids and pressure atrophy in the adjacent hepatic lobules" in a lizard (*Uromastix hardwicki*) infected with cysticercoids of *Joyeuxiella echinorhynchoides*.

Diagnosis The larva is easy to recognize. Dupouy and Kechemir (1973) listed the following hosts and sites for larvae:

Joyeuxiella	from *Cerastes vipera*	(mesenteries and intestinal wall)
Acanthotaenia	from *Cerastes vipera*	(mesenteries and duodenum)
Ophiotaenia	from *Cerastes vipera*	(mesenteries)
Oochoristica	from *Agama mutabilis*	(three larvae at different stages of development in the liver)

B. Subphylum Nemathelminthes (Aschelminthes)

(1) Class Nematodes (Roundworms)

Parasitic nematodes of reptiles vary in length from a few millimetres to 30 cm or more. Petter and Brygoo (1972) postulated a relationship between the size of nematodes and that of their hosts. Nematodes of five species from the tortoise *Testudo yniphora* were found to be considerably larger than the same species from *Testudo radiata*. *Testudo yniphora* lives in an isolated region of Madagascar and has no contact with other chelonians. Whether this difference in size of parasites is attributable to evolutionary causes or whether it could be reproduced artificially is as yet unknown. Taxonomists, however, should bear these observations in mind so as not to overburden the already long list of nematodes with new but invalid species.

Most parasitic nematodes inhabit either the digestive tract or organs which connect with the gut or the environment; as such they ensure that their progeny can be passed out with faeces, urine or mucus. A few groups, such as the Dracunculoidea and the Filarioidea, live entirely outside the intestine; escape from the host in these cases must be effected either through a break in the skin or by aspiration of embryos or larvae by blood-sucking arthropods.

The life-cycle of nematodes may be direct (without an intermediate host), as in the Oxyuroidea, or indirect, with one or several intermediate hosts, as in the Dracunculoidea and in the Filarioidea. Occasionally, as in the Gnathostomatoidea, paratenic or transport hosts are included in the life-cycle.

The developmental modes of nematodes vary. In most cases the young do not develop within the original host but have either to be transmitted to a fresh host or undergo a phase of differentiation outside a host before the next phase of their development. Self-infection occurs in some species of *Rhabdias* where parthenogenetic females are the only parasitic stages.

In many species larval moults occur directly in the intestinal canal while in others moulting takes place during a complicated migration through the body of the host. This "histiotropic" phase may damage internal organs or even kill the host.

Subclass Adenophora (Aphasmida)

Representatives of this subclass are few in number and all belong to the order Enoplida (Chabaud, 1974). Only a few genera of the three superfamilies (Dioctophymatoidea, Trichuroidea and Muspiceoidea) occur as adults in reptiles. Incidentally and exceptionally reptiles may harbour larval stages of the Dioctophymatoidea.

Superfamily Trichuroidea

Family Trichuroidea
The only representatives of this family belong to the genus *Capillaria*. The life-cycle is direct but a few species use paratenic hosts. In some capillariids these transport hosts have become mandatory.

The species of *Capillaria* were listed by Yamaguti (1961) and Skrjabin *et al* (1970).

Most species inhabit the intestinal tract but they may also be found in other organs. Telford (1971), for example, reported *Capillaria* infections in the liver of lizards and snakes and Pence (1970) *Capillaria colubra* in the oviducts of the snake *Coluber constrictor priapus*. A particularly interesting species is *C. recurva* which lays its eggs in the lamellar layer of the stratum corneum of the American crocodile (*Crocodylus acutus*) although the sexually mature stages live in the crocodile's intestine (Elkan, 1974).

Biology

Transmission of *Capillaria* spp. is probably direct. It is uncertain as to what extent paratenic or transport hosts are needed. Telford (1971) pointed out that "little is known of the host specificity, the life-cycles or modes or transmission of the reptilian capillariids" but most of them appear to be species specific.

Clinical signs   None reported.

Pathology   There are very few relevant publications but infestation appears to be serious if vital organs, such as the liver, are heavily parasitized (Telford, 1971).

Capillaria colubra appears to produce no gross pathological changes but, as in other capillariids, the heads of the worms are found embedded into the mucosa (Pence, 1970).

In the case of *C. recurva* in *Crocodylus acutus* Elkan (1974) could not detect any pathological lesions associated with the migration of worms. Nor were changes noted in the neighbourhood of the eggs in the epidermis.

Diagnosis   *Capillaria* infection may be diagnosed by the detection of eggs which have characteristic plugs at each pole.

Other members of the Trichuroidea

Trichinella spiralis may be transmitted experimentally to reptiles. Matoff (1953) succeeded in rearing larvae in tortoises if the latter were kept at appreciably higher temperatures than normal. Merkushev (1955) identified necrophagous tropical beetles or their larvae as paratenic hosts for *Trichinella spiralis* and these could be ingested by reptiles.

Superfamily Dioctophymatoidea

Biology

Lichtenfels and Lavies (1976) reported deaths in the snake *Thamnophis sirtalis parietalis* which were fed on killifish (*Fundulus diaphanus*) caught in the wild. The larval nematodes were identified as *Eustrongylides* spp. Seven out of 25 snakes died from the infection. The others showed a variety of clinical features including subcutaneous swellings, violent contortions and a sanguineous exudate from the nares. Nematodes collected at necropsy were found beneath the skin, in the lungs, in the body cavity and along the spinal column. This account emphasizes that the Dioctophymatoidea are able to survive oral ingestion of the intermediate hosts (fish) by animals which are unsuitable as definitive hosts; the snakes serve a paratenic role.

Subclass Secernentea (Phasmida)

ORDER RHABDITIDA

Biology

The most important characteristic of these small nematodes is their appearance in two phases, one parasitic (parthenogenetic) the other free-living (dioecious). Goodey (1924) determined the life-cycle of *Rhabdias fuscovenosa*; transmission to new hosts is affected by oral ingestion of the free-living third-stage larvae.

Superfamily Rhabditoidea

Representatives of this superfamily are important parasites of reptiles. The parthenogenetic stage mainly inhabits the lungs. The worms are oviparous with thin-shelled eggs which, at the time of deposition, contain either blastomere cells or fully developed larvae. The latter may develop in the lungs. First-stage larvae may be found in faeces or in oral mucus. These larvae produce a free-living generation (males and females), the larvae of which infect new hosts. Some species may use facultative intermediate hosts such as snails or earthworms.

Reptiles are mainly infected by the genera *Rhabdias*, *Entomelas* and *Strongyloides*. *Rhabdias* occurs only in snakes whereas *Entomelas* is found in chameleons and legless lizards (*Anguis*). The preferred habitats are the lungs (*Rhabdias*) or, more rarely, the pericardial and pleural cavities (*Entomelas*). *Strongyloides* mainly inhabits the intestinal tract (Little, 1966).

The best known species of *Rhabdias* is *R. fuscovenosa*, which is common in snakes. The hosts reported for this species include snakes of the genera *Natrix, Coluber, Thamnophis, Lampropeltis, Elaphe, Naja* and *Bitis*.

Biology

Although worms of the genus *Rhabdias* are not infrequently encountered, little is known of their life-cycle. One mainly relies on the work of Goodey (1924) on *R. fuscovenosa*. The parthenogenetic females in the lungs deposit thin-shelled eggs with many blastomeres which, after a short time, develop into first-stage larvae. These leave the lungs and are expelled either via oral mucus or with the faeces. Goodey observed direct development from the rhabditiform to the filariform third-stage infectious larva without the intermission of a sexually differentiated free-living generation. Normally, however, rhabditiform larvae change after two moults into sexually mature males and females of a smaller size than parasitic generations. Free-living generations produce fewer and larger eggs which, if ingested, give rise to infective larvae after two moults. In a terrarium with a high humidity these nematodes can pose a problem and may kill snakes.

A similar mode of transmission is assumed for *Entomelas* and *Strongyloides* but definite observations on these genera are not available. Holt *et al* (1978) suggested that the transmission of *Strongyloides* in snakes might be similar to that in mammals.

Clinical signs Infective larvae penetrate the host skin or oral mucosa, migrate by the blood stream to the lungs and thence, via the trachea, to the mouth and the intestinal canal. This migration, in particular the passage through the respiratory system, may cause respiratory distress. Other clinical signs can include anorexia, loss of weight and diarrhoea. The clinical picture will be aggravated if a bacterial infection supervenes.

If snakes are heavily parasitized they can be seen to gasp and to expel mucus from the mouth. Breathing is rapid and irregular and there may be anorexia with consequent loss of weight. Diarrhoea may be a feature of *Strongyloides* infestation (Holt *et al*, 1978).

The author has observed intense oedema and inflammation of the oral mucosa in several species of *Thamnophis* infected with a *Rhabdias* sp. deeply embedded in the dental pockets.

Pathology Since the worms penetrate deeply into the pulmonary tissue pathological damage is to be expected. In captive snakes the damage may be sufficient to cause death. Zwart (1968, 1974) compared cases in reptiles with *Metastrongylus* infections in mammals. The pathological picture has been described as "pneumonia verminosa". The pulmonary septa gradually lose their respiratory epithelium and become fibrotic; as a result gaseous exchange is impaired. Bacteria may complicate the infection and cause pneumonitis. Holt *et al* (1978) attributed the death of a *Lampropeltis getulus holbrooki* infested with *Strongyloides* spp. to loss of fluids and electrolytes but could find no pathological changes in the intestinal tract.

Diagnosis Pulmonary *Rhabdias* infection is diagnosed by the demonstration of free larvae in the faeces. However, the latter may easily be mistaken for intestinal Rhabditoidea (*Strongyloides* spp.). A safer diagnostic procedure is to search for the thin-shelled eggs or free first-stage larvae in the oral mucus, and this also applies to the eggs or first-stage larvae of *Strongyloides* (Holt *et al*, 1978).

ORDER STRONGYLIDA

These medium-sized or small worms are of relatively little importance in reptiles. Those of most importance in snakes and lizards are the Diaphanocephaloidea which parasitize the intestinal tract. Skrjabin *et al* (1961) gave a detailed description of the species concerned. Of the Trichostrongyloidea only a few species occur in reptiles (Skrjabin *et al*, 1954).

Superfamily Diaphanocephaloidea
These nematodes are 1–1·5 cm long and usually inhabit the anterior sector of the small intestine of snakes (rarely lizards). They can be recognized by their dark brown intestinal canal which is visible through the transparent cuticle. Low magnification also shows the typical tripartite configuration of the head.

Like other Strongylida the diaphanocephalids feed mainly on the blood of their hosts. They are oviparous and the thin-shelled eggs show early developmental stages (4–14 blastomeres) when shed in the faeces or oral mucus. Their life-cycle is direct. Ingestion with drinking water is a possibility but skin penetration is probably more common (Schad, 1956).

The only family, the Diaphanocephalidae, contains the genera *Diaphanocephalus* and *Kalicephalus*. Of the former only a few species are known but more than 50 *Kalicephalus* species have been described. Schad (1962) reduced this number to 23 including a few new species. The various species show a marked intra-specific variation and a low host specificity.

Biology

The transmission of all *Kalicephalus* species seems to be similar; in work performed by Schad (1956) there were a few differences in three N. American species studied. The eggs of *K. parvus* and those of *K. agkistrodontis* hatched after 24 hours, whereas those of *K. rectiphilus* needed four days at room temperature. Third-stage exsheathed larvae of *K. parvus* were found encapsulated in the mucosa of the stomach for up to 130 days while those from *K. rectiphilus* remained in the duodenal wall for up to 33 days and *K. agkistrodontis* developed free in the intestinal lumen. The prepatent period varied depending on host and parasite species—for example, between 58 days for *K. agkistrodontis* and 115 days for *K. parvus*.

Schad's results may be applicable to other species. Ingestion of the infective third-stage larva takes place during drinking, while, according to Yamaguti (1961), "Introduction through the tongue or the possibility of skin penetration is considered likely". This mode of transmission facilitates infection in captive animals and may result in severe parasitism. Heavy infestations have, however, also been recorded in free-living snakes (Cooper, 1973).

Clinical signs and pathology Species living in the oesophagus may occasionally be expelled from the mouth with mucus. Telford (1971), did not consider these worms pathogenic in snakes but this was not supported by Cooper (1971) who described large burdens of nematodes in freshly captured snakes and reported that the adult *Kalicephalus* "attach to the upper intestinal tract and can cause erosive lesions with haemorrhage and a build-up of cellular debris". Ulceration of this kind facilitates bacterial invasion, particularly by such organisms as *Arizona*, *Pseudomonas* and *Salmonella* spp.

Diagnosis

The thin-shelled eggs with only a few blastomeres are easily recognized in freshly deposited faeces. The larvae may also be detected.

ORDER OXYURIDA

Superfamily Oxyuroidea
Yamaguti (1961) distinguished seven families in this superfamily but Petter and Quentin (1976) recognized only three. Of these only the Pharyngodonidae parasitize reptiles. Certain species, such as *Skrjabinodon* and *Thelandros*, show great similarity to the Thelastomatidae,

which are parasites of invertebrates. Petter and Quentin therefore suggested that the Pharyngodonidae of lower vertebrates may have arisen from insect oxyurids.

The main hosts of oxyuroid nematodes are tortoises and turtles of the genera *Terrapene, Testudo, Geochelone, Gopherus, Emys, Clemmys, Podocnemis, Kinixys, Chrysemys* and *Trionyx*. Many genera of lizards may also be infected including *Lacerta, Calotes, Agama, Chalcides, Uromastix, Mabuya, Tarentola, Trachysaurus, Iguana, Ctenosaura, Ameiva, Tupinambis, Sceloporus, Conolophus* and others.

Well over a hundred different oxyurids have been described from reptiles (Yamaguti, 1961). Detailed descriptions may be found in Skrjabin *et al* (1974, 1976). There have been a number of additions and new descriptions.

The valid genera are:

Pharyngodon	Carnivorous hosts.
Skrjabinodon	Carnivorous hosts.
Spauligodon	Carnivorous hosts.
Veversia	Carnivorous hosts.
Thelandros	Carnivorous and herbivorous hosts.
Paralaeuris	Herbivorous Iguanidae.
Ortleppnema	Testudinidae (Madagascar).
Ozolaimus	Herbivorous Iguanidae.
Alaeuris	Herbivorous Testudinidae and Iguanidae. Rarely carnivorous hosts.
Mehdiella	Testudinidae.
Tachygonetria	Testudinidae and lizards—*Uromastix* only.
Thaparia	Testudinidae.

Biology

Sexually mature oxyurids are usually small and often pin-shaped. They inhabit the posterior part of the alimentary tract and large numbers may be present. In some captive animals large whitish clumps consisting of thousands of oxyurids have been recorded.

The life-cycle is direct (Telford, 1971). Most species are oviparous. In many species the eggs are ellipsoid and asymmetrically flattened. The shell is often thick with typical surface markings. Operculated eggs occur and in a few species the eggs are extremely pointed at both ends (Fig. 9.10). A few species of the genera *Mehdiella* and *Tachygonetria* are viviparous while those of *Thaparia* are ovoviviparous. Petter (1968a) studied the life-cycle of two species in Madagascan chameleons (*Spinicauda inglisi* and *S. freitasi*). Ingested eggs develop in the digestive tract of reptiles. The larvae develop as far as the immature adult stage in the anterior gut and migrate to the rectum as mature adults. The complete cycle takes about forty days.

The host specificity in the Oxyuridae is very marked and it is doubtful whether cross infections ever occur (Telford, 1971). Large worm burdens are often seen at necropsy of both land tortoises and iguanas but there is no evidence that cross infections occur among captive reptiles.

Clinical signs The author has observed that heavily parasitized tortoises are reluctant to resume feeding when they awake from hibernation and that those specimens may subsequently die.

Pathology If the number of worms is not excessive their pathogenicity is generally low. Telford (1971) suggested that, in their natural environment, these worms live as commensals and "perhaps they serve some useful role to the host by breaking up faecal masses, thus preventing constipation by chitinous insect remains and undigested cellulose".

Kane *et al* (1976) found a large palpable abdominal mass in a Fiji island iguana (*Brachylophus fasciatus*). At necropsy "the mass was found to involve the large intestine and to contain a mass of nematode parasites. The nematodes were identified as *Alaeuris brachylophi*."

In the author's opinion a case of this severity must be regarded as exceptional.

ORDER ASCARIDIDA

Superfamily Ascaridoidea

Genera and Species

According to Hartwich (1974) only two families in this order, the Anisakidae and the Ascarididae, parasitize reptiles. Compared with other intestinal nematodes of reptiles these worms are large and stout, many species reaching a length of 10 cm or more. They are oviparous and the eggs are thick-shelled—some of them ball-like, others ellipsoid—and they usually have an ornamental surface (Fig. 9.10). They are excreted with the faeces, undeveloped or with only a few blastomeres. Most species develop via intermediate hosts which form part of the food chain of the final host. The worms are found in crocodiles, chelonians, lizards and, particularly, snakes. They may cause extensive damage and can cause death (see later).

Over 50 species of ascaridoid worms have been described and classified into two families and 12 genera. In this chapter the author follows the systematics established by Hartwich (1974).

Table 9.1

Family/genus	Hosts	Comments
Anisakidae		
Goezia	Teleost fishes	Accidentally in reptiles?
Terranova	Crocodilia	—
Sulcascaris	Turtles	—
Ascarididae		
Thyphlophorus	Crocodilia	—
Multicaecum	Crocodilia	—
Hartwichia	Crocodilia	—
Dujardinascaris	Crocodilia	Thin-shelled eggs
Angusticaecum	Tortoises	—
Amplicaecum	Snakes	Intermediate hosts: rodents
Ophidascaris	Snakes, lizards	Intermediate hosts: rodents and amphibia
Polydelphis	Snakes, lizards	Intermediate hosts: rodents and amphibia
Hexametra	Snakes, lizards	Intermediate hosts: rodents

It is not possible here to discuss single species; for this reference should be made to Yamaguti (1961) and subsequent publications—for example, those by Petter (1968b) and Sprent (1969a,b).

Biology

The ecology and the phylogeny of the Ascaridoidea have been extensively reviewed by Osche (1958). The ability of ascaridoid larvae to develop in various hosts is particularly marked in those species whose life-cycle includes an obligatory intermediate host. There are few reports on this but the investigations of Kutzer and Grünberg (1965b) and Kutzer and Lamina (1965) show that various vertebrates can serve as intermediate hosts—for example, rodents for *Ophidascaris baylisi* and frogs for *O. labiatopapillosa*. Cold-blooded vertebrates appear to be unsuitable hosts for species found as adults in mammals, such as *Toxocara*: Merdivenci and Sezen (1965) were not able to raise larvae of this species in *Testudo graeca*. On the other hand, Kutzer and

Grünberg (1965b) and Petter *et al* (1967) showed that larvae of ascarids from snakes can infect primates and produce severe pathological damage to internal organs, including the central nervous system.

The host specificity of adults is low. *Ophidascaris* spp. can be found in many species of snakes (Ash and Beaver, 1962). Some ascaridoid species have a wide geographical distribution and host range.

The biology of many species is as yet unknown; there are, however, reports both of direct life-cycles and others with obligatory intermediate hosts. Araujo (1971) published interesting material, accompanied by photographs, of three species—*Ophidascaris sprenti, Polydelphis quadrangularis* and *Hexametra quadricornis*—and showed that the larvae moult twice, not once, while still in the egg. Araujo concluded "Thus the larvae are in the third stage, and not in the second, when they infect the intermediate host."

Detailed accounts of the development of some species of the genera *Ophidascaris, Polydelphis, Hexametra* and *Amplicaecum* have been published by Walton (1936), Hörchner (1962), Ash and Beaver (1962), Sprent (1963, 1970), Kutzer and Grünberg (1965b), Kutzer and Lamina (1965), Petter (1968b) and Araujo (1971, 1972).

Araujo's investigations (1972) showed that the development of adult worms in the definitive host depends on the time the third-stage larvae spend in the intermediate host. The eggs of *Polydelphis quadrangularis*, parasitic in *Crotalus durissus terrificus*, contain third-stage larvae after seven days if kept at 25°C. If these eggs are given to mice, the infective larvae may be found in the liver after three days. Although they remain at the same stage, their organs continue to develop; this allows the differentiation of the sexes after another 15 days. After 28 days these stages are infectious to snakes; the optimal time, however, amounts to about 173 days.

If third-stage larvae of less than 173 days' age are used to infect snakes, they migrate and cause gastric ulceration. Only older larvae complete their development in the stomach. This different behaviour of the larvae, depending on the time spent in the intermediate host, may explain the variety of pathological changes seen in cases of ascaridoid infections.

Third-stage larvae of *P. quadrangularis* pass their third moult either in the tissues or in the intestinal lumen, depending on their age; the fourth moult always takes place in the lumen. Immature adults may be found either after 232 days (78 in mice, 154 in snakes), or after 248 days (173 in mice, 75 in snakes). Compared with nematodes in naturally infected snakes, the adults reach their full size only after 539 days (173 in mice, 366 in snakes).

Sprent's investigations (1963) on *Amplicaecum robertsi* demonstrated the relationship between the development of the larvae and the species of intermediate host. The eggs of this species needed 2–3 weeks to become infective for mice. In the liver they reached a length of 79 mm in about 28 weeks. Development in rats was much slower; larvae which were younger than 12 weeks produced encapsulated stages in the definitive host in various tissues, particularly in the aorta where they remained coiled up in cysts filled with coagulated blood. Larvae older than 12 weeks from rats and 8 weeks from mice underwent their next moult in the wall of the oesophagus and the stomach.

In another study Sprent (1970) found larval stages of *Ophidascaris moreliae* in the lung of 25 out of 165 experimentally infected snakes, *Morelia spilotes variegatus*. Embryonated eggs fed directly to snakes resulted in second-stage larvae (cf. Araujo, 1971) but only in the tissues; no further development could be observed. These results, which are similar to those of Araujo (1972), show clearly how the mode of development in the definitive host depends upon the degree of maturity of the transferred stages.

Apart from the age of the larvae the amount of food in the snake's stomach is also of importance. Sprent (1970) found ascarids (*O. moreliae*) free among items of food; in the empty stomach, however, he found about 50 worms embedded in a crater-like ulceration. Ash and Beaver (1962) did not mention food but recorded that in *Ophidascaris labiatopapillosa* "adults threaded into or through the stomach wall with the anterior and posterior ends extending into the lumen while the middle of the body either is buried deep within the tissues or forms a loop between the stomach and the serosa. Occasionally, especially when the worms are numerous and large, a loop of the body may extend 1 cm or more into the supporting mesenteries".

Ascaridoid larvae develop in various organs—for example, *Ophidascaris moreliae* in subcutaneous tissue (mice and rats), *Amplicaecum robertsi* in the liver (mice) (Sprent, 1970), *Hexametra quadricornis* in the abdominal cavity (Hörchner, 1962) and *Ophidascaris labiatopapillosa* in the liver or the mesenteries (Ash and Beaver, 1962).

Studies on species of *Polydelphis* from a sea snake (*Laticauda colubrina*) from the Philippines, however, demonstrated that other modes of development are possible (Schmidt and Kuntz, 1972).

Clinical signs Regurgitation of half digested food in snakes can be a feature of an ascarid worm infestation. When the worms are associated with gastric lesions digestion is impeded and the food may not pass on to the mid-gut. Sometimes nematodes are expelled when the snake regurgitates.

Severe anorexia over several months may also indicate heavy parasitism. The characteristic eggs are always present in the faeces (Fig. 9.10).

Pathology Pathological lesions may be severe in infected snakes and the mortality rate can be high.

However, there is a paucity of detailed descriptions of such cases and those that exist tend to be based on snakes kept in captivity (Kutzer and Grünberg, 1965b).

Kutzer and Grünberg were the first to publish detailed investigations on the lesions caused by ascarid worms. Other reports of ulceration with central necrosis have since appeared (Cooper, 1973; Frank, 1971, 1975, 1976b, 1978; Frank and Loos-Frank, 1977; Grünberg *et al*, 1963; Ippen, 1971). The description given by Kutzer and Grünberg was probably a typical example; pathological changes caused by migrating third-stage larvae could be seen in all organs. Sprent (1963) even recorded deaths in the snake *Morelia spilotes variegatus* due to stages of *Amplicaecum robertsi* in the wall of the aorta (*aortitis verminosa*). The main pathological changes are those of gastroenteritis with necrotic and ulcerative destruction and inflammatory reaction in the stomach and the intestinal wall; thickening of the wall as a result of granulomatous growths frequently occurs. Such lesions may reach the size of an apple with central necrosis and the formation of abscesses filled with pus (Fig. 9.5). Elbihari and Hussein (1973) found identical pathological changes in a free-living specimen of *Python sebae*.

Other lesions may include intestinal perforation while the ability of ascarids to enter bile and pancreatic ducts can lead to obstruction followed by pancreatic or hepatic necrosis. Jaundice may occur as a result of bile-duct obstruction (Frank, unpublished). An overabundance of ascarids may lead to intestinal obstruction and infarction of the small gut.

Recently captured reptiles, particularly snakes, may carry large burdens of worms but it is less certain whether single worms have any deleterious effect (Cooper, 1973). Allison *et al* (1973) found "several hundred specimens" of *Sulcascaris* (syn. *Porrocaecum*) *sulcatum* in the stomach of a turtle, *Chelonia mydas*, caught off the coast of North Carolina, but no pathological damage was mentioned in their report. On the other hand Elbihari and Hussein (1973) reported gastric

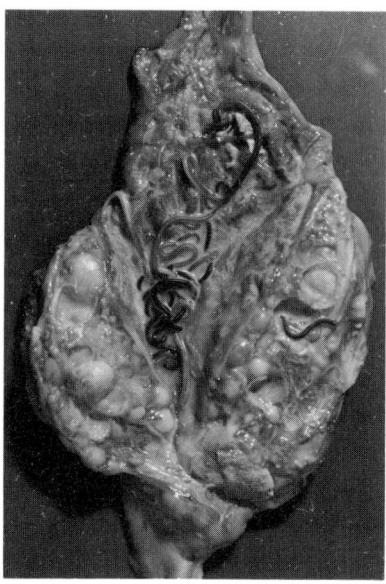

Fig. 9.5. Purulent abscesses in the stomach of a snake (*Morelia argus*) caused by a *Nocardia* sp. The heads of many nematodes (Ascaridida) are visible.

lesions in a free-living python (*Python sebae*) caused by *Ophidascaris filaria*.

Pathological changes due to ascarid infestation may be classified as follows:

(1) Mechanical destruction of the epithelium causing digestive insufficiency and providing a portal of entry for bacteria. Perforation causes peritonitis.
(2) Secretion of toxic metabolites by the nematodes and a possible noxious effect on serum protein (Will, 1975a).

Diagnosis Characteristic eggs may be seen in the faeces. Kutzer and Grünberg (1965b) maintained that the eggs of *Ophidascaris, Polydelphis, Hexametra* and *Amplicaecum* may be distinguishable on the basis of their surface structure. (See Fig. 9.10.)

Superfamilies Cosmocercoidea and Heterakoidea

Views on the taxonomy of these groups vary.

Biology

These nematodes are medium or small and mainly parasitize the posterior part of the large intestine. The hosts are small lizards, iguanids and, rarely, snakes or tortoises. The life-cycle is direct. Eggs shed with the faeces are either undeveloped or in the earliest stages of development.

These worms are probably of little importance in reptiles. No accounts of any damage caused by these worms have been published but a build-up of infestation in captivity would seem possible.

ORDER SPIRURIDA

Suborder Camallanina

Superfamily Camallanoidea
Members of this superfamily have a life-cycle which includes an intermediate host—crustaceans such as *Cyclops* and *Asellus*. The worms are found in the intestinal tract: clinical signs of damage have not been reported. MacDonald and Litchford (1974) observed unusual pathology (cystic degeneration of the pancreas) in a terrapin, *Pseudemys scripta troosti*, infected with the species *Camallanus trispinosus*.

A detailed review of this order has been published by Skrjabin (1969) and by Skrjabin *et al* (1971).

Superfamily Dracunculoidea

Biology

The dracunculid worms known from reptiles are relatively small (10–40 cm long) with the exception of *Dracunculus dahomensis* where the females may reach a size of 80 cm. The life histories of only a few species have been examined and they are probably similar to that of *D. medinensis*. The dracunculids parasitize the body cavity, the serous membranes, connective tissue and subcutaneous tissue.

The taxonomy of the reptilian dracunculids is complicated; many physical features vary considerably and this casts doubt on the validity of a number of species. Mirza (1957) and Mirza and Roberts (1957) considered several of the species synonymous but Yamaguti (1961) opposed this view and established two separate subfamilies. The present author follows the classification of Chabaud (1975a) who placed all species in the genera *Dracunculus* (Dracunculidae) and *Micropleura* (Micropleuridae). Approximately 15 of the former and three of the latter are recognized and their respective hosts include several species of snake, monitor lizards (*Varanus* spp.), crocodiles and chelonians.

Development

The males are considerably smaller than the females. The latter produce a large number of larvae which can be recognized by their long tails. The larvae must reach water where they remain viable for up to 12 days. They will only develop further if they find suitable crustaceans such as *Cyclops*, *Macrocyclops* or other copepods.

Liberation from vertebrates involves a complicated procedure. Observations on *Eunectes murinus* have shown that when gravid females lie in the subcutaneous tissue the epidermis softens on contact with water and becomes oedematous, thus allowing the larvae to emigrate (Frank, unpublished). Moravec (1966) reported similar multiple swellings on the back of a *Eunectes murinus*; these burst and released a milky fluid consisting of innumerable larvae. In another case, an infested specimen of *Claudius angustatus*, 1–3 mm large lesions could be seen in the cloaca, caused by gravid females in the subcutaneous tissue. Emigration of larvae would have been quite possible from this site (Frank, unpublished).

In the haemocoel of the intermediate host the first-stage larvae develop into second and third-stage larvae.

Mackin (1928) observed that "cyclops were not inconvenienced by the presence of the worms (*D. globocephalus*) except when a very heavy infection occurred in which cases the alimentary canal became so lacerated as to cause death. It is probable that over-infection in nature would rarely or never occur".

Reptiles become infected by accidentally or intentionally ingesting copepods.

Clinical signs   Dermal lesions are seen.

Pathology   Histological reports on the skin lesions are not yet available.

Diagnosis   Examination of skin lesions may reveal larvae.

Suborder Spirurina

Superfamily Spiruroidea

Biology

These are small to medium-sized nematodes of fish, amphibians, reptiles and mammals. In mature specimens the posterior end is spirally coiled. The life-cycle includes one or two intermediate hosts and one or more facultative transport hosts may also be used. Reptiles may either act as hosts of the larvae (in which case the final hosts are birds or mammals) or may serve as final hosts. The parasites prefer the anterior digestive tract but there are no reports of associated lesions.

Larvae can survive in unsuitable vertebrate hosts and may be consumed in raw or insufficiently cooked fish, amphibian or reptile meat.

According to Chabaud (1975b) only members of the family Spiruridae parasitize reptiles, the two genera concerned being *Paraspirura* and *Spirura*.

Superfamilies Gnathostomatoidea, Physalopteroidea, Thelazioidea, Rictularioidea and Habronematoidea

Biology

All these small to medium-sized nematodes are able to anchor themselves in the intestinal mucosa or to penetrate deeper into the tissues. Some have been found to cause papillomata in the oesophagus and the stomach. Their definite hosts can be reptiles but these can also act as obligatory second intermediate or paratenic hosts. Arthropods, particularly insects, serve as first intermediate hosts. Definite hosts are larger reptiles which prey on smaller species, birds of prey or mammals.

Larvae penetrate the intestinal wall and settle in various organs.

Reports of gnathostomiasis have mainly come from Eastern Asia. Daengsvang (1949), Miyazaki (1960) and Nitidandhaprabhas *et al* (1975) reported that they can invade the urinary bladder. Eye damage can also occur.

Ash (1962) investigated obligatory intermediate hosts for the species *Gnathostoma procyonis*. His list of hosts included snakes, turtles and alligators. Such secondary intermediate hosts do not, however, necessarily fit into the food chain of the definitive host, in this case the raccoon (*Procyon lotor*)—but the larvae are able to survive in unsuitable species. Larvae of some species whose second intermediate hosts should be fish, amphibians or aquatic reptiles have been found in human patients; the larvae were probably acquired as a result of ingestion of insufficiently cooked meat.

The adults are dioecious. They are frequently deeply embedded in the tissue where they cause destruction and the formation of granulomata. The eggs are passed out in the faeces; they must then be taken up by an intermediate host, usually an arthropod.

Second intermediate hosts which feed on arthropods are frequently necessary. In some reptiles gastric nematodes of the genus *Physaloptera* are commonly found. Since the host specificity of this species is low, infection can occur in captivity, ants serving as intermediate hosts (Lee, 1957). Even under natural conditions, the infection may be high, particularly in *Phrynosoma* spp. which prey on ants, but the pathogenicity is low (Telford, 1970). In many cases paratenic hosts are involved in the cycle thereby broadening the field for the definitive hosts. Cawthorn and Anderson (1976), for example, reported the survival of third-stage larvae of *Physaloptera maxillaris* for 21 days in the snake *Thamnophis sirtalis*. The larvae remained in the lumen of the gut and did not penetrate the intestinal wall. Even after this time they remained infectious for skunks (*Mephitis mephitis*).

Clinical signs None reported.

Pathology A detailed account has been published (Pflugfelder, 1947/49) of a species of *Tanqua*, resembling *T. tiara*, found in *Varanus salvator*. The pathological lesions reported are probably applicable to the whole group and are therefore summarized here.

The infective larvae penetrate the gastric mucosa and settle in the submucosa. Here they become surrounded by foreign-body giant cells and a loose connective tissue capsule. It is assumed that the change to four-stage larvae takes place in this site. The parasite metabolizes the granuloma material and eventually breaks through to the intestinal lumen where it adheres to the mucosa. The anterior end of the young mature worms probably penetrates deeply with the aid of the cervical bulbs (head bulbs) the latter being a typical feature of the Gnathostomatidae. At the site of attachment the muscularis mucosae of the host is ruptured. Efficient wound closure is facilitated by the production of coagulating enzyme by the host, the balloon-shape of the worm's head and the expansion of the parasite's cervical collar. Furthermore, anchorage is perfected by the ring-shaped structure of the head bulbs which, when sectioned longitudinally, are seen to be sharp ridges armed with barbed hooks.

Four zones of reaction develop in response to the head bulbs. The first of these is exudate. This connects with zone 2, a layer of dead cells which are, according to Pflugfelder (1977), acidophilic granulocytes. Will (1977) defined these cells as heterophilic cells. Together with detached mucosal cells and connective tissue they serve to nourish the nematodes. Connective tissue comprises zone 3 and provides a connection with zone 4 where capillaries offer optimal nutritive conditions for the parasite.

Diagnosis Differentiation of eggs is difficult. Spirurids should be suspected if they are thick-shelled and embryonated but some species have eggs with polar opercula and others have ornamented thin shells and incompletely developed embryos. If larvae can be isolated from subcutaneous abscesses a search should be made for such typical features as head bulbs and thorns.

Superfamily Diplotriaenoidea

Biology
These large nematodes, formerly classified with the Filarioidea, are distinguished by the production of thick-shelled eggs, containing fully differentiated first-stage larvae. The worms parasitize birds and reptiles. Normally the eggs are shed with the faeces or with the respiratory mucus. Arthropods which ingest the eggs can act as intermediate hosts in which the infective (third-stage) larvae develop. Only members of one subfamily live in reptiles.

Subfamily Dicheilonematinae

Biology
The only representatives are species of *Hastospiculum*. These large, thick-bodied worms live in the serous membranes of large reptiles (Varanidae, *Boa*, *Python* and *Crotalus*). Sexual dimorphism is marked; while the females of some species may be 30 cm long the males usually only attain a few centimetres. The thick-shelled eggs are normally found close to the females and they are embryonated. Eggs of species living in the lung tissue are excreted via the trachea, but it is not known how they are liberated if the worms are situated in serous membranes of the abdominal cavity. In the neighbourhood of the females the tissues may become waterlogged and oedematous and this

may be advantageous for the distribution and transport of the eggs. The whole life-history of these worms is as yet unknown but the author's observations suggest that development does not take place in water.

Assuming that the eight species mentioned by Yamaguti (1961) are valid one must now add a ninth described by Baruš and Sonin (1971) who found *Hastospiculum cubaense* in two species of Cuban snakes.

Superfamily Filarioidea
Anderson and Bain (1976) established the superfamily Filarioidea with the exclusion of the Diplotriaenoidea and the Aproctoidea and this approach is accepted by the author. The common feature of the superfamily is the production of microfilariae in place of eggs.

All filariae share the following characteristics: a small oral aperture, no oral capsule, no pharynx, partition of the oesophagus into an anterior muscular and a posterior glandular part, a cuticle (usually smooth or slightly annulated) and two unequal spicula. The males are usually considerably smaller than the females. Another characteristic is the localization of the mature worms (macrofilariae) outside the intestinal lumen of the definitive host, usually in the lungs, the blood vessels and in other tissues.

Microfilariae are commonly seen in the blood. Transmission from one definitive host to another necessitates blood-sucking arthropods. Intermediate hosts are mainly mosquitoes (Culicidae) and ticks.

Lavoipierre (1958b) described only two life-cycles of species parasitizing reptiles. Other experimental life-cycles have been described subsequently but for none of the species involved has the natural intermediate host been established. In Australia, Johnston and Mawson (1943) assumed that *Culex fatigans* was the natural intermediate host for *Oswaldofilaria chlamydosauri*.

Of the large number of species described by Yamaguti (1961), Skrjabin (1969) and Sonin (1974) only those accepted by Anderson and Bain (1976) are mentioned in this chapter.

Only one family, the Onchocercidae, needs to be discussed here.

Family Onchocercidae
Anderson and Bain (1976) mentioned eight subfamilies, only five of which are found in reptiles.

Oswaldofilariinae (Parasites of crocodilians and lacertilians)
Befilaria   *Piratuba*
Conofilaria   *Piratuboides*
Oswaldofilaria   *Solafilaria*

Dirofilariinae (Parasites of lacertilians and chameleons)
Foleyella

Onchocercinae (Parasites of ophidians and lacertilians)
Macdonaldius

Splendidofilariinae (Parasites of chelonians and lacertilians)
Cardianema (In the heart of turtles)
Madathamugadia (Lizards, Madagascar)
Pseudothamugadia (Lizards)
Thamugadia (Subcutaneous tissues of geckos)

Lemdaninae (Parasites of lacertilians)
Saurositus

Biology

Female macrofilariae produce thousands of well developed embryos (microfilariae) each day. The latter are either enveloped in a "sheath", the stretched vitelline membrane (ovoviviparous species) or they are free "unsheathed" (viviparous species). Microfilariae are only equipped with primordial cells, not with organs.

The nocturnal or diurnal periodicity which is typical of several microfilariae of man, some mammals and birds appears to have no parallel in reptiles (Hawking, 1962). Telford (1965a) confirmed such aperiodicity in respect of the circadian cycle in *Macdonaldius oschei* Chabaud and Frank (1961) but was able to show variation in the density of microfilariae in the blood of a *Boa constrictor mexicanus* every two days.

Only if the microfilariae are ingested by a suitable blood-sucking arthropod intermediate host does further development occur. The infective stage (third-stage larva) is reached after two moults within 7–25 days. These larvae are transmitted to a new vertebrate host in one of the next blood meals of the arthropod (Frank, 1964c). The transmission of infective stages to reptiles is similar to that in mammals (Lavoipierre, 1958a,b; Bain and Philippon, 1969).

Unsuitable intermediate hosts suffer severe damage. The microfilariae reach the haemocoel via the intestinal wall and destroy the epithelial cells. Heavy burdens of microfilariae cause the death of the arthropods (Frank, 1964b; Telford, 1965b) but it should be borne in mind that many microfilariae die in suitable hosts (Nelson, 1963). Bain and Philippon observed this phenomenon in *Anopheles stephensi* infected with the microfilariae of *Foleyella furcata* while Pflugfelder (1977) reported that the microfilariae of *F. philistinae* in the haemocoel of the intermediate hosts are surrounded by granulomatous material and giant cells.

Although most filariae of reptiles have been described from only a few hosts, several accounts suggest that they are not very host specific. Frank (1964a), working with *Macdonaldius oschei*, was able to show that members of the Boinae and Pythoninae from different geographical regions could be infected experimentally. Equally, Telford (1965b) showed that Colubridae and Viperidae from Mexico were naturally infected with the same parasite species and in 1977 Frank and Loos-Frank demonstrated the same phenomenon in the snake *Elaphe guttata*, bred in captivity in Europe. For the latter species at least, the chance of spreading seems to depend on the availability of suitable intermediate hosts, a point emphasized by Telford (1965b).

Relatively little is known of the vectors of reptilian species. Mackerras (1953, 1962) found *Oswaldofilaria chlamydosauri* in two species of mosquitoes (*C. fatigans*, *C. annulirostris*), and Bain and Chabaud (1975) inculpated several species (*Culex* and *Aedes*) as suitable vectors for *Oswaldofilaria petersi*, *O. belemensis* and *O. spinosa*.

Suitable vectors are the prerequisite for filarial transmission amongst captive reptiles. Since many of these reptiles originate from tropical or subtropical countries the vectors must be species which can develop at the temperature in which the reptiles are kept. Acarines may play an important role in this connection, particularly laelaptid mites (*Ophionyssus* spp.). The argasid tick (*Ornithodoros talaje*) proved to be a suitable vector for *Macdonaldius oschei* (Frank, 1964b,c). These results were obtained from reptiles kept in captivity in Europe, but Telford (1965a) thought it very likely that ticks also function as vectors in the wild and in 1971 he suggested that an ixodid tick *Amblyomma dissimile* may play this role in Mexico. Similarly, Smith (1910) found a filaria in *Heloderma suspectum* and described developmental stages in a tick found attached to the same reptile. This "*Filaria mitchelli*" may well be identical to *Macdonaldius andersoni* described by Chabaud and Frank (1961a,b) and it may be reasonable to regard ticks as frequent vectors for *Macdonaldius* species. Other investigations show that mosquitoes play an important part in the experimental transmission of filariae to reptiles. Specificity for these arthropods seems to be small and probably several species may serve as hosts for filariae in nature.

Clinical signs Observations are at present limited to accidentally infected pythons and boas. This applies especially when there are large numbers of filariae in the large arteries, particularly in the abdomen.

For example, in a *Python molurus bivittatus*, several hundred were found clustered in this site; this led to an interruption of the blood supply with subsequent gangrene of the tail tip and the gradual development of dermal ulcers which spread cranially (Frank, 1964a).

Similar lesions to those described above have been seen in *Python reticulatus*. Telford (1965b), on the other hand, never observed such a clinical picture in Mexican snakes naturally infected with *M. oschei*. It may be that snakes from the same environment as the filariae are well adapted to the infection. A similar situation may apply to other New World snakes; Frank and Loos-Frank (1977) examined heavily infected North American snakes of the species *Elaphe guttata* which had been bred in captivity and these too showed no clinical signs.

There is a paucity of clinical and pathological reports in the literature. Hull and Camin (1959) ascribed the death of a *Pituophis catenifer* to an obstruction of the portal vein with *Macdonaldius seetae* without being able to observe any clinical signs *ante mortem*. A report by Elkan (in Reichenbach-Klinke, 1977) demonstrated clearly that reptiles may live for long periods in spite of a filarial infection. In Elkan's case, a *Physignathus lesueuri* which had lived for nine years in captivity in Britain showed an intense filarial infection *post mortem*. The lizard must have been infected in Australia before being imported, but it showed no sign of illness before its sudden death. A similar case was seen by Telford (1965b) who kept a *Trimorphodon biscutatus* for 21 months during which time the snake continuously showed 30 000 microfilariae per ml of blood.

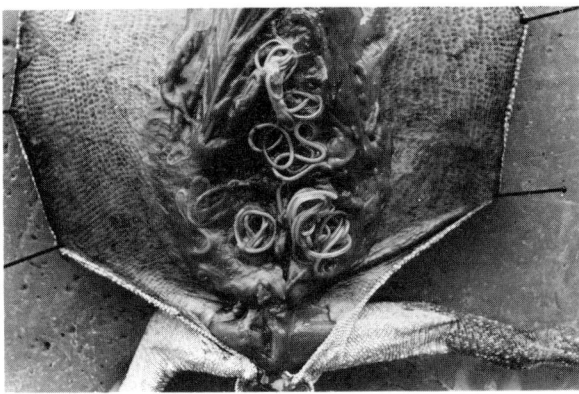

Fig. 9.6 Heavy filarial burden (*Foleyella furcata*) in a chameleon (*Chamaeleo oustaleti*). At the time of examination the filariae were yellow-orange in colour.

Pathology Filarial infestations may severely damage the viscera of reptiles. Frank (1964a) demonstrated that pathological changes, similar to aneurysms, around balls of filarial worms and arterial granulomata containing filaria did not arise *post mortem* but in life.

Such an accumulation of filariae produces a picture of thrombarteritis verminosa (Fig. 9.7). Telford (1965b) found calcified worms in cases where the microfilaraemia rose to more than 200 microfilariae per ml of blood. These dead worms were always located in the distal portions of the aneurysms or behind living adults.

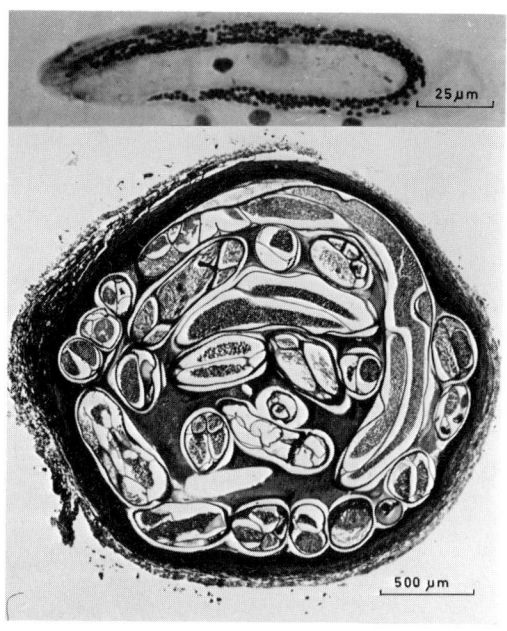

Fig. 9.7. Section of an obstructed artery of *Python reticulatus* infected with filariae (*Macdonaldius oschei*). Above is a microfilaria of this species showing its typical ovoid sheath.

Nelson (1966) reviewed the pathology of filarial infections and emphasized the importance of the number of filariae. This is also valid for reptiles but Nelson's supposition that the relatively minor reaction seen in animals compared with that in humans is linked with their shorter life-span is not necessarily correct. The nine year infection period quoted by Elkan represents only half the time cited by Nelson for human infections with *Onchocerca volvulus* in which there were severe complications.

Frank (1964a) reported in detail on the pathological changes in the skin of snakes which became accidentally infected with filariae.

It is not yet known whether the filariae deprive the host of important nutrients. However, it should be noted that some filariae accumulate large amounts of carotenoids, and these are derived from the host's food (Frank and Fetzer, 1968).

Diagnosis Microfilariae can be found in fresh blood in physiological saline preparations, in stained blood smears or, best of all, in "thick drop" preparations. During autopsy only a careful search will reveal the macrofilariae, particularly the males which are much smaller than the females.

C. Subphylum Acanthocephala (Spiny-headed worms)

Biology

The adult worms live in the alimentary tract of vertebrates. They are rarely seen in reptiles but immature stages may be encountered in the mesenteries or embedded in the intestinal wall. Their life-cycles involve aquatic or terrestrial invertebrates. In many species vertebrate intermediate hosts have only a paratenic function and in such cases reptiles may play an important role.

The main characters of these worms are the presence of a protrusible proboscis at the anterior end, armed with spines or hooklets of various sizes, and the lack of a digestive tract. Nutrients are absorbed through the surface and, in the case of lipids, via the "lemnisci" (Pflugfelder, 1949). Details of these parasites may be found in Nicholas (1967) and Crompton (1970).

The Acanthocephala are divided into three orders, the Archiacanthocephala, Palaeacanthocephala and Eoacanthocephala.

All species known up to 1963 were catalogued by Yamaguti (1963b). The few species which parasitize reptiles fall largely within the last two orders.

Semi-aquatic or aquatic reptiles may be heavily infested. During investigations where, amongst other species, 125 terrapins (*Pseudemys scripta*) were killed in a search for helminths, Martin (1972) found Acanthocephala in 123 animals.

It is generally accepted that the original life-cycle of the Acanthocephala included a single invertebrate intermediate host and fish as final hosts. In many instances juvenile acanthocephalans have been found encapsulated in the tissues of vertebrates which feed on invertebrates, the latter functioning as first intermediate hosts. Often these hosts, unsuitable for the further development of the larvae, are merely paratenic. It may be assumed that acanthocephalans found encapsulated in reptilian tissue, particularly in snakes, represent re-encapsulated stages which originated as juveniles in another unsuitable vertebrate. Such surviving juveniles assist in the infestation of vertebrates such as reptiles. *Neoechinorhynchus emydis* normally develops in a small crustacean (*Ostracoda*) and infects turtles, but it can also survive in certain snails if these feed on infected ostracods. Only if these snails are eaten by turtles can the adults complete their development in the chelonian intestine. Paratenic hosts are not required but they may serve as links in the food chain and carry the larval stages to the suitable definitive host. The stages in the development of the Acanthocephala are as follows: egg, acanthor, acanthella (juvenile), cystacanth and adult male and female.

Clinical signs   None reported.

Pathology   Only the developmental stages of the acanthocephalans are of importance in reptiles. The few parasitizing reptiles as adults are usually only present in small numbers. They may damage the intestinal tract producing lesions similar to those found in birds and mammals. Such lesions are caused by the spines of the protrusible proboscis of the worm.

Bullock (1963) described the histopathology of fishes infested by acanthocephalans and his pictures are similar to those seen in turtles infested with *Neoechinorhynchus emydis*. Pflugfelder (1956) reported extensive connective tissue proliferation around dead acanthocephalans and granulomata were present on the serosa of the gut. Humoral reactions to these worms are recognized in fish (Harris and Cottrell, 1974) and in rats (Andreassen, 1974a,b) and may reduce superinfection. It could be relevant to reptiles living permanently in the same aquatic environment.

Occasionally Acanthocephala whose normal definitive hosts are amphibians are found in snakes and chelonians. These worms can apparently survive some time in normally unsuitable hosts but cannot stay there permanently. *Acanthocephalus ranae*, for example, has been found in *Natrix natrix* and *A. anthuris* in turtles. Nicholas (1967) mentioned "a remarkable lack of specificity" with regard to definitive hosts.

Even the larvae have a great ability to survive in unsuitable hosts. Ingested cystacanths which fail to establish themselves in the gut of a definitive host may migrate into the tissue where they remain viable and infective. The hosts thereby become potential transport or paratenic vectors. This lack of specificity enlarges the choice of further hosts to such an extent that new records are constantly reported. Encapsulated juveniles are commonly found around the intestinal wall in reptiles but they may also occur in the liver of lizards (*Lacerta* spp.) (Frank, unpublished). Histological observations on similar lesions were published by Bogitsh (1961). Juvenile acanthocephalans can become so numerous in snakes as to impede the passage of food. Elkan (1974) recorded a case where there were masses of acanthellae in the body-cavity and embedded in the wall of the gut of a snake (*Dryophis prasina*). The acanthellae belonged to a species of *Sphaerechinorhynchus* and had an average length of 25 mm. Each was enclosed in a tough capsule of collagenous fibres and situated both intra- and extraperitoneally. Elkan reported that "In the present case their number was 48 but with their comparatively large size they took up all the available space in the snake's body and would have made feeding impossible". Although the present author has seen many similar cases he has been less confident that the effect was anorexia due to mechanical obstruction.

Diagnosis Detection of eggs in the faeces is usually relatively easy. Juveniles encapsulated in the host tissues cannot be diagnosed unless some of them form nodules under the skin.

V. Phylum Arthropoda

The main characters of this phylum are dealt with in Chapter 10.

A. Subphylum Pentastomida (syn. Linguatulida) (Tongue worms)

The pentastomids live exclusively as endoparasites. Osche (1963), on the basis of embryological investigations, grouped them close to the Myriapoda, while Doucet (1965), who carried out comparative neurological examinations of adults, concluded that the Annelida, Arthropoda and Pentastomida had a common origin but that no group could have been derived from another. This view was also supported by a number of other authors including Trainer (1974) and Trainer *et al* (1975). Other authors who have discussed their origin include Haffner (1977), Wingstrand (1972, 1974) and Riley *et al* (1978).

The Pentastomida can be divided into two groups; the more primitive Cephalobaenida and the parasitic Porocephalida (Haffner, 1977).

The Pentastomida vary in size from a few millimetres (*Railliettiella* spp.) to 14 cm (*Armillifer armillatus*). The usual colour of the worms is whitish-yellow. The eggs are embryonated when shed. The primary larvae of all species are equipped with four truncated articulated limbs, usually with a terminal claw. These larvae have an anterior perforating apparatus which facilitates hatching and further migration through the tissues of the host. Detailed descriptions of the eggs and the primary larvae may be found in Esslinger (1962a, 1968).

The infectious larvae (nymphs) of most species perforate the intestinal wall of the definitive host, travel through the body and enter the lungs. This migration may cause severe pathological damage (Fain, 1966).

The morphology and anatomy of the Pentastomida have been dealt with by various authors (Heymons, 1926, 1935; Fain, 1961; Self, 1969); the essential characters may also be found in certain text books (Cheng, 1973; Frank, 1976a). Monographs on the pentastomes include those by Sambon (1922), Heymons (1932, 1935, 1938), Heymons and Vitzthum (1935), Hill (1948), Fain (1961) and Nicoli (1963).

About 70 pentastomid species are known from all parts of the world. Reptiles, particularly snakes, are their preferred definitive hosts.

As yet there is no unanimity on the life-cycles of these peculiar parasites. Most species probably require an intermediate host. The number of larval or nymph stages quoted in the literature varies. For example, in *Linguatula serrata*, found in mammals, 9–10 skin changes are recorded while Esslinger (1962a,b,c) described seven stages in *Porocephalus crotali*. Lavoipierre and Lavoipierre (1966) and Lavoipierre and Rajamanickam (1973), however, reported two larval stages in *Railliettiella hemidactyli*.

Recent observations by the author confirm that larvae may occur in definitive hosts as well as mature worms. For example, in the lungs of a *Bothrops atrox* a total of 246 *Railliettiella* spp. of all stages was seen. Such an accumulation of parasites is probably an auto-infection and cannot be compared with a natural direct infection; the condition

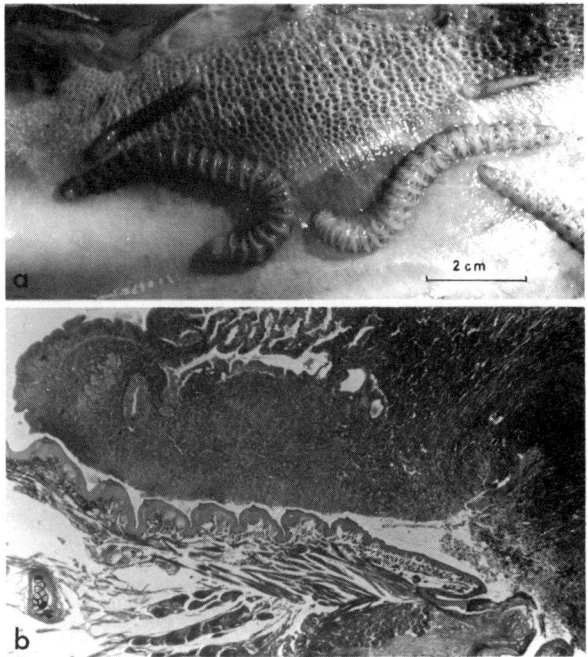

Fig. 9.8. (a) *Armillifer armillatus* pentastomids in the lung of a Gaboon viper (*Bitis gabonica*). (b) An undetermined pentastomid deeply inserted into the lung (which shows pathological lesions) of an Australian elapid snake.

probably resulted from a reduction in body defences of the particular snake. A similar situation may apply to the findings reported by Fain and Mortelmans (1960). If auto-infection with pentastomids is accepted the wide variation in results when larvae have been fed to a variety of definitive hosts remains to be explained (Lavoipierre and Rajamanickam, 1973). It should be noted in this context that Banaja et al (1975), working with *Railliettiella hemidactyli* (Cephalobaenida), showed experimentally that invertebrates are an essential part of the life-cycle.

The presence of both larvae and mature worms of the same species in one and the same host is not evidence *per se* of direct development since primary larvae may start their development in many different hosts which are of no significance in perpetuating the life-cycle (Heymons and Vitzthum, 1935; Fain, 1961; Haffner et al, 1967). Even in aberrant hosts, eggs swallowed accidentally may develop into infective larvae. This lack of specificity in pentastomes was further demonstrated when Nadakal and Nayar (1968) successfully transplanted larvae and adults obtained from reptiles to amphibians.

Biology

In their final hosts the Pentastomida inhabit the respiratory passages or, in a few cases, the oral or pharyngeal regions. In some species only parasites of one sex are found in one host. Female pentastomids produce a large number of eggs but their numbers are not comparable with those of the helminths. When shed the eggs usually contain a well developed primary larva. They reach the oral cavity in pulmonary mucus and are either coughed up or swallowed and excreted with the faeces. The shape of the egg is characteristic. They are mostly spherical and contain an embryo (larva) in a separate shell. In *Railliettiella* spp. the outer shell may be absent and in other species which are aquatic (*Subtriquetra*) the sclerotized shell is missing and there remains only a flexible membrane which is easily ruptured by the movements of the larva (Vargas, 1974). The morphology, in particular the extremities, is easily recognizable through the egg membranes. Further development of the eggs can only occur if they are ingested by a suitable host. As was emphasized earlier, these are not always genuine intermediate hosts and may be biologically useless because they are outside the food chain of the definitive hosts. Some pentastomids, however, seem to have the capacity to develop in a great variety of such aberrant hosts and in this way even species which only migrate through certain regions may become infected. For example, Heymons and Vitzthum (1935) found *Armillifer armillatus* in a number of mammals and birds and described larvae in a honey buzzard (*Pernis apivorus*), a bird which inhabits Africa only for a few months of the year and spends the rest of its time in Europe.

The development of fully mature worms occurs if the eggs gain access to suitable intermediate hosts which are part of the food chain of the definitive hosts. The question of direct development, i.e. the ingestion of eggs by host animals already infected by mature pentastomids, was discussed earlier. It has not yet been proved.

Because of their low host specificity and the variety of potential definitive hosts, the pentastomids are relatively common in areas where reptiles still exist in some numbers. For example, Nadakal and Nayar (1968) found 60 per cent of reptiles to be infected.

Data on the life span of these parasites are uncertain and are based entirely on conditions in captivity. Species living in small hosts appear to have a life span of only about one year. Varanid lizards, on the other hand, have been observed to excrete eggs over a period of several years. The larger *Armillifer* species which inhabit snakes in Asia and Africa may live in their hosts for years unless they become sufficiently numerous to be pathogenic. The incidence of infection in captivity is uncertain but transmission is by no means unlikely where intermediate hosts (cockroaches) have free access to cages. Even rodents may act as intermediate hosts if they are not kept hygienically and entirely separated from reptiles. There is also some potential danger to the personnel looking after these animals (Cooper, 1973); human cases of this kind have not yet been reported, however.

Clinical signs Specific clinical signs have not yet been described. In the author's experience a heavy infestation may be detected by noisy respiration and the production of viscous oral mucus.

Pathology Insofar as reptiles are concerned the damage caused by adult worms is of the greatest interest but in human patients larvae may play an equally serious role. These two stages will be discussed separately.

(a) *Adults*

The pulmonary damage caused by pentastomids is characteristic. Occasionally the cellular response is so great as to lead to complete encapsulation of the anterior end and to a heavy fibrous degeneration of the pulmonary parenchyma. The latter reduces both the elasticity and the respiratory function of the lung. Eventually the worms may penetrate through the lung into the body cavity (Frank, 1975).

In spite of their apparently firm attachment to the lung pentastomes may leave this site and be regurgitated (Self and Kuntz, 1967; Deakins, 1971).

Pentastomids may cause severe tissue damage. Deakins (1971) ascribed the death of several alligators *Alligator mississippiensis* to an infestation with *Sebekia oxycephala*, in spite of a concomitant steatitis. The immediate cause of death seemed to be pulmonary damage with additional intestinal haemorrhage in two cases.

In many cases of pentastomid infestation the author has seen chronic pneumonia with muco-purulent foci on the pulmonary epithelium filling the alveoli and the air-sacs. However, the relationship of such lesions to the pentastomid infestation is difficult to establish. Possibly the infestation aggravates an already existing chronic pulmonary infection since the pentastomid hooks may facilitate the entry of bacteria into the tissues. (See Fig. 9.9).

346 W. FRANK

Apart from mechanical damage the influence of pentastomids on their hosts seems to be small. Reptiles examined immediately after capture rarely show pentastomid damage. Self and Kuntz (1967) found over 100 *Porocephalus crotali* in an otherwise healthy *Crotalus adamanteus* and reported no specific lesions.

The author's experiences are similar but attention should be drawn to an observation by Awachie (1974) who found heavy pulmonary destruction, inflammation, haemorrhage and necrosis in freshly caught geckos (*Hemidactylus angulatus*) caused by the pentastome *Raillietiella affinis*.

(b) *Larvae*

Young migrating stages and moribund larvae may on occasion produce severe reactions, as reported by Self *et al* (1972) in mice infected with *Porocephalus*.

The severe damage reported in laboratory rodents by Fülleborn (1919) has yet to be reproduced. The author had no deaths in a batch of four *Mus musculus*, five *Meriones unguiculatus* and thirteen *Mastomys natalensis* each of which was given 150 eggs of *Armillifer armillatus*. After several months 54 fully developed larvae were found in one of the *Mus musculus*; most of these larvae were free in the pleural cavity or the coelom but a few were in the lung or liver (Frank, unpublished).

Some batches of non-human primates imported for biomedical

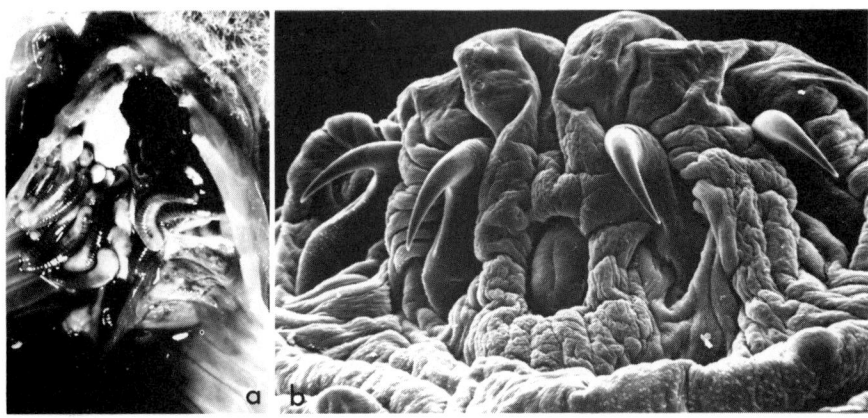

Fig. 9.9. (a) Infectious larvae of *Armillifer armillatus* in the pleural cavity of the rodent *Mastomys natalensis* 6 months after oral administration of eggs. Up to 42 larvae—size 1·5–2·0 cm—were found in a single rodent. (b) Anterior end of a larva of *A. armillatus* with two pairs of hooks and mouth opening between them. SEM-micrograph by F. R. Matuschka.

work are heavily infected with pentastomes but the lesions are not severe (Kuntz, 1974). These findings were supported by the work of Thurston (1972) who found a bush genet (*Genetta tigrina*) infested with about 2000 larvae of *Armillifer armillatus*. 1500 of these larvae were free in the body cavities but they were not considered responsible for the death of the animal. Some authors have reported "tumours" containing innumerable larvae of *Armillifer* in hosts which are unlikely prey for snakes. Fain (1961) reported such a case in an antelope. The "tumour" weighed 320 g and contained about 5000 *A. armillatus* larvae.

There are some reports of cases where intermediate hosts were severely affected. Boch (1957) working with rhesus monkeys (*Macaca mulatta*), reported a thick capsule of host tissue around the larvae of *Armillifer moniliformis*; this capsule was the product of a reactive inflammation with lymphocytes, histiocytes, macrophages and eosinophils. Where the larvae had died the tissue was necrotic. The lungs apart from a lobar bronchopneumonia, were emphysematous. Similar lesions may also occur in reptiles as observed by Zwart (1963) who found encysted nymphs of a *Porocephalus* sp. just under the renal capsule and between the renal tubules of a *Boa constrictor*. The capsule consisted of well vascularised connective tissue and a few mononuclear inflammatory cells. *Porocephalus* nymphs are of parasitological interest but appear to be of only minor pathological significance. Connective tissue encapsulation was seen by Awachie (1974) in the gecko *Hemidactylus angulatus* which contained larval stages of *Raillietiella affinis*.

Humoral reactions against pentastome larvae are also recognized (Self, 1974). Antibodies against *Armillifer armillatus* can be demonstrated by immunofluorescence or immunoprecipitation (Ranque *et al*, 1972, 1974a,b). The production of such antibodies may be protective; challenge after infection with larvae produced abscess formation around the dead larvae (Self, 1974).

Intermediate hosts react only moderately to live larvae, but the response may be severe when the larvae die (Haffner *et al*, 1967; Ranque *et al*, 1974a,b).

Reactions against pentastomid larvae appear to be a feature of infection of accidental intermediate hosts but are usually absent in natural hosts (Fain, 1966).

Special reference should, perhaps, be made to the situation in man.

Often human infections occur without any symptoms yet at autopsy a high infection rate may be found. Fain (1960) reported an 8–20 per cent prevalence and Buchanan (1967) 5–23 per cent. Prathap *et al* (1969) found pentastomids in liver or lung of 45·4 per cent of 30

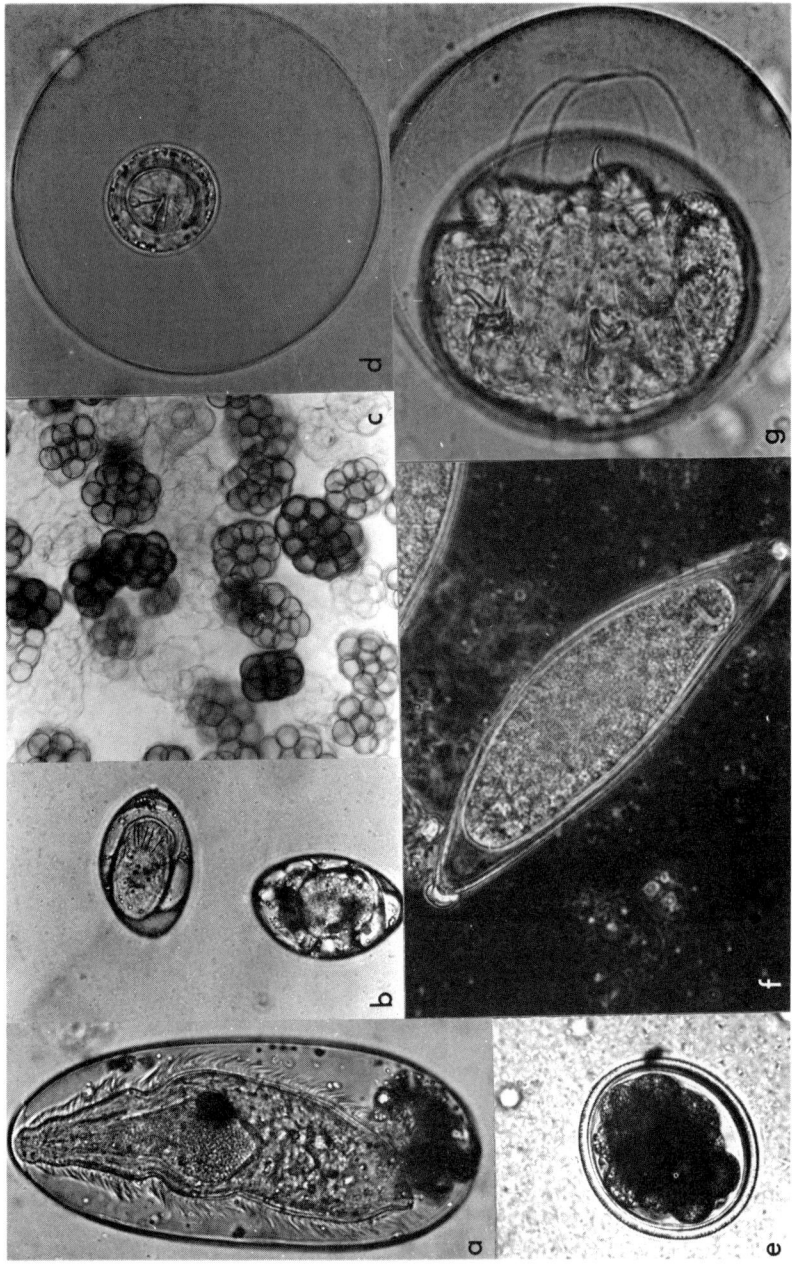

autopsies but did not relate these findings to the cause of death. They concluded that these infestations are very common in primitive societies. As in experimental animals, the living larvae usually elicit few reactions but the dead larvae can produce severe damage. Ranque *et al* (1974a,b) even suggested that pentastomiasis (porocephaliasis) might be a common cause of hepatic cirrhosis in Africans.

Occasionally, however, even living larvae may produce severe complications, particularly if the infestation is extensive (Buchanan, 1967). A particularly serious problem is aberrant invasion of the eyes (Reid and Jones, 1963; Lazar and Traub, 1967). Even fatalities have been reported; Canon (1942), recorded a case of a Nigerian woman who died from intestinal occlusion caused by large numbers of encysted larvae of *Armillifer armillatus* in the wall of the colon. From a careful review of the literature Cannon quoted a number of cases where pentastomid larvae have caused pneumonitis, peritonitis, meningitis, pericarditis and obstructive jaundice due to bile-duct occlusion (see also Bouckaert and Fain, 1959).

The multitude of reports on pentastomid infestation in humans emphasizes the importance of this disease in certain geographic regions, such as Asia and Africa (Amy, 1973). The larvae calcify rapidly in human patients and can then be located radiographically (Steinbach and Johnstone, 1957; Lechner, 1965; De Coster *et al*, 1967; Burns-Cox *et al*, 1969; Coulibaly *et al*, 1972; Browne, 1975; Rail, 1967). Pentastomid lesions can usually be distinguished from other parasitic foci or pathological processes by their number, size and density. They may, however, be confused with calcified dracunculids (Dönges, 1966; Goldsmid and Melmed, 1973).

It is uncertain as to which species of pentastomids are most likely to affect humans. This may be due to difficulties in identification and to poor preservation of specimens found during surgery or necropsies. Fain (1966, 1974) pointed out that of those larvae which become mature in reptiles only the *Armillifer* group affects humans, and he

---

Fig. 9.10. Examples of typical trematode, cestode, nematode and pentastomid eggs. (a) *Gogatea serpentium* from *Erpeton tentaculatum*. A typical trematode egg with operculum and fully developed miracidium. ($\times$ 265) (b) *Bothridium* sp. from *Elaphe radiata*. The eggs are in different stages of development. One egg shows the oncosphere with 6 hooklets. ($\times$ 210) (c) *Kapsulotaenia* sp. from *Varanus komodoensis*. Fully developed egg clusters are dark coloured. ($\times$ 150) (d) *Ophiotaenia* sp. from *Natrix n. persa*. Three of the 6 hooklets of the oncosphere are clearly seen. ($\times$ 40) (e) *Ophidascaris* sp. from *Bitis gabonica*. Eggs of ascarids often have an ornamented surface on the thick-walled shell. ($\times$ 230) (f) *Pharyngodon* sp. (Oxyuridae) from *Gekko gecko*. ($\times$ 360) (g) Egg of an undetermined pentastomid with fully developed larva; note the stumpy extremities with two claws. ($\times$ 300)

refuted the validity of statements by Sambon (1922) regarding *Porocephalus crotali* in America and *P. subulifer* in Africa. The following species have to date been found in humans in larval form:

Armillifer armillatus	Africa	Very frequently
Armillifer moniliformis	E. Asia, Australia	Not frequently
Armillifer grandis	Africa	Rarely
Leiperia cincinnalis	Africa	One case
Railliettiella gehyrae	Vietnam	Extremely rarely

Sexually mature pentastomids of species with reptiles as natural definitive hosts are very rare in humans. In some countries—for example, Vietnam—people eat large numbers of live lizards for various medicinal purposes and many of these reptiles are infected with pentastomids. In such circumstances transmission to humans can occur. Dollfus and Canet (1954) recorded one such case where adults of a *Railliettiella* species were found in a human patient.

The distribution of pentastomiasis varies considerably and several factors are responsible for this. The most important prerequisite is an abundance of snakes capable of harbouring the two species most important for humans (*Armillifer armillatus* and *A. moniliformis*). The second point is that the populace must be involved in such activities as the consumption of snake meat or the catching, preparation or sale of snakes. An additional factor may be climatic conditions; the drying-up of most water sources in the summer may force man and beasts—including snakes—to drink at the same place and the transmission of the parasite may then occur (Self *et al*, 1975).

References

Allison, V. F., Webster, R. W., Ubelaker, J. E. and Riddle, J. M. (1973). *Trans. Am. microsc. Soc.* **92**, 291–297.
Allroggen, R. and Allroggen, L. (1959). *Kleintier-Praxis* **4**, 138–139.
Amy, D. (1973). "La Pentastomose à Armillifer armillatus. Étude biologique, immunologique et radiologique". Thèse Doctorat en Médecine, Marseille.
Anderson, R. C. and Bain, O. (1976). *In* "CIH Keys to the Nematode Parasites of Vertebrates". (R. C. Anderson, A. G. Chabaud and S. Wilmott, eds). pp. 59–116. Commonwealth Agricultural Bureaux, Farnham Royal, Bucks, England.
Andreassen, J. (1974a). *III Int. Congr. Parasit. (München)* **2**, 1068–1069.
Andreassen, J. (1974b). *III Int. Congr. Parasit. (München)* **2**, 1057–1058.
Araujo, P. (1971). *Annls. Parasit. hum. comp.* **46**, 605–611.
Araujo, P. (1972). *Annls Parasit. hum. comp.* **47**, 91–120.

Ash, L. R. (1962). *J. Parasit.* **48,** 298–305.
Ash, L. R. and Beaver, P. C. (1962). *J. Parasit.* **48,** No. 2, Section 2 (Suppl.) 41/Abstract 85.
Awachie, J. B. E. (1974). *III Int. Congr. Parasit. (München)* **2,** 1024.
Bain, O. and Chabaud, A. G. (1975). *Annls. Parasit. hum. comp.* **50,** 209–221.
Bain, O. and Philippon, B. (1969). *C. R. Acad. Sci. (D) (Paris)* **269,** 1081–1083.
Banaja, A. A., James, J. L. and Riley, J. (1975). *Parasitology* **71,** 493–503.
Barus, V. and Sonin, M. D. (1971). *Fol. Parasit. (Prague)* **18,** 187–189.
Boch, J. (1957). *Z. Parasitenk.* **17,** 424–429.
Bogitsh, B. J. (1961). *Proc. Helminth. Soc. Wash.* **28,** 75–81.
Bouckaert, L. and Fain, A. (1959). *Ann. soc. belge Med. trop.* **39,** 793–797.
Browne, D. (1975). *Med. biol. Illus. (London)* **25,** 20.
Buchanan, G. (1967). *Trans. R. Soc. trop. Med. Hyg.* **61,** 746–747.
Bullock, W. L. (1963). *J. Morphol.* **112,** 23–44.
Burns-Cox, C. J., Prathap, K., Clark, E. and Gillman, R. (1969). *Trans. R. Soc. trop. Med. Hyg.* **63,** 409–411.
Bychowsky, B. E. (1962). "Monogenetic Trematodes. Their Systematics and Phylogeny". (Translation of the 1957 Russian edition) (W. J. Hargis, ed.). *Amer. Inst. Biol. Sci.* (Washington D.C.).
Cannon, D. A. (1942). *Ann. trop. Med. Parasit.* **36,** 160–166.
Cawthorn, R. J. and Anderson, R. C. (1976). *Can. J. Zool.* **54,** 313–323.
Chabaud, A. G. (1974). *In* "CIH Keys to the Nematode Parasites of Vertebrates". (R. C. Anderson, A. G. Chabaud and S. Wilmott, eds). pp. 1–17. Commonwealth Agricultural Bureaux, Farnham Royal, Bucks, England.
Chabaud, A. G. (1975a). *In* "CIH Keys to the Nematode Parasites of Vertebrates". (R. C. Anderson, A. G. Chabaud and S. Wilmott, eds). pp. 1–17. Commonwealth Agricultural Bureaux, Farnham Royal, Bucks, England.
Chabaud, A. G. (1975b). *In* "CIH Keys to the Nematode Parasites of Vertebrates". (R. C. Anderson, A. G. Chabaud and S. Wilmott, eds). pp. 29–58. Commonwealth Agricultural Bureaux, Farnham Royal, Bucks, England.
Chabaud, A. G. and Frank, W. (1961a). *Annls. Parasit. hum. comp.* **36,** 127–134.
Chabaud, A. G. and Frank, W. (1961b). *Annls. Parasit. hum. comp.* **36,** 804–805.
Cheng, T. C. (1973). "General Parasitology". Academic Press, New York and London.
Cho, S. Y. and Seo, B. S. (1972). *Korean J. Parasit.* **10,** 122–123.
Cho, S. Y., Hwang, K. I. and Seo, B. S. (1973). *Korean J. Parasit.* **11,** 87–94.
Cooper, J. E. (1971). *Vet. Rec.* **89,** 385–388.
Cooper, J. E. (1973). *Br. J. Herpet.* **5,** 368–374.
Cooper, J. E. (1974). *Br. J. Herpet.* **5,** 431–438.
Coulibaly, N., Delporte, P., Delormas, P., Saracino, E. and Doucet, J. (1972). *Ann. Univ. Abidjan, Med.* **6,** 236–238.

Crompton, D. W. T. (1970). "An Ecological Approach to Acanthocephalan Physiology". Cambridge University Press, London.
Daengsvang, S. (1949). *J. Parasit.* **35,** 116–121.
Deakins, D. E. (1971). *J. Parasit.* **57,** 1197.
De Coster, P., Andrien, J. M. Prevot, H. and Parent, M. (1967). *Annls. Soc. belge Méd. trop.* **47,** 257–264.
Dollfus, R. Ph. (1957). *Arch Inst. Pasteur Maroc.* **5,** 300–328.
Dollfus, R. Ph. (1958a). *Ann. Parasit. hum. comp.* **33,** 305–395.
Dollfus, R. Ph. (1958b). *Arch. Inst. Pasteur Maroc.* **5,** 540–546.
Dollfus, R. Ph. and Canet, J. (1954). *Bull. Soc. Path. Exot.* **47,** 401–407.
Dönges, J. (1966). *Z. Tropenmed. Parasit.* **17,** 252–256.
Doucet, J. (1965). *Mem. Off. Rech. Sci. Techn. Outre-Mer Paris* **14,** 1–150.
Dupouy, J. and Kechemir, N. (1973). *Bull. Soc. Hist. nat. Afr. Nord Alger.* **64,** 47–98.
Eckert, J., v. Brand, Th. and Voge, M. (1969). *J. Parasit.* **55,** 241–249.
Elbihari, S. and Hussein, M. F. (1973). *J. Wildl. Dis.* **9,** 171–173.
Elkan, E. (1974). *Bull. N. Y. Herpet. Soc.* **2,** 9–18.
Esslinger, J. H. (1962a). *J. Parasit.* **48,** 457–462.
Esslinger, J. H. (1962b). *J. Parasit.* **48,** 452–456.
Esslinger, J. H. (1962c). *J. Parasit.* **48,** 631–638.
Esslinger, J. H. (1968). *J. Parasit.* **54,** 411–416.
Fain, A. (1960). *Bull. Acad. R. Med. Belg. Ser. 6,* **25,** 516–532.
Fain, A. (1961). *Mus. Roy. Afr. Centr. Tervuren Belg. Ann. Ser. Sci. Zool.* **92,** 1–115.
Fain, A. (1966). *Mem. Inst. Butantan.* **33,** 167–174.
Fain, A. (1974). *III Int. Congr. Parasit. (München)* **2,** 1028.
Fain, A. and Mortelmans, J. (1960). *Bull. Acad. R. Belg. Ser 5,* **46,** 518–531.
Frank, W. (1964a). *Z. Parasitenk.* **24,** 249–275.
Frank, W. (1964b). *Z. Parasitenk.* **24,** 319–350.
Frank, W. (1964c). *Z. Parasitenk.* **24,** 415–441.
Frank, W. (1966a). *Z. Parasitenk.* **27,** 90–98.
Frank, W. (1966b). *In* "Erkrankungen der Zootiere." Verh. Ber. VIII Int. Symp. Erk. der Zootiere, Leipzig, pp 184–196. Akademie Verlag, Berlin.
Frank, W. (1971). *Aquarien Magazin.* **5,** 244–250.
Frank, W. (1975). *Tierärztl. Praxis* **3,** 343–363.
Frank, W. (1976a). "Parasitologie". E. Ulmer Verlag, Stuttgart.
Frank, W. (1976b). *In* "Zootierkrankheiten". (H. G. Klös and E. M. Lang, eds). pp. 290–305. P. Parey Verlag, Berlin and Hamburg.
Frank. W. (1978). "Schlangen im Terrarium; Haltung und Pflege ungiftiger Schlangen". Franckh'sche Verlagshandlung, Stuttgart.
Frank, W. and Fetzer, U. (1968). *Z. Parasitenk.* **30,** 199–206.
Frank, W. and Loos-Frank B. (1977). *In* "Erkrangungen der Zootiere." Verh. Ber. XIX Int. Symp. Erk. der Zootiere, Poznań, pp. 31–44. Akademie Verlag, Berlin.
Frank, W. and Reichel, K. (1977). *In* "Erkrankungen der Zootiere." Verh. Ber. XIX Int. Symp. Erk. der Zootiere, Poznań, pp. 107–114. Akademie Verlag, Berlin.

Freeman, R. S. (1973). *Adv. Parasitol.* **11**, 481–557.
Freze, V. I. (1965). *In* "Essentials of Cestodology". (K. I. Skrjabin, ed.) Vol. V, pp 1–597. (English translation 1969). Israel Programme for Scientific Translations, Jerusalem.
Frye, F. L. (1973). "Husbandry, Medicine and Surgery in Captive Reptiles". VM Publishing Inc., Kansas.
Fülleborn, F. (1919). *Arch. Schiffs. Trop. Hyg.* **23**, Beiheft **1**, 1–36.
Goldsmid, J. M. and Melmed, M. H. (1973). *Centr. Afr. J. Med.* **19**, 213–216.
Goodey, T. (1924). *J. Helminth.* **2**, 51–64.
Grenot, C. and Vernon, R. (1973). *C. R. Soc. Biogéogr.* **433**, 96–112.
Grünberg, W. and Kutzer, E. (1964). *Zbl. Vet. Med. B.* **11**, 190–199.
Grünberg, W., Kutzer, E. and Otte, E. (1963). *Berl. Münch. Tierärztl. Wschr.* **76**, 90–95.
Haffner, K. v. (1977). *Zool. Anz. (Jena).* **199**, 353–370.
Haffner, K. v., Sachs, R. and G. Rack. (1967). *Z. Parasitenk.* **29**, 329–355.
Harris, J. E. and Cottrell, B. J. (1974). *III Int. Congr. Parasit. (München)* **2**, 1045–1046.
Hartwich, G. (1974). *In* "CIH Keys to the Nematode Parasites of Vertebrates". (R. C. Anderson, A. G. Chabaud and S. Wilmott, eds). pp. 1–15. Commonwealth Agricultural Bureaux, Farnham Royal, Bucks, England.
Hawking, F. (1962). *Ann. N.Y. Acad. Sci.* **98**, 940–953.
Herde, K. E. (1938). *Trans. Am. microsc. Soc.* **57**, 282–291.
Heymons, R. (1926). *In* "Handbuch der Zoologie; eine Naturgeschichte der Stämme des Tierreichs". (W. Kükenthal and T. Krumbach, eds). pp. 69–128. W. de Gruyter, Berlin.
Heymons, R. (1932). *Z. Parasitenk.* **4**, 409–430.
Heymons, R. (1935). *In* "Klassen und Ordnungen des Tierreichs". (H. G. Bronns, ed.). Bd. 5, Abt. 4, 1. Teil 1–268. Akademie Verlagsgesellschaft, Leipzig.
Heymons, R. (1938). *Z. Parasitenk.* **10**, 675–690.
Heymons, R. and Vitzthum, H. Grat (1935). *Z. Parasitenk.* **8**, 1–103.
Hill, H. R. (1948). *Bull. S. Calif. Acad. Sci.* **47**, 56–73.
Hörchner, F. (1962). *Z. Parasitenk.* **21**, 187–194.
Holt, P. E., Brown, A. and Brown, B. (1978). *Vet. Rec.* **102**, 404–405.
Hubbard, W. E. (1933). *Am. Midl. Nat.* **19**, 617–618.
Hull, R. W. and Camin, J. H. (1959). *Trans. Am. microsc. Soc.* **78**, 323–329.
Ippen, R. (1965). *Zbl. allg. Path.* **107**, 520–529.
Ippen, R. (1971). *In* "Erkrankungen der Zootiere." Verh. Ber. XIII Int. Symp. Erk. der Zootiere, Helsinki, pp. 173–186. Akademie Verlag, Berlin.
Jackson, O. F. and Muller, T. A. (1976). *Vet. Rec.* **99**, 375–376.
Johnston, T. H. and Mawson, P. M. (1943). *Trans. R. Soc. S. Aust.* **67**, 183–186.
Joyeux, C. and Baer, J. G. (1932). *Bull. Soc. Path. Exot.* **25**, 993–1010.
Joyeux, C. and Baer, J. G. (1933). *C. R. Acad. Sci.* **196**, 1838–1839.
Joyeux, C. and Baer, J. G. (1936). *C. R. Soc. Biol.* **121**, 67–68.
Joyeux, C., Baer, J. G. and Martin, R. (1933). *C. R. Soc. Biol.* **114**, 1179–1180.

Kane, K. K., Corwin, R. M. and Boever, W. J. (1976). *VM/SAC* **71**, 183–184.
Kazacos, K. R. and Fisher, L. F. (1977). *J. Am. vet. med. Ass.* **171**, 876–878.
Kumada, N., Mizuno, S., Kato, Y., Mizuno, T., Oya, H., Suzuki T. and Hattori, T. (1972). *Jap. J. Parasit.* **21**, 336–345.
Kuntz, R. E. (1974). *III Int. Congr. Parasit. (München)* **2**, 1027.
Kutzer, E. and Grünberg, W. (1965a). *Z. Parasitenk.* **26**, 24–28.
Kutzer, E. and Grünberg, W. (1965b). *Zbl. Vet. Med.* B **12**, 155–175.
Kutzer, E. and Lamina, J. (1965). *Z. Parasitenk.* **25**, 211–230.
Lavoipierre, M. M. J. (1958a). *Ann. trop. Med. Parasit.* **52**, 103–121.
Lavoipierre, M. M. J. (1958b). *Ann. trop. Med. Parasit.* **52**, 326–345.
Lavoipierre, M. M. J. and Lavoipierre, M. (1966). *Nature* **210**, 845–846.
Lavoipierre, M. M. J. and Rajamanickam, C. (1973). *J. med. Ent.* **10**, 301–302.
Lazar, M. and Traub, Z. (1967). *Am. J. Ophthalmol.* **63**, 1799–1800.
Lee, S. H. (1957). *J. Parasit.* **43**, 66–75.
Lechner, G. (1965). *Deutsch. Med. Wschr.* **90**, 488–491.
Lichtenfels, J. R. and Lavies, B. (1976). *Lab. Anim. Sci.* **26**, 465–467.
Little, M. D. (1966). *J. Parasit.* **52**, 85–97.
Loos-Frank, B. (1980). *Z. Tropenmed. Parasit.* **31**, 2–14.
MacDonald, D. M. and Litchford, R. G. (1974). *J. Tenn. Acad. Sci.* **49**, 58–59.
Mackerras, M. J. (1953). *Parasitol.* **43**, 1–3.
Mackerras, M. J. (1962). *Austr. J. Zool.* **10**, 400–457.
Mackin, J. G. (1928). *J. Parasit.* **14**, 91–94.
Magath, T. B. (1929). *Ann. trop. Med. Parasitol.* **23**, 121–127.
Marcus, L. C. (1968). *Curr. Vet. Therap.* **3**, 335–442.
Martin, D. R. (1972). *Trans. Ill. Acad. Sci.* **65**, 61–67.
Matoff, K. (1953). *Acta Veterinaria (Budapest)* **3**, 329–335.
Mazaud, R., Audebaud, G., Brumpt, V., Imbert, X. and Goube, P. (1973). *Bull. Soc. Pathol. Exot.* **66**, 320–324.
Meggitt, F. J. (1927). *Parasitol.* **19**, 420–448.
Merdivenci, A. and Sezen, Y. (1965). *Z. Parasitenk.* **25**, 387–392.
Merkushev, A. V. (1955). *Med. Parazitol. Parazit. Bolez.* **24**, 125–130.
Mirza, M. B. (1957). *Z. Parasitenk.* **28**, 44–47.
Mirza, M. B. and Roberts, L. S. (1957). *Z. Parasitenk.* **18**, 40–43.
Miyazaki, I. (1960). *Exp. Parasit.* **9**, 338–370.
Moravec, F. (1966). *Fol. Parasit. (Prague)* **13**, 281–283.
Mueller, J. F. (1937). *Science* **85**, 519–520.
Mueller, J. F. (1974). *J. Parasit.* **60**, 3–14.
Nadakal, A. M. and Nayar, K. K. (1968). *J. Parasit.* **54**, 189–190.
Nelson, G. S. (1963). *In* "Host–Parasite Relationships in Invertebrate Hosts". (A. E. R. Taylor, ed.) Vol. 2, pp. 75–119. Blackwell Scientific Publications, Oxford.
Nelson, G. S. (1966). *Helm. Abstr.* **35**, 311–336.
Nicholas, W. L. (1967). *Adv. Parasitol.* **5**, 205–246.
Nicoli, R. M. (1963). *Annls. Parasit. hum. comp.* **38**, 483–516.

Nitidandhaprabhas, P., Sirikarna, A., Harnsomburana, K. and Thepsitthar, P. (1975). *Amer. J. trop. Med. Hyg.* **24,** 49–51.
Odening, K. (1960). *Monatsber. deutsche Akad. Wiss. Berlin* **2,** 438–445.
Odening, K. (1961). *Monatsber. deutsche Akad. Wiss. Berlin* **3,** 59–69.
Odening, K. and Bockhardt, J. (1976). *Angew. Parasit.* **17,** 9–14.
Olsen, O. W. and Haas, W. R. (1976). *Hawaii Med. J.* **35,** 261–263.
Osche, G. (1958). *Z. Parasitenk.* **18,** 479–572.
Osche, G. (1963). *Z. Morph. Ökol. Tiere.* **52,** 487–596.
Page, L. A. (1966). *Bull. Wildl. Dis. Assoc.* **2,** 111–126.
Pence, D. B. (1970). *J. Parasit.* **56,** 261–264.
Petter, A. J. (1968a). *Annls. Parasit. hum. comp.* **43,** 693–704.
Petter, A. J. (1968b). *Annls. Parasit. hum. comp.* **43,** 655–691.
Petter, A. J. and Brygoo, E. R. (1972). *Annls. Parasit. hum. comp.* **47,** 581–583.
Petter, A. J. and Quentin, J-C. (1976). *In* "CIH Keys to the Nematode Parasites of Vertebrates." (R. C. Anderson, A. G. Chabaud and S. Wilmott, eds). Commonwealth Agricultural Bureaux, Farnham Royal, Bucks, England.
Petter, A. J., Bain, O. and Orcel, L. (1967). *Annls. Parasit. hum. comp.* **42,** 207–210.
Petter, C. (1960). *Annls. Parasit. hum. comp.* **35,** 118–137.
Pflugfelder, O. (1947/49). *Wilhelm Roux Arch. EntwMech. Tiere.* **143,** 304–331.
Pflugfelder, O. (1949). *Z. Parasitenk.* **14,** 274–280.
Pflugfelder, O. (1956). *Z. Parasitenk.* **17,** 371–382.
Pflugfelder, O. (1977). "Wirtstierreaktionen auf Zooparasiten". G. Fischer Verlag, Jena.
Prathap, K., Lau, K. S. and Bolten, J. M. (1969). *Am. J. trop. Med. Hyg.* **18,** 20–27.
Price, C. E. (1967). *Riv. Parassit.* **28,** 249–260.
Rail, G. A. (1967). *Trans. Roy. Soc. trop. Med. Hyg.* **61,** 715–717.
Ranque, Ph., Mattei, X. and Quilici, M. (1972). *C. R. Acad. Sci. Paris Série D.* **275,** 437–439.
Ranque, Ph., Amy, D., Discamps, G. and Quilici, M. (1974a). *III Int. Congr. Parasit. (München)* **2,** 1025.
Ranque, Ph., Amy, D., Discamps, G., Mattei, X. and Quilici, M. (1974b). *Z. Parasitenk.* **44,** 329–338.
Rees, G. (1963). *Parasitology* **53,** 201–215.
Rees, G. (1967). *Helm. Abstr.* **36,** 1–23.
Rego, A. A. (1973). *Atas. Soc. Biol. Rio de Jan.* **16,** 97–129.
Reichenbach-Klinke, H. (1977). "Krankheiten der Reptilien". G. Fischer, Stuttgart and New York.
Reichenbach-Klinke, H. and Elkan, E. (1965). "The Principal Diseases of Lower Vertebrates". Academic Press, London.
Reid, A. M. and Jones, D. W. E. (1963). *Br. J. Ophthal.* **47,** 169–172.
Riley, J., Banaja, A. A. and James, J. L. (1978). *Int. J. Parasit* **8,** 245–254.
Rohde, K. (1972). *Adv. Parasitol.* **10,** 77–151.
Rolón, P. A. (1976). *Bull. Soc. Path. Exot.* **69,** 351–359.

Sambon, L. W. (1922). *J. trop. Med. Hyg.* **25,** 186–206 and 391–428.
Schad, G. A. (1956). *Canad. J. Zool.* **34,** 425–452.
Schad, G. A. (1962). *Canad. J. Zool.* **40,** 1035–1165.
Schmidt, G. D. and Kuntz, R. E. (1972). *Trans. Am. microsc. Soc.* **91,** 63–66.
Self, J. T. (1969). *Exp. Parasitol.* **24,** 63–119.
Self, J. T. (1974). *III Int. Congr. Parasit. (München)* **2,** 1026.
Self, J. T. and Kuntz, R. E. (1967). *J. Parasit.* **53,** 202–206.
Self, J. T., Hopps, H. C. and Williams, A. O. (1972). *Exp. Parasitol.* **32,** 117–126.
Self, J. T., Hopps, H. C. and Williams, A. O. (1975). *Trop. Geogr. Med.* **27,** 1–13.
Seo, B. S. and Cho, S. Y. (1972). *Korean J. Parasit.* **10,** 132.
Shinde, G. B. (1968). *Riv. Parassitol.* **29,** 115–118.
Shoop, W. L. and Janovy, J. (1978). *J. Parasit.* **64,** 561–562.
Singh, M. D. and Pande, B. P. (1972). *Ind. J. animal Sci.* **42,** 207–213.
Skrjabin, K. I. (1947–1964) "Trematodes of Animals and Man". (Russian) Moscow. Vol. 1–22.
Skrjabin, K. I. (1969). "Key to Parasitic Nematodes. Vol. 1 Spirurata and Filariata". Israel Programme for Scientific Translations, Jerusalem.
Skrjabin, K. I., Shikobalova, N. P. and Logadovskaya, E. A. (1974 and 1976). *In* "Essentials of Nematodology." (K. I. Skrjabin, ed.). Israel Programme for Scientific Translations, Jerusalem.
Skrjabin, K. I., Shikobalova, N. P. and Orlov, I. V. (1970). *In* "Essentials of Nematodology." (K. I. Skrjabin, ed.). Israel Programme for Scientific Translations, Jerusalem.
Skrjabin, K. I., Shikobalova, N. P. and Schulz, R. S. (1954). *In* "Essentials of Nematodology." (K. I. Skrjabin, ed.). Israel Programme for Scientific Translations, Jerusalem.
Skrjabin, K. I., Sobolev, A. A. and Ivashkin, V. M. (1961). *In* "Essentials of Nematodology." (K. I. Skrjabin, ed.). Israel Programme for Scientific Translations, Jerusalem.
Skrjabin, K. I., Shikobalova, N. P., Schulz, R. S., Popova, T. I., Boer, S. N. and Delyamure, S. L. (1961). *In* "Key to Parasitic Nematodes. Vol. III Strongylata." (K. I. Skrjabin, ed.). Israel Programme for Scientific Translations, Jerusalem.
Šlais, J. (1973). *Adv. Parasit.* **11,** 395–480.
Smith, A. J. (1910). *Univ. Pennsylv. Med. Bull.* **23,** 487–497.
Soldatova, A. P. (1944). *Dokl. Akad. Nauk. SSSR* **45,** 310–312.
Soler, P. M. (1945). *Rev. Ibér. Parasitologia* Tomo Extraordinario, 67–72.
Solomon, S. G. (1932). *J. Helminth.* **10,** 67–74.
Sonin, M. D. (1974). *In* "Essentials of Nematodology." (K. I. Skrjabin, ed.). Israel Programme for Scientific Translations, Jerusalem.
Spasskii, A. A. (1951). *In* "Essentials of Cestodology." (K. I. Skrjabin, ed.). Israel Programme for Scientific Translations, Jerusalem.
Specht, D. and Voge, M. (1965). *J. Parasit.* **51,** 268–272.
Sprent, J. F. A. (1963). *Parasitology* **53,** 7–38.

Sprent, J. F. A. (1969a). *Parasitology* **59**, 129–140.
Sprent, J. F. A. (1969b). *Parasitology* **59**, 937–959.
Sprent, J. F. A. (1970). *Parasitology* **60**, 97–122.
Steinbach, H. L. and Johnstone, H. G. (1957). *Radiology (Syracuse)* **68**, 234–237.
Telford, S. R. (1964). "A Comparative Study of Endoparasitism among some Southern California Lizard Populations". Ph.D. Thesis. University of California.
Telford, S. R. (1965a). *Jap. J. exp. Med.* **35**, 291–300.
Telford, S. R. (1965b). *Jap. J. exp. Med.* **35**, 565–586.
Telford, S. R. (1965c). *Jap. J. exp. Med.* **35**, 301–303.
Telford, S. R. (1970). *Amer. Midl. Nat.* **83**, 516–554.
Telford, S. R. (1971). *J. Am. vet. med. Ass.* **159**, 1644–1652.
Thomas, L. J. (1934). *Anat. Rec.* **60**, 79–80.
Thomas, L. J. (1941). *Rev. Med. Trop. y Parasit. Bact. Clin. y Lab.* **7**, 74–78.
Thurston, J. P. (1972). *East Afr. med. J.* **49**, 791–792.
Trainer, J. E. (1974). *III Int. Congr. Parasit. (München)* **2**, 1019.
Trainer, J. E., Self, J. T. and Richter, K. M. (1975). *J. Parasit.* **61**, 753–758.
Tury, E. and Kobulej, T. (1973a). *Acta. vet. acad. sci. hung.* **23**, 167–175.
Tury, E. and Kobulej, T. (1973b). In "Erkrankungen der Zootiere". Verh. Ber. XV Int. Symp. Erk. der Zootiere, Kolmarden, pp. 343–345. Akademie Verlag, Berlin.
Vargas, V. M. (1974). *III Int. Congr. Parasit. (München)* **2**, 1021.
Voge, M. (1953). *Am. Midl. Nat.* **49**, 249–251.
Voge, M. (1967). *Adv. Parasitol.* **5**, 247–297.
Voge, M. (1973). *Adv. Parasitol.* **11**, 707–730.
Wallach, J. D. (1969). *J. Am. vet. med. Ass.* **155**, 1017–1034.
Walton, A. C. (1936). *J. Parasit.* **22**, 525–537.
Wardle, R. A. and McLeod, J. A. (1968). "The Zoology of Tapeworms". Hafner Publ. Comp., New York and London.
Wardle, R. A., McLeod, J. A. and Radinovsky, S. (1974). "Advances in the Zoology of Tapeworms 1950–1970". University of Minnesota Press, Minneapolis.
Webster, J. D. (1949). *J. Parasit.* **35**, 83–90.
Wiesenhütter, E. (1964). *Z. Parasitenk.* **24**, 80–82.
Will, R. (1975a). *Zbl. Vet. Med. B* **22**, 626–634.
Will, R. (1975b). *Zbl. Vet. Med. B* **22**, 635–655.
Will, R. (1977). "Hämatologische und serologische Untersuchungen bei Lacertiden (Reptilia, Squamata)". Thesis, University of Hohenheim.
Wingstrand, K. G. (1972). *Biol. Skrifter (København)* **19**, (4) 1–72.
Wingstrand, K. G. (1974). *III Int. Congr. Parasit. (München)* **2**, 1018–1019.
Witenberg, G. (1932). *Z. Parasitenk.* **4**, 542–584.
Witenberg, G. (1934). *Arch. zool. ital.* **20**, 467–509.
Yamaguti, S. (1935). *Jap. J. Zool.* **6**, 233–246.
Yamaguti, S. (1958). "Systema Helminthum, Vol. I. The Digenetic Trematodes of Vertebrates". Interscience Publ. Inc., New York and London.

Yamaguti, S. (1959). "Systema Helminthum, Vol. II. The Cestodes of Vertebrates". Interscience Publ. Inc., New York and London.
Yamaguti, S. (1961). "Systema Helminthum, Vol. III. The Nematodes of Vertebrates". Interscience Publ. Inc., New York and London.
Yamaguti, S. (1963a). "Systema Helminthum, Vol. IV. Monogenea and Aspidocotylea". Interscience Publ. Inc., New York and London.
Yamaguti, S. (1963b). "Systema Helminthum, Vol. V. Acanthocephala". Interscience Publ. Inc., New York and London.
Yamaguti, S. (1971). "Synopsis of Digenetic Trematodes of Vertebrates". Keigaku Publ. Comp., Tokyo.
Yamaguti, S. (1975). "A Synoptical Review of Life Histories of Digenetic Trematodes of Vertebrates, with Special Reference to the Morphology of their Larval Forms". Keigaku Publ. Comp., Tokyo.
Zwart, P. (1963). "Studies on Renal Pathology in Reptiles". Thesis, University of Utrecht.
Zwart, P. (1968). *In* "Erkrankungen der Zootiere". Verh. Ber. X Int. Symp. Erk. der Zootiere, Salzburg, pp. 45–48. Akademie Verlag, Berlin.
Zwart, P. (1972). *Lacerta* **30**, 41–48, 72–79, 121–127.
Zwart, P. (1973). *Lacerta* **31**, 26–30, 116–120, 177–182.
Zwart, P. (1974). *Zoo Anvers* **39**, 152–158; **40**, 14–22, 63–70.

10 Ectoparasites

W. FRANK*

Universität Hohenheim, Abteilung Parasitologie, D 7000 Stuttgart 70, Emil-Wolff Strasse 34, West Germany

I. Phylum Parenchymia (Parenchymatic Worms)

—see also Chapter 9 (Endoparasites)
   Subphylum Platyhelminthes (Flatworms)
     Class Turbellaria
       Order Neorhabdocoela
         Suborder Temnocephalida

Most of the 35 species of the suborder Temnocephalida live in the Southern hemisphere but have spread to a number of new areas. Their original hosts are a group of decapod crustaceans (Parastacidae). These parasites are similar to the turbellarians, but they differ in details (Nichols, 1975).

The temnocephala vary in size between 0·1–2 mm; they live *on* their hosts (crustaceans, molluscs and chelonians) and there spend their whole life-cycle. They feed on protozoa, rotifers, annelids and small crustaceans or share the food taken up by their host. Some of the European species are truly parasitic and feed on fluid extracted from the host. Most are species specific. A few can survive in the absence of a host if they are supplied with foods but others die within hours. The interaction between these ectocommensals or ectoparasites and their hosts is as yet only partly understood (Jennings, 1971).

Certain species, notably in America, are found on chelonians. They adhere to these hosts with the aid of a sucking disc and the preferred sites are the axillary and caudal regions. *Temnocephala brevicornis* is known from several reptilian hosts; Cordero (1946) and Boettger (1957) listed *Hydromedusa tectifera, H. maximiliani, H. platanensis,*

---

* Dedicated to the author's most esteemed teacher Prof Dr O. Pflugfelder on the occasion of his 75th birthday (15.2.79).

Platemys radiolata and *Mesoclemmys gibba*. Further reports may be found in Baer (1931) and Bresslau and Reisinger (1933).

Clinical signs and pathology   None reported.

II. Phylum Annelida

Class Hirudinea

The Hirudinea (leeches) parasitize semi-aquatic and aquatic reptiles in both fresh and salt water.

Biology   Leeches are commonly found in fresh water but some marine and a few terrestrial species are known. Many are predatory while others are scavengers; they can be temporary ectoparasites on vertebrates.

The Hirudinea can be divided into the following three Orders:

Order Rhynchobdellida
Order Gnathobdellida
Order Pharyngobdellida

Of these only the first two include ectoparasitic species. Reports of parasitism usually refer to chelonians and crocodilians. Most leeches have no particular host preference; only a few appear to be specific. *Ozobranchus jantseanus* is only found on the aquatic turtle *Clemmys japonica* but it may also live freely in fresh water. This particular host–parasite relationship depends upon the ability of the leech to remain in a state of anabiosis for several days, an adaptation necessary if it is to survive regular exposure to the air when the turtles leave the water (Cheng, 1973).

Significance of Leeches

Reports of reptiles being damaged by leeches are rare. Affected animals may become anaemic and die, but for this to happen the number of leeches must be large. Schwartz (1974) reported such cases in the USA in sea turtles (*Caretta caretta*, loggerhead turtle and *Chelonia mydas*, the green turtle) which were kept in a tank of sea water which was not filtered. The turtles succumbed to a heavy infestation of *Ozobranchus margoi*. The plastrons of the green turtles were covered with sheets of leech eggs and some of the leeches had worked themselves an entry under the scales; most were found around the throat and the axillary region of the legs. The eyes of the largest loggerhead turtle were destroyed in their sockets and the leeches had penetrated the nostrils, the mouth and the cloaca.

O. margoi also occurs in the Bay of Naples and in the Indian Ocean. Davies and Chapman (1974) found it in a sea-water aquarium.

Cases of the severity described above are exceptional. Smith *et al* (1976) reported a 40 per cent infestation rate with leeches (*Placobdella papillifera*) in *Alligator mississippiensis*. In two animals over 100 leeches were found in the mouth, particularly in the pits corresponding to the mandibular teeth. Others were found in traumatized areas of the body. There were, however, no obvious signs of disease. *Placobdella multilineata* also invades the mouth, the neck and the axillae of *Alligator mississippiensis* (Forrester and Sawyer, 1974).

Infestation with leeches deserves close attention since they may transmit bacteria and protozoa. This aspect has not been sufficiently explored since the natural hosts of most species are as yet unknown (Herter, 1968). For example, it remains to be clarified whether there is a connection between leech infestation and the appearance of fibro-epithelial tumours, as reported by Nigrelli and Smith (1943) for *Chelonia mydas*. Leeches might also transmit the herpesvirus-like agent which causes the "gray-patch disease" in *Chelonia mydas* (personal comment) since, according to Rebell *et al* (1975) this agent is easily transmitted in green turtles. The same considerations may be valid for a herpesvirus-like infection found by Frye *et al* (1977) in pacific pond turtles (*Clemmys marmorata*) (see Chapter 5).

The following leeches are known as intermediate hosts for protozoa, transmitting them to aquatic turtles:

Table 10. 1. Leeches which are intermediate hosts for protozoa of reptiles.

Leech	Protozoon	Reptile affected
Placobdella (syn. *Haementeria*) *costata*	*Haemogregarina stepanowi*	*Emys orbicularis*
Placobdella multilineata	*Haemogregarina* sp.	*Alligator mississippiensis*, Forrester and Sawyer (1974).
Ozobranchus shipleyi	*Haemogregarina nicoriae*	*Geoemyda nicoriae*
Placobdella parasitica	*Trypanosoma chrysemydis*	*Trionyx ferox* *Chrysemys picta* *Chelydra serpentina*

It is possible, but not yet proven, that *Aeromonas* and other bacteria may be transferred by leeches (Frank, 1976). In 1936 Autrum compiled a list of the leeches known to infest reptiles while Herter (1968) and Reichenbach-Klinke (1977) mentioned additional species parasitizing reptiles but without author citations. Sawyer and Shelley (1976) listed species found in the USA. The taxonomy was discussed by Sóos (1965, 1969).

III. Phylum Arthropoda

Of the arthropods only representatives of the Pentastomida (see Chapter 9), the Chelicerata and the Insecta serve as ecto- or endoparasites of reptiles.

A. Subphylum Chelicerata

Class Acarina (Acari) Mites and ticks.
The taxonomy of the Acarina is still disputed.

ORDER PARASITIFORMES
Suborder Metastigmata
Superfamily Ixodoidea (Ticks)

Family Ixodidae (Hard-bodied ticks)
Arthur (1962) divided these ticks (of which over 500 species are known) into three groups:

(1) Species-specific
(2) Group-specific
(3) Non-specific

The preferential hosts of certain species are known and some include reptiles. Frequently only larvae or nymphs are found on reptiles while the mature stages infest mammals. A few ticks are only found on reptiles, sometimes preferentially on particular species (Bull and Smith, 1973; Smith, 1973). *Aponomma hydrosauri* from S. Australia has been recorded as only infecting reptiles, particularly the sleepy lizard *Trachydosaurus rugosus* (Roberts, 1970; Smith, 1973; Bull and Sara, 1976). However, species of the same genus may parasitize different hosts. In many geographical regions ixodids have become specialized parasites of reptiles. *Aponomma exornatum* usually attacks the monitor lizard *Varanus niloticus* and, exceptionally, other reptiles. Very large numbers of ticks may be found in the axillae of the forelegs, on the cranial aspect of the elbow joint and between the toes. Others occupy the nostrils and the cloacal region. Another *Aponomma* species, *A. transversale*, is both host and site specific in that it confines itself to the eye sockets of pythons. Other large African snakes may become infested by *A. latum. A. gervaisi*, in Sri Lanka, shows an interesting type of adaptation: the ticks are found on old specimens of *Testudo elegans* and are of an identical colour to that of their hosts (Deraniyagala, 1939). Investigations by Hunt (1957) confirmed that these ticks become darker as the colour of their hosts gradually changes.

The genus *Amblyomma* also shows a number of host adaptations. *A. sylvaticum, A. nuttali* and *A. marmoreum* feed on tortoises. *A. marmoreum* is split into three subspecies, each with its individual preferences. *A. sparsum* of Central Africa infests both tortoises and warm-blooded animals. Other *Amblyomma* species such as *A. tholloni* and *A. rhinocerotis*, have only accidentally been found on reptiles.

Merdivenci (1967) failed in an attempt to transfer *Hyalomma aegyptium*, a tick which regularly infests the tortoise *Testudo graeca* in Turkey, to rabbits and rats. Hoogstraal and Kaiser (1958a,b) found this tick regularly on *Testudo graeca ibera* and rarely on the lizard *Agama stellio*. It can, however, be found on hedgehogs (*Erinaceus europaeus concolor*).

A detailed investigation by Hoogstraal and Kaiser (1958a,b) revealed several species of *Hyalomma* which parasitize reptiles. In Egypt they found lizards, *Acanthodactylus boskianus asper, A.s. scutellatus* and *Agama mutabilis* infested by immature stages of *Hyalomma impeltum, H. franchinii* and *H. dromedarii*. Adults of *H. franchinii* were only found on land tortoises in Libya.

It was, however, shown that reptilian blood can have a toxic effect on ticks. When the rare African tick *Cosmiomma hippopotamensis* was transferred to turtles all the former died within a few days irrespective of whether the host animals had access to water or not (Bezuidenhout and Schneider, 1972).

Since they live close to the ground reptiles may act as accidental hosts for the larvae of many ticks. On such accidental hosts one may also find nymphs but no adults. Hoogstraal (1959) found larvae and nymphs of *Ixodes festai* attached to the head, the lower jaw and the axillae of various lizards (*Chalcides ocellatus, Agama bibroni, Eumeces algeriensis* and *Psammodromus algirus*). Some lizards were infested by more than 20 ticks but females were seen very rarely. Hoogstraal and Kaiser (1958a,b; 1960) encountered both *Haemaphysalis otophila* and (in one case) *Hyalomma dromedarii* on lizards.

It is probable that about 60 per cent of the larger lizards and snakes are infested by some type of tick in the wild. If one omits those species which are unsuitable for ticks because they live underground or are aquatic the figure may, in some areas, reach 100 per cent (Dunn, 1918). However, Vercammen-Grandjean (1965) found that ticks may even attack certain aquatic species such as the marine iguana (*Amblyrhynchus cristatus*) on the Galapagos islands. Likewise sea snakes, *Laticauda* spp., are commonly infested and have a specific tick, *Amblyomma nitidum*. There is one report of both *A. nitidum* and an *Aponomma* sp. on the same snake (*Laticauda colubrina*) in New Guinea (Zann *et al*, 1975).

New species of Ixodidae are regularly described from freshly caught lizards and snakes (Kohls, 1969; Keirans, 1972). Terrestrial tortoises, with well protected recesses between plastron and carapace, offer excellent sites for ticks during the long act of blood sucking. All three stages of hard ticks (larva, nymph and adult) need many days, sometimes weeks, to become replete. It has been shown, for example, that *Amblyomma tuberculatum* females, feeding on the gopher tortoise (*Gopherus polyphemus*) need between 40 and 74 days to ingest a full meal. As many as 19 ticks may be found on one free-living tortoise. Each female tick increases its weight during this time from 2·1 to 3·7 grammes; the weight of unfed, newly emerged female ticks is only 88 mg (Cooney and Hays, 1972).

The time required to become replete seems to be longer when ticks feed on reptiles rather than on mammals. Small species appear only able to survive an attack by several female ticks because the process is prolonged and can be compensated for by haemopoiesis. The males of many species do not feed on blood but they may often be found on the same hosts where they seek a mate. Copulation usually takes place on the host. Not only physiological factors but also the structure of the mouthparts appears to determine whether a particular tick will attack a certain reptile. Unpublished work by the author suggests that species with a long, slender hypostome are better able to anchor themselves among the hard, horny structures of the reptilian skin than those with short, blunt hypostomata.

In summary, the genera of hard-bodied ticks which affect reptiles are *Amblyomma*, *Aponomma*, *Hyalomma*, *Ixodes* and *Haemaphysalis* (Arthur, 1962; Radchenko, 1973). It is impossible to mention all the species described. Useful reviews are to be found in Arthur (1962) and in the numerous papers by Hoogstraal and his co-workers.

Family Argasidae (Soft-bodied ticks)
The Argasidae comprise approximately 85 species and are found worldwide. They may infest snakes, lizards and chelonians. It is probable that the distribution of the Argasidae amongst reptiles is

greater than at present known. For *Ornithodoros talaje*, for example, reptiles seem to be the preferred hosts as shown by the higher number of eggs they lay when feeding on reptiles. The quality of the blood seems to be of minor importance for larvae and nymphs (Frank, 1964a).

Those six-legged larvae which feed at all do so for a few days and then leave the host to moult. Both the nymphs and the adult argasids are very active creatures; they engorge themselves with blood during the night and leave the reptile host after 10–30 minutes. The females feed several times and produce 30–300 eggs after each meal (the Ixodidae, on the other hand, lay only once but may produce thousands of eggs).

The genus *Ornithodoros* comprises about 50 species, some of which infest reptiles. *O. turicata*, an American species, is found on reptiles (rattlesnakes and turtles) as well as on a great variety of other hosts. Hoogstraal and Kaiser (1960) reported *O. foleyi* in Egypt in small caves in the company of geckos and agamids. The statement by Arthur (1962) that *O. moubata*, the African relapsing fever tick, also attacks tortoises, seems to be incorrect. According to Walton (1962) *O. moubata* should be divided into four distinct species and one subspecies. Only one of these, *O. compactus*, attacks tortoises. Recently, European zoological gardens and amateur herpetologists have encountered *Ornithodoros talaje* (Frank, unpublished); this species has a host preference for reptiles (Frank, 1964a). Only a few records exist of *Argas* spp. on reptiles; *A. brumpti* is found occasionally on lizards in East Africa.

Pathology

Intensive infestation of reptiles by ixodid ticks may prove fatal (Walker and Bezuidenhout, 1973). The main cause of death is anaemia from loss of blood.

Local damage through tick bites has been reported. Roth and Schneider (1974) recorded that all stages of the South American tick *Amblyomma testudinis* may cause paralysis when they infest the snake *Natrix natrix*. The condition is characterized by muscular degeneration in the region of the bite; there is vacuolation of the muscle and atrophy of the muscle fibrils. Gothe (1971a,b; 1972) and Gothe *et al* (1970) reported similar lesions in chickens bitten by *Argas* (*Persicargas*) *persicus*.

Ticks are also of great importance because they can transmit viruses although as yet little is known of the role of reptile ticks in this context. The investigations of Sekeyová *et al* (1970) are relevant.

These authors showed that *Lacerta agilis* and *L. viridis* produced antibodies against tick-borne encephalitis only if the temperature was raised to over 30°C. At normal temperatures no antibodies were produced, although the lizards were infested by virus-bearing ticks, and the same lizards developed viraemia later on in the laboratory. It can probably be assumed that the chance of virus transmission by ticks is greater in hot climates than in temperate. Doherty *et al* (1970) detected antibodies against a virus (MRM 4059) in *Ablepharus boutonii virgatus*, a species from which this virus had originally been isolated. Other aspects of this subject were discussed by Ahne (1977). Protozoa too may be transmitted by ixodid ticks. For example, Brumpt (1938) isolated *Haemogregarina mauretanica* from the tick *Hyalomma syriacum*; this protozoon is identical to *Hepatozoon mauretanicum* from *Hyalomma aegyptium* (Reichenbach-Klinke, 1977). Garnham (1954) found stages of a haemogregarine in *Argas brumpti*.

However, of greater importance, especially to captive reptiles, is the possibility that certain filariae (*Macdonaldius oschei*) may be transmitted to snakes (Boidae) by *Ornithodoros talaje* (Frank, 1964a,b).

Suborder Mesostigmata

Mites of this suborder commonly parasitize vertebrates but in this chapter only those families and genera which are of importance to reptiles are discussed.

Family Laelaptidae (Laelapidae—Fain and Yunker, 1972)
This family of about 50 genera contains most of the parasitic species, some of which can be pathogenic to reptiles. Their developmental cycle involves egg, larva, protonymph, deutonymph and adult. At optimal humidity and temperature the whole cycle requires only 8–28 days. The species of most importance to reptiles is *Ophionyssus natricis* Gervais, 1844. A number of other names (*O. serpentium, O. arabicus, Ichoronyssus serpentium, Liponyssus natricis, L. serpentium, L. arabicus, Serpenticola easti, S. serpentium, Steatonyssus arabicus* and *Dermanyssus natricis*) are now considered to be synonyms and invalid (Camin, 1949; Till, 1957). This mite is of world-wide distribution and its main hosts are snakes, with minor differences between American and African types (Till, 1957). Saurians are rarely affected. The mite is occasionally found on freshly caught reptiles (Till, 1957; Blanc and Ascione, 1959).

The species occurs in zoological gardens throughout the world. It has always been regarded as a most unwelcome pest since it reduces the vitality of the exhibits and heavy infestations may cause death.

A monograph by Camin (1953) described the life-cycles and the sensory behaviour. Under optimal conditions (30°C and 95 per cent relative humidity) development is complete in about 3 weeks. The larvae do not suck blood. Each female produces 60–80 eggs. Egg laying begins on the host while the females are feeding, but it also continues afterwards. The snake is affected by the loss of blood and the toxic effect of the mite's saliva and severe anaemia and death may occur (Wallach, 1969; Elkan, 1973).

In severe cases 10 000–20 000 mites may live on one captive snake. In the author's experience such an infestation manifests itself by a rough and ugly looking skin and incomplete skin shedding.

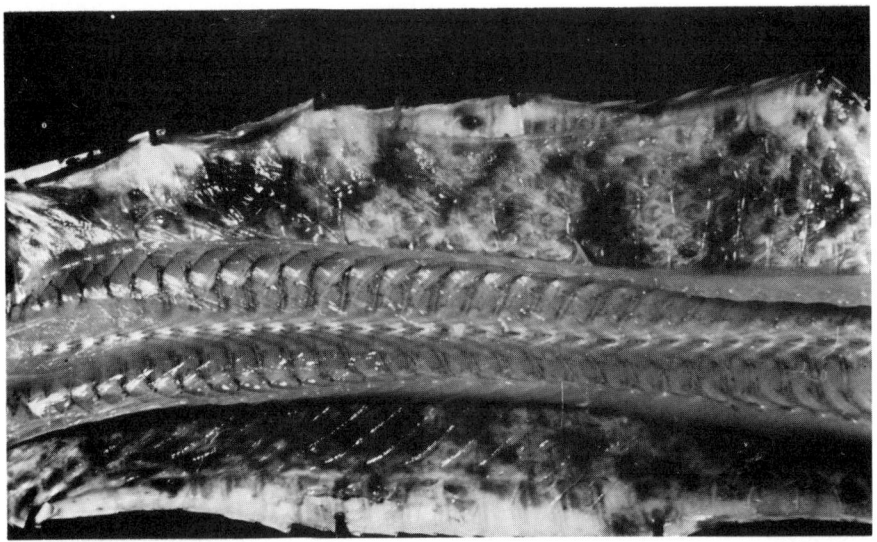

Fig. 10.1 Numerous haemorrhages under the skin of a colubrid snake caused by large numbers of *Ophionyssus* mites.

Relatively little is known of the role of *O. natricis* in the dissemination of bacteria although Camin (1948) demonstrated the transmission of *Aeromonas hydrophila*.

Humans may become infested with *Ophionyssus natricis* if the snakes are heavily parasitized. The clinical features are a papular–vesiculo-bullous dermatitis (Schultz, 1975).

Other species described include *Ophionyssus mabuyae* from South Africa and *O. lacertinus* from Europe.

The following genera have been described from reptiles: *Ophionyssus*, *Ophidilaelaps*, *Neoliponyssus*. *Neoliponyssus saurarum* is of interest in that it can act as vector for coccidia (*Schellackia*) which parasitize the gut of lizards.

Family Entonyssidae
These mites usually live in the trachea and lungs of their hosts but the genus *Mabuyonyssus* inhabits the nasal cavity of skinks in Africa. The females are ovoviviparous. The life-cycle consists of egg, larva, protonymph, deutonymph and adult. The mode of transmission has not been investigated. There are few reports of the role of these mites although in some areas they affect 2 per cent of all snakes (Fain, 1961a).

Family Ixodorhynchidae
These mites have only been reported from snakes; the single female found on a bat by Fain and Yunker (1972) was accidental. They are known from America, Africa and Asia, but recent discoveries in the Philippines suggest a much wider distribution (Voss, 1967). The family is divided into several genera (Fain, 1961b,c, 1962) but it seems possible that not all are valid.

Only freshly caught reptiles have so far been found infested. No specific clinical or pathological features have been reported.

ORDER ACARIFORMES

Suborder Prostigmata (syn. Trombidiformes)

Superfamily Cheyletoidea
This interesting group of mites includes transitional types. Apart from one family which lives on insects (Heterocheylidae) they only parasitize vertebrates. Some of them have become true parasites but only two families occur on reptiles. These are:
Family Ophioptidae—under scales of snakes
Family Cloacaridae—in the cloaca of turtles

The family Cloacaridae, established by Camin *et al* (1967), shows great modifications to parasitism. The reduction of the legs suggests that they would hardly be able to move off their host's body. Further, the hypertrophy and claw-shaped modification of the leg setae and the fang-like development of the pedipalps make these effective holdfast and burrowing structures. The mites are only about 300 μm long. Cloacarids appear only to occur on mature turtles; they are probably venereally transmitted. The adult mites are found embedded under a thin layer of the mucosa. The immediate environment shows no pathological damage. The nymphs, on the other hand, are aggregated in minute pustules which may develop into lesions on the surface of the cloacal mucosa. Only two species have been described:

Cloacarus faini—from *Chelydra serpentina* in the USA
Cloacarus beeri—from *Chrysemys picta* in the USA

Family Trombiculidae (Chiggers or Chigger mites)
These differ from other ectoparasites in that they only infest vertebrates as larvae. Nymphs (1 stage only) and adults are free-living and predaceous. Trombiculid larvae feed on lymph or ingest externally digested host tissue, but they do not suck blood. The six-legged larvae, which measure only 250–600 μm, are often overlooked. In countries where reptiles are fairly numerous, new species or new reptilian hosts are still occasionally reported. For example, until the investigations by Lawrence (1949) only one species was known from South African snakes. Lawrence alone, however, discovered 35 new species from lizards and 2 from snakes. The total number of species may be very large if one considers the many new species described by Taufflieb (1958) and Audy and Vercammen-Grandjean (1961).

Trombiculid larvae appear to have predilection sites on the host. They prefer areas around joints and it is here that they feed for 2–10 days. Some species infest several hosts (Cheng, 1973). For example, *Trombicula batatas* in the USA is known to attack 100 different vertebrates, including reptiles and amphibians. Frequently, however, the same species may be found on the same hosts.

The Trombiculidae are particularly important insofar as they may transfer rickettsiae pathogenic to humans. The larvae of one generation pick up the rickettsiae when they feed on rodents which serve as reservoir hosts, and transmit them transovarially to the next generation. The larvae of the new generation may transmit the rickettsiae when parasitic on humans. The role of reptiles in such a cycle is unknown.

There are reports of Trombiculidae infesting reptiles from Europe, N. and S. America, the Near East, India, Malaysia, Australia, the Maldive Islands, Taiwan and Africa.

It is impossible to catalogue here the large numbers of species which parasitize reptiles as larvae. For details the reader should consult Lawrence (1949, 1951), Audy (1954, 1956a,b; 1957, 1959), Audy and Domrow (1957) and Vercammen-Grandjean (1956). There are also valuable data in the checklist of world chiggers by Wharton and Fuller (1952). Other details may be found in the checklist of the Oriental and Australasian regions by Audy (1957) and in an illustrated key and synopsis of the chiggers of the Far East by Vercammen-Grandjean (1968). More recent publications are those by Nadchatram and Kethley (1974) and Hadi et al (1974).

Biology

Little is known of the biology of the trombiculid species which infest reptiles with the exception of the genus *Vatacarus* (Nadchatram and Kethley, 1974). The cycle in reptiles probably differs little from that in birds and mammals infested by the same species. Kulkarni (1974) studied the biology of 36 Indian species. The duration of the life-cycles of larvae varied from 68 to 338 days between temperatures of 20 to 30°C, depending on species, temperature and humidity. Most trombiculids deposit their eggs singly on a moist substance. The shell breaks after 4–8 days but the larvae remain inside the shell for another 5–7 days within a special layer, the deutovum. The hexapod larva then escapes, and seeks a host. Without food it can only survive for two weeks. It is probable that any vertebrate living in the environment may be infested but there are possibly preferred hosts (Nadchatram and Kethley, 1974). Preferences also seem to exist in respect of the site of invasion. Nadchatram and Kethley, working in the Far East, investigated *Herpetacarus leprochaeta* and *Microtrombicula chamlongi* from the skink *Riopa bowringi*, and *H. cadignani* from the gecko *Phyllodactylus siamensis*. The hexapod larvae do not suck blood but ingest lymph and dissolved host tissue. The larvae secrete a lytic substance which dissolves the epidermal cells and only this fluid matter can be ingested. An interesting structure, the stylostome, forms in the host's tissue in response to the lytic process and the reaction of the host. The larvae gorge themselves for 2–10 days with the digested tissues and then drop off and become semi-dormant. They now are what some authors call 'protonymphs'. Accordingly, when after a short while they moult, the next stage must be that of 'deutonymphs'. These live for 3–7 weeks as predators on insects and spiders. After this period the nymphs moult again to reach the sexually mature free-living stage. As adults they live for about six weeks.

Family Pterygosmidae

These are a highly specialized group of mites, divided into 9 genera. They are limited to lizards of the families Geckonidae, Agamidae, Zonuridae, Gerrhosauridae and, exceptionally, Iguanidae (*Geckobiel-*

la). Only a few live on invertebrates such as insects and scorpions. Various species seem to prefer different areas on their host's body. They may be found in the periocular skin folds, on the tympanum, under scales, between the toes and in the axillae (Womersly, 1941). They are flattened mites, usually broader than they are long. They have typical broad, sometimes spatulate, bristles which may even be branched (*Geckobiella*). They usually occur in small numbers and the blood loss they cause is too small to damage the host. With a few exceptions these mites do not survive long in captivity and a heavy infestation is not to be expected.

Goodwin (1954) investigated the biology of *Geckobiella*. Larvae, nymphs and adults (males as well as females) feed on blood. The development of the females from the egg to gravid adult requires 42–85 days. The females go through the following stages: egg, deutovum, larva, nymphochrysalis, nymph, imagochrysalis and adult. In the males the stages of nymph and nymphochrysalis are omitted. Parthenogenetic development is possible but the few eggs thus produced all develop into males. These mites are probably vectors of a haemogregarine often found in *Sceloporus undulatus* in Georgia, United States of America. The species more commonly seen on reptiles belong to the following genera:

Geckobia	Particularly on geckos.
Pterygosoma	Particularly on Agamidae.
Zonurobia *Scaphothrix* *Ixodiderma*	Preferably on Zonuridae.
Geckobiella	Iguanidae (*Sceloporus floridianus, S. undulatus*.)
Pimeliaphilus *Hirstiella*	Geckonidae—most species live on invertebrates (insects and scorpions).

Occasionally mites belonging to other families are found on reptiles but these infestations are probably accidental. Many of the species involved parasitize invertebrates and it seems possible that mites become transferred when their hosts are eaten by reptiles. For example, species of the genus *Ophiomegistus* (Family Paramegistidae) have been found on snakes and skinks but the majority of the genera parasitize only insects and myriapods (Voss, 1966).

Elkan (1977) reported the circumocular region of a slow-worm (*Anguis fragilis*) heavily infested with a *Caloglyphus* sp. (Astigmata, syn. Sarcoptiformes). This was possibly another case of where a reptile functions as a transport host for the non-feeding larval stages of a mite (Reichenbach-Klinke, 1977).

B. Subphylum Insecta (Insects)

Class Pterygota (Winged insects)

Only a few species of insects are of any importance to reptiles. The Heteroptera include the true bugs, some of which are known to suck blood from vertebrates, including reptiles. Of greater importance are certain Diptera. Reports of fleas (Siphonaptera) are extremely rare and attributable to accidental infestations (Jäth, 1952).

ORDER HETEROPTERA (True bugs)

Only members of one family, the Reduviidae, are known to suck blood from reptiles.

Family Reduviidae
4000 different species are known of which only a few attack man and vertebrate animals. These bugs have frequently been reported feeding on reptiles and have been used to obtain small amounts of reptilian blood for experimental purposes (Will, 1977). Reichenbach-Klinke (1977) reported the finding of developmental stages of *Hepatozoon triatomae* (*Haemogregarina triatomae*—Osimani, 1942) in *Eutriatoma rubrovaria*.

ORDER DIPTERA (Sand flies, mosquitoes, midges, gnats, flies etc.)

This order embraces 85 000–100 000 species, many of which are recognized vectors of disease in man and animals. Their mouth-parts are modified for piercing and sucking or rasping and lapping-up of blood. The systematics can be simplified as follows:

Suborder Nematocera

Family Psychodidae
   Phlebotominae (Sand flies)

A few of these species, like *Sergentomyia bedfordi* in Africa, regularly feed on reptiles while others, like *P. longipes*, never utilize these hosts (Foster *et al*, 1972). Thatcher and Hertig (1966) observed *P. panamensis*, *P. trapidoi*, *P. sanguinarius*, *P. gomezi*, *P. shannoni* (syn. *Lutzomyia*), *P. ylephiletrix* (syn. *Lutzomyia*), *P. vexillarius* and *P. ovalesi* in Panama but found no evidence that they fed on *Boa constrictor*. However, Tesh *et al* (1971), using the precipitin test, showed that 4 per cent of 126 *P. ylephiletrix* in the same areas had fed on reptiles.

Higher figures were obtained from other species—for example, *Lutzomyia micropyga* (50 per cent of 4 specimens), *L. trinidadensis* (76 per cent of 25), *L. rorotaensis* (57 per cent of 7) and *Warileya nigrosacula* (13 per cent of 8). Sand flies can transmit *Leishmania* species to reptiles as demonstrated for *L. adleri* from *Latastia longicauda revoili*, a lacertid lizard, the vector being *Phlebotomus clydei* (Adler, 1964; Southgate, 1967). There are also reports on the presence of crithidial forms in the mid-gut of psychodid flies. However, the latter may be developmental stages of trypanosomes although no such flagellates were found in the specimens examined (Chaniotis and Anderson, 1968). Problems in interpretation may also arise when there are developmental stages in the gut since the relationship between the intestinal and the extraintestinal stages which occasionally occur in the blood is uncertain.

Cheng (1973) believed that the *Leishmania* species found in reptiles should be regarded as primitive forms which have not as yet adapted themselves to intracellular life. The extent to which sand flies play a part in transmission remains to be investigated. Ayala and Lee (1970) described a particularly interesting example of the transference of malaria parasites (*Plasmodium mexicanum*) to *Sceloporus* in California although this group of protozoons is usually transmitted exclusively by Culicidae. Haemogregarines may also be transmitted to lizards and snakes by sand flies. Ayala (1970a,b), working with *Phlebotomus vexator occidentis*, was able to infect *Thamnophis sirtalis* and *Sceloporus occidentalis* with a *Hepatozoon* sp. Reichenbach-Klinke (1977) mentioned the transmission of *Bartonella* (*Haemobartonella*).

It is probable that further examples of transmission will come to light in due course. This is reasonable since reptiles are preferred hosts for some Phlebotominae. Chaniotis (1967) examined *P. vexator occidentis*, *P. stewarti* and *P. californicus* in the laboratory and found that these were feeding exclusively on cold-blooded hosts. Both lizards and snakes were bitten but the former tended to eat the flies. Bogdanow (1956) working in Central Asia showed that well known species like *P. papatasii*, *P. sergenti*, *P. caucasicus* and *P. chinensis* attack not only mammals but also reptiles.

The role of the Phlebotominae in transmitting arthropod-borne viruses is uncertain. However, Doherty *et al* (1973), surveying Australian arboviruses, isolated a new viral type 'Ch 9924' (Charlesville virus) from *Phlebotomus* spp. and from the gecko *Gehyra australis*.

Family Culicidae (Mosquitoes)
These flies may suck blood from reptiles and there are a number of reports of this in the wild (Henderson and Senior, 1961; Gebhardt *et al*, 1964; Hayes, 1965; Nolan *et al*, 1965).

Although some species, like *Aedes aegypti*, are mainly anthropophilous, turtles, lizards and geckos can be hosts under laboratory conditions and this mosquito was used by MacDonald (1967) and Yuill (1969) to obtain blood from small lizards for virological investigations. De Foliart (1967) reported that the preferred host for *Aedes canadensis* under natural conditions was probably Blanding's turtle (*Emydoidea blandingii*). With the use of the precipitin test Boreham and Snow (1973) demonstrated that a number of ornithophilic species (*Culex decens* and *C. invidiosus*) occasionally attack reptiles. Other species too, which normally prefer birds or mammals, feed occasionally on reptiles. Edman (1974) detected snake blood in 0·7 per cent of *Deinocerites cancer* and reptile–amphibian blood in a further 0·7 per cent. Christopher and Reuben (1971) reported small percentages of engorged blood meals of *Culex* (*Mochthogenes*) sp. and *Culex gelidus* which were positive to reptilian antiserum by the precipitin test. Surveys in Panama, based on the capillary precipitin test, on approximately 3000 blood meals confirmed that reptiles are the preferred hosts of a number of Culicidae. *Culex egcymon, C. tecmarsis, C. dunni* and *C. elevator* showed a strong preference for lizards. *C. aikenii, C. apanastasis* and *C. amazonensis*, also took a number of blood meals from poikilothermic animals (Tempelis and Galindo, 1975).

The feeding behaviour of the Culicidae is influenced by temperature, humidity, smell, CO_2 concentration and visual stimuli but not all these factors need necessarily play a part every time (McIver, 1968). McIver showed that the colour of lizards plays no part in attracting culicids. Further, she was able to demonstrate that *Culex tarsalis* and *Aedes aegypti* neglected reptiles if warm-blooded vertebrates were available.

The suitability of reptile blood for mosquitoes is still uncertain. It is interesting to note that in *Culex tarsalis* snake and chicken blood is digested faster than that of guinea-pigs (Downe and Archer, 1975). Egg production, on the other hand, is significantly higher in mosquitoes fed on chickens than in those fed on snakes. The ability of the eggs to hatch is not influenced by the host.

Although reptiles can be directly debilitated by mosquitoes, the main importance of the latter lies in their ability to transmit protozoa, filariae and, probably, arthropod-borne viruses.

It has been known for some time that *Culex, Anopheles* and *Aedes* species may function as vectors for various species of *Hepatozoon*. Ball et al (1967), and Chao and Ball (1969) were able to transmit *Hepatozoon rarefaciens* to various snake species by feeding them *Culex tarsalis* infected from indigo snakes (*Drymarchon corais*). After 20 days the mosquitoes were fed to snakes of quite different families (*Boa constrictor* and *Pituophis catenifer*) and both became infected 7 weeks later. Similarly, Booden *et al* (1970) succeeded in transferring a species of *Hepatozoon* from a *Boa constrictor* to a lizard (*Anolis carolinensis*).

The complicated life-cycle of *Hepatozoon* was only elucidated for *Hepatozoon domergui* by Landau *et al* in 1972. Other *Hepatozoon* species are assumed to have a similar life history (Ball *et al*, 1967; Chao and Ball, 1969; Booden *et al*, 1970). In the case of *Hepatozoon domergui* it is not sufficient for the infection to be transmitted from one snake (*Madagascarophis colubrina*) to another snake. The cycle includes not only mosquitoes but also a lizard (*Oplurus sebae*) on which these snakes feed.

Plasmodium species may also be transmitted by Culicidae although other vectors are suspected (Garnham, 1966; Walliker, 1966; Lainson and Shaw, 1969a; Ayala, 1970a,b; Telford, 1970, 1973a,b; Lainson *et al*, 1971, 1974a,b). In Brazil *Culex pipiens* was found to be the vector for *Saurocytozoon tupinambi* from *Tupinambis nigropunctatus*, (Lainson and Shaw, 1969b; Landau *et al*, 1973) but Culicidae are unusual vectors for the Leucocytozoidae (Landau, 1973).

Culicidae may also function as vectors of filariae to reptiles. The life-cycle has been investigated for a number of species.

Reptiles may be of great significance as reservoir hosts for viruses and Culicidae may serve as vectors. Taylor (1967), who reviewed these viruses, reported the isolation of Charco-Marco and Timbo viruses from *Ameiva ameiva ameiva* from Brazil which could be transmitted by *Aedes aegypti*. Such reptilian infections are, however, uncommon since only two animals showed the Chaco strain, two the Marco strain and three the Timbo strain while nothing was found in 4000 further reptiles.

Reptiles may harbour WEE (western equine encephalitis) viruses or their antibodies (see Chapter 5). They may even act as virus reservoirs during the period of hibernation (Burton *et al*, 1966; Prior and Agnew, 1971). It has been shown experimentally that Texas tortoises (*Gopherus berlandieri*) whose WEE virus strains had been injected subcutaneously, showed a prolonged viraemia of up to 105 days. The duration of this viraemia was markedly influenced by the environmental temperature. 30°C shortened the pre-viraemic period as well as the duration of the viraemia.

Lower temperatures had the opposite effect. This suggests that tortoises may act as winter reservoirs for the virus (Bowen, 1977). The isolation of EEE (eastern equine encephalitis) virus from the blood of lizards (iguanas endemic in Cuba) is suggestive of the role certain cold-blooded vertebrates may play in the ecology of this agent (Berezin, 1977). Gebhardt et al (1966) demonstrated transmission of WEE virus to snakes by *Culex tarsalis*. A similar modus may operate in the case of the VEE (Venezuelan equine encephalitis) virus (Grayson and Galindo, 1969). The Japanese encephalitis (JE) virus may also be carried by lizards (*Tachydromys tachydromoides*) (Doi et al, 1968). Recent results obtained by Shortridge et al (1977) showed the presence of antibodies in cold-blooded animals against JE virus. The most important review on this subject is that of Ahne (1977).

Family Ceratopogonidae (Midges)
Midges also bite cold-blooded animals and may transmit protozoa. They have been incriminated in respect of *Haemoproteus* (syn. *Plasmodium*) *gonzalezi* whose hosts are lizards and for *H. mesnili* where the hosts are snakes. Lainson et al (1974b) also assumed that *Culicoides* transmitted *Saurocytozoon mabuyi*.

There are no data available on the transmission of arbo-viruses although these have been isolated from *Culicoides* spp. in Australia (Doherty et al, 1973) and midges are known to suck blood from reptiles.

Suborder Brachycera

Adult flies may damage reptiles by their blood-sucking activity and by transmitting pathogens. Some of the species cause myiasis in the larval stage.

Family Glossinidae (Tsetse flies)
Since the beginning of this century it has been known that reptiles may form important food sources for certain species of the family Glossinidae; for example *Glossina palpalis*, *G. fuscipes* and *G. tachinoides* (Bruce et al, 1910). Simpson (1918) showed that in the laboratory *G. tachinoides* fed readily on puff adders (*Bitis arietans*), black cobras (*Naja nigricollis*), the yellow spotted monitor (*Varanus niloticus*) and crocodiles (*Crocodylus niloticus*). Reptile blood was found in the intestinal contents of tsetse flies but it was not possible to determine its exact reptilian origin (Weitz, 1963, 1970). Boreham and Gill (1972, 1973) produced immune sera against reptile blood from several families and examined 672 *Glossina fuscipes*. 18·8 per cent had taken up reptile blood exclusively and Varanidae (monitor lizards), snakes (possibly

pythons) and tortoises had served as donors. These workers also showed (1973) that, in the two districts of Uganda where they worked, of 1212 *Glossina fuscipes* examined 93 per cent fed on monitor lizards (*Varanus niloticus*), 6 per cent on snakes (probably *Python sebae*) and 0·6 per cent on tortoises. Only six out of 373 *G. pallidipes* and two out of 655 *G. brevipalpis* had taken blood from *Varanus niloticus*. The animals bitten by *Glossina* in any district depends on the availability of host animals and also on the preference of the various *Glossina* species.

Family Tabanidae (Horse flies)
Flies of this family also use reptiles as sources of food. There are few observations published but the work of De Giusti and Dobrzechowski (1974) showed that turtles may be bitten by horse flies. The development of *Simondia* (syn. *Haemoproteus*) *metchnikovi* includes a change of host from *Chrysemys picta* to *Chrysops callidus*. A host–parasite relationship of this kind could only develop because *Chrysops callidus* seeks out the turtles for feeding. Other horse flies may also transmit pathogens like protozoa or act as intermediate hosts.

Family Calliphoridae (Blow and Flesh flies)
Larvae of some brachyceran diptera may cause myiasis in reptiles. The author's own observations and those in the literature refer only to chelonians. The flies responsible for these cases are, so far as can be judged, not obligatory but facultative parasites. The larvae belong to two subfamilies of the Calliphoridae, the Calliphorinae (blow flies) and the Sarcophaginae (flesh flies). Zumpt (1965) distinguished between benign and malignant myiasis. The reptilian cases so far observed probably belong to the former category. Normally the fly larvae develop on carcasses, rarely in wounds or in areas heavily soiled by excreta. However, experimentally, adult *Chrysomyia megacephala* may lay their eggs on unbroken reptilian skin where the eggs hatch and the larvae produce myiasis (Roy and Das Gupta, 1971). This would correspond with the malignant form. There are a number of records from North America to the effect that larvae of the flesh fly *Sarcophaga cistudinis* parasitize box turtles of the genus *Terrapene*. Specimens of *T. ornata* were found infested with larvae in subcutaneous pockets on the legs and under the loose skin ·which attaches the neck to the plastron (Rainey, 1953). Other reports mention the discovery of larvae of these flies in *T. carolina, T. carolina triunguis* and *T. c. bauri* (Peters, 1948). Further information may be obtained from Jackson *et al* (1969).

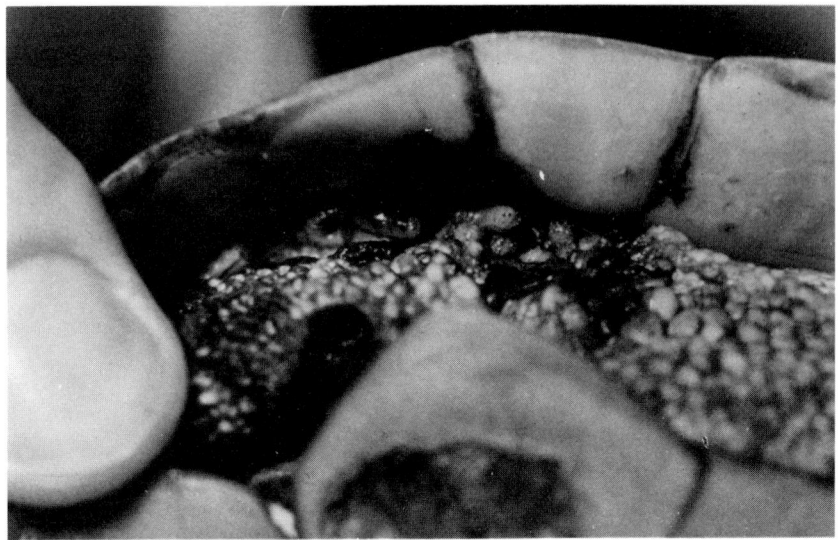

10.2 Many fly maggots of the genus *Lucilia* under the carapace of a live tortoise (*Testudo hermanni*).

Areas around the cloaca of chelonians attract flies which then lay their eggs around the base of the tail (Graham-Jones, 1961). The author has removed 37 third instar larvae of an undetermined *Lucilia* species from a pocket dorsal to the tail base under the carapace of a *Testudo hermanni* which had lived for many years in captivity in Germany. Das Gupta and Roy (1969) found that other *Lucilia* species, for example *L. illustris*, may experimantally infest wounded reptiles and cause myiasis. This has also been demonstrated for *Chrysomya megacephala* and *Hemipyrella ligurriensis* and the larvae of these caused a fatal myiasis. The larvae of *C. megacephala* mentioned earlier penetrated the healthy skin of lizards (*Hemidactylus fluviviridis*), fed on their tissues and ultimately killed them. The larvae of *H. ligurriensis*, on the other hand, were not able to penetrate the skin and could only invade the underlying tissue through pre-existing wounds. Having done this, however, they killed the hosts.

There is as yet no information on the exact mode of tissue destruction and on any reactions on the part of the hosts. Roy and Das Gupta (1971) noted that the larvae of the three species they used seemed to have a particular affinity for brain tissue, a feature which may add to the pathogenicity of these flies if they become parasites.

References

Adler, S. (1964). *Adv. Parasit.* **2,** 35–96.
Ahne, W. (1977). *In* "Krankheiten der Reptilien." (H. Reichenbach-Klinke, ed.) pp. 13–19. G. Fischer, Stuttgart and New York.
Arthur, D. R. (1962). "Ticks and Disease". Int. Series of Monographs on Pure and Applied Biology. Pergamon Press, Oxford, London, New York, Paris.
Audy, J. R. (1954). *Stud. Inst. med. Res. Malaya* **26,** 123–170.
Audy, J. R. (1956a). *Bull. Raffles Mus.* **28,** 5–26.
Audy, J. R. (1956b). *Bull. Raffles Mus.* **28,** 27–80.
Audy, J. R. (1957). *Parasitology* **47,** 217–294.
Audy, J. R. (1959). *Med. J. Malaya.* **14.**
Audy, J. R. and Domrow, R. (1957). *Stud. Inst. med. Res. Malaya* **28,** 121–152.
Audy, J. R. and Vercammen-Grandjean, P. H. (1961). *Ann. Natal Mus.* **15,** 135–140.
Autrum, H. (1936). *In* "Klassen und Ordnungen des Tierreichs." (H. G. Bronns, ed.). Akademie Verlagsgesellschaft, Leipzig.
Ayala, S. C. (1970a). *J. Parasit.* **56,** 417–425.
Ayala, S. C. (1970b). *J. Parasit.* **56,** 387–388.
Ayala, S. C. and Lee, D. (1970). *Science* **167,** 891–892.
Baer, J. G. (1931). *Bull. biol. Fr.* **65,** 1–57.
Ball, G. H., Chao, J. and Telford, S. R. (1967). *J. Parasit.* **53,** 897–909.
Berezin, V. V. (1977). *Vopr. Virusol.* 62–70.
Bezuidenhout, J. D. and Schneider, H. P. (1972). *J. S. Afr. vet. med. Ass.* **43,** 301–304.
Blanc, G. and Ascione, L. (1959). *Arch. Inst. Pasteur Maroc.* **5,** 666–668.
Boettger, C. R. (1957). *Abh. Braunschw. wiss. Ges.* **9,** 26–35.
Bogdanow, O. P. (1956). Cited in Reichenbach-Klinke (1977).
Booden, Th., Chao, J. and Ball, G. H. (1970). *J. Parasit.* **56,** 832–833.
Boreham, P. F. L. and Gill, G. S. (1972). *Trans. R. Soc. trop. Med. Hyg.* **66,** 324–325.
Boreham, P. F. L. and Gill, G. S. (1973). *Acta trop.* **30,** 356–365.
Boreham, P. F. L. and Snow, W. F. (1973). *Trans. R. Soc. trop. Med. Hyg.* **67,** 724–725.
Bowen, G. S. (1977). *Amer. J. trop. Med. Hyg.* **26,** 171–175.
Bresslau, E. and Reisinger, E. (1933). *In* "Handbuch der Zoologie." (W. Kükenthal, ed.) II Bd. 1. Hälfte 294–308, 319–320. W. de Gruyter, Berlin and Leipzig.
Bruce, D., Hamerton, A. E., Bateman, H. R. and Mackie, F. P. (1910). *Proc. R. Soc. B London* **82,** 490–497.
Brumpt, E. (1938). *Annls. Parasit. hum. comp.* **16,** 350–361.
Bull, M. and Sara, G. J. (1976). *J. Med. Ent.* **13,** 137–142.
Bull, M. and Smith, M. (1973). *Aust. J. Zool.* **21,** 103–110.
Burton, A. N., McLintock, J. and Rempel, J. G. (1966). *Science* **154,** 1029–1031.

Camin, J. H. (1948). *J. Parasit.* **34**, 345–354.
Camin, J. H. (1949). *J. Parasit.* **35**, 583–589.
Camin, J. H. (1953). *Chicago Acad. Sci. Spec. Publ.* **10**, 1–75.
Camin, J. H., Moss, W. W., Oliver, J. H. and Singer, G. (1967). *J. Med. Ent.* **4**, 261–272.
Chaniotis, B. N. (1967). *J. Med. Ent.* **4**, 221–233.
Chaniotis, B. N. and Anderson, J. R. (1968). *J. Med. Ent.* **5**, 273–292.
Chao, J. and Ball, G. H. (1969). *J. Parasit.* **55**, 681–682.
Cheng, Th. C. (1973). "General Parasitology". Academic Press, New York and London.
Christopher, S. and Reuben, R. (1971). *J. Med. Ent.* **8**, 314–318.
Cooney, J. C. and Hays, K. L. (1972). *J. Med. Ent.* **9**, 239–245.
Cordero, E. H. (1946). *Comm. zool. Mus. hist. nat. Montevideo II* **34**, 1–12.
Das Gupta, B. and Roy, P. (1969). *Parasitol.* **59**, 299–304.
Davies, R. W. and Chapman, C. G. (1974). *J. Fish. Res. Board Can.* **31**, 104–106.
De Foliart, G. R. (1967). *J. Med. Ent.* **4**, 31.
De Giusti, D. L. and Dobrzechowski, D. (1974). *ICOPA III*, **1**, 80–81.
Deraniyagala, P. E. P. (1939). "The Tetrapod Reptiles of Ceylon, Testudinates and Crocodilians." Vol. I. Dulau and Co., London.
Doherty, R. L., Whitehead, R. H., Wetters, E. J., Gorman, B.M. and Carley, J. G. (1970). *Trans. Roy. Soc. trop. Med. Hyg.* **64**, 748–753.
Doherty, R. L., Carley, J. G., Standfast, H. A., Dyce, A. L., Kay, B. H. and Snowdon, W. A. (1973). *Trans. R. Soc. trop. Med. Hyg.* **67**, 536–543.
Doi, R., Oya, A. and Telford, S. R. (1968). *Jap. J. Med. Sci. Biol.* **21**, 205–207.
Downe, A. E. R. and Archer, J. A. (1975). *J. Med. Ent.* **12**, 431–437.
Dunn, L. H. (1918). *J. Parasit.* **5**, 1–10.
Edman, J. D. (1974). *J. Med. Ent.* **11**, 105–107.
Elkan, E. (1973), *Br. J. Herpet.* **5**, 344–346.
Elkan, E. (1977). Cited in Reichenbach-Klinke (1977).
Fain, A. (1961a). *Bull. Inst. r. Sci. nat. Belg.* **37**, 1–135.
Fain, A. (1961b). *Rev. Zool. Bot. Afr.* **64**, 175–182.
Fain, A. (1961c). *Rev. Zool. Bot. Afr.* **64**, 283–296.
Fain, A. (1962). *Bull. Inst. r. Sci. nat. Belg.* **38**, 1–149.
Fain, A. and Yunker, C. E. (1972). *J. Med. Ent.* **9**, 482–484.
Forrester, D. J. and Sawyer, R. T. (1974). *J. Parasit.* **60**, 673.
Foster, W. A., Boreham, P. F. and Tempelis, C. H. (1972). *Ann. trop. Med. Parasitol.* **66**, 433–443.
Frank, W. (1964a). *Z. Parasitenk.* **24**, 415–441.
Frank, W. (1964b). *Z. Parasitenk.* **24**, 319–350.
Frank, W. (1976). "Parasitologie". E. Ulmer Verlag, Stuttgart.
Frye, F. L., Oshiro, L. S., Dutra, F. R. and Carney, J. D. (1977). *J. Am. vet. med. Ass.* **171**, 882–884.
Garnham, P. C. C. (1954). *Riv. Parassit.* **15**, 425–435.
Garnham, P. C. C. (1966). "Malaria Parasites and other Haemosporidia". Blackwell, Oxford.

Gebhardt, L. P., Stanton, G. J., De, S. T. and Jeor, S. (1966). *Proc. Soc. exp. Biol. Med.* **123**, 233–235.
Gebhardt, L. P., Stanton, G. J., Hill, D. W. and Collett, G. C. (1964). *New Engl. J. Med.* **271**, 172–177.
Goodwin, M. H. (1954). *J. Parasit.* **40**, 53–59.
Gothe, R. (1971a). *Z. Parasitenk.* **35**, 298–307.
Gothe, R. (1971b). *Z. Parasitenk.* **35**, 308–317.
Gothe, R. (1972). Pathogenitätsmechanismen bei Zeckenparalysen. Paper presented at Kongress Deutschsprachiger Tropenmedizinischer Gesellschaften. Montreux, Switzerland.
Gothe, R., Kunze, K. and Alt, H. (1970). *Z. Parasitenk.* **34**, 31.
Graham-Jones, O. (1961). *Vet. Rec.* **73**, 313–321.
Grayson, M. A. and Galindo, P. (1969). *J. Am. vet. med. Ass.* **155**, 2141–2145.
Hadi, T., Carney, W. P., Peenen, P. F. D. van and Sulianti Saroso, J. (1974). *ICOPA III* **2**, 982.
Hayes, J. (1965). *Mosquito News* **25**, 344.
Henderson, B. E. and Senior, L. (1961). *Mosquito News* **21**, 29–32.
Herter, K. (1968). "Der medizinische Blutegel und seine Verwandten". A. Ziemsen Verlag, Wittenberg Lutherstadt.
Hoogstraal, H. (1959). *Arch. Inst. Pasteur Maroc.* **5**, 710–713.
Hoogstraal, H. and Kaiser, M. N. (1958a). *Ann. Ent. Soc. Amer.* **51**, 7–12.
Hoogstraal, H. and Kaiser, M. N. (1958b). *Ann. Ent. Soc. Amer.* **51**, 397–400.
Hoogstraal, H. and Kaiser, M. N. (1960). *Ann. Ent. Soc. Amer.* **53**, 445–457.
Hunt, T. J. (1957). *Herpetologica* **13**, 19–23.
Jackson, C. G., Jackson, M. M. and Davis, J. D. (1969). *Bull. Wildl. Dis. Assoc.* **5**, 114.
Jäth, H. (1952). *Die Aquarien u. Terrarien Zeitschrift* **5**, 276.
Jennings, J. B. (1971). *Adv. Parasit.* **9**, 1–32.
Keirans, J. E. (1972). *J. Med. Ent.* **9**, 138–139.
Kohls, G. M. (1969). *J. Med. Ent.* **6**, 439–442.
Kulkarni, S. M. (1974). *ICOPA III* **2**, 979.
Lainson, R. and Shaw, J. J. (1969a). *Parasitology* **59**, 163–170.
Lainson, R. and Shaw, J. J. (1969b). *Parasitology* **59**, 159–162.
Lainson, R., Landau, I. and Shaw, J. J. (1971). *Int. J. Parasitol.* **1**, 241–250.
Lainson, R., Landau, I. and Shaw, J. J. (1974a). *Parasitology* **68**, 117–125.
Lainson, R., Landau, I. and Shaw, J. J. (1974b). *Parasitology* **69**, 215–223.
Landau, I. (1973). Development of *Saurocytozoon tupinambi*, parasite of Brazilian lizards in an unexpected vector for the Leucocytozoidae, *Culex pipiens*. Paper presented at 4th International Congress of Protozoology. Clermont-Ferrand, France.
Landau, T., Michel, J. C., Chabaud, A. G. and Brygoo, E. R. (1972). *Z. Parasitenk.* **38**, 250–270.
Landau, I., Lainson, R., Boulard, Y., Michel, J-C. and Shaw, J. J. (1973). *C. R. Acad. Sc. Paris, Série D* **276**, 2449–2452.
Lawrence, R. F. (1949). *Ann. Natal Mus.* **11**, 405–486.
Lawrence, R. F. (1951). *Ann. Transvaal Mus.* **21**, 447–459.

MacDonald, W. W. (1967). *Bull. Wld. Hlth. Org.* **36,** 597–599.
McIver, S. B. (1968). *J. Med. Ent.* **5,** 422–428.
Merdivenci, A. (1967). *Türk Hijiyen oe Tecrübi Biyoloji Dergisi* **27,** 65–72.
Nadchatram, M. and Kethley, J. (1974). *J. Med. Ent.* **11,** 581–587.
Nichols, K. C. (1975). *Int. J. Parasit.* **5,** 245–252.
Nigrelli, R. F. and Smith, G. M. (1943). *Zoologica* **28,** 107–108.
Nolan, M. P., Moussa, M. A. and Hayes, D. E. (1965). *Mosquito News* **25,** 218–219.
Osimani, J. J. (1942). *J. Parasit.* **28,** 147–154.
Peters, J. A. (1948). *Amer. Midl. Nat.* **40,** 472–474.
Prior, M. G. and Agnew, R. M. (1971). *Can. J. comp. Med.* **35,** 40–43.
Radchenko, N. M. (1973). *Zoologičeskij žurnal (Akademija nauk SSSR), Moskau* **52,** 1398–1400.
Rainey, D. G. (1953). *Herpetologica* **9,** 109–110.
Rebell, G., Rywlin, A. and Haines, H. (1975). *Amer. J. vet. Res.* **36,** 1221–1224.
Reichenbach-Klinke, H. (1977). "Krankheiten der Reptilien". 2nd edition. G. Fischer, Stuttgart and New York.
Roberts, F. H. S. (1970). Australian ticks. 267 pp. C.S.I.R.O., Melbourne.
Roth, B. and Schneider, C. C. (1974). *ICOPA III* **3,** 1667–1668.
Roy, P. and Das Gupta, B. (1971). *S. Afr. J. med. Sci.* **36,** 85–91.
Sawyer, R. T. and Shelley, R. M. (1976). *J. nat. Hist.* **10,** 65–97.
Schultz, H. (1975). *Br. J. Derm.* **93,** 695–697.
Schwartz, F. J. (1974). *J. Parasit.* **60,** 889–890.
Sekeyová, M., Grešiková, M. and Leško, J. (1970). *Acta virol.* **14,** 87.
Shortridge, K. F., Oya, A., Kobayashi, M. and Duggan, R. (1977). *Trans. R. Soc. trop. Med. Hyg.* **71,** 261–262.
Simpson, J. J. (1918). *Bull. ent. Res.* **8,** 193–214.
Smith, E. N., Johnson, C. R. and Voigt, B. (1976). *Copeia* 1976, 842.
Smith, M. (1973). *Aust. J. Zool.* **21,** 91–101.
Soós, Á. (1965). *Acta zool. acad. sci. hung.* **11,** 417–463.
Soós, Á. (1969). *Acta zool. acad. sci. hung.* **15,** 397–454.
Southgate, B. A. (1967). *J. trop. Med. Hyg.* **70,** 33–36.
Taufflieb, R. (1958). *Arch Inst. Pasteur Maroc* **5,** 619–634.
Taylor, R. M. (1967). "Catalogue of Arthropod Viruses of the World. A Collection of Data on Registered Arthropod-borne Animal Viruses." Publ. Health Ser. Publ. 1760 (1967) U.S. Department of Health, U.S. Government Printing Office, Washington, D.C.
Telford, S. R. (1970). *J. Protozool.* **17,** 566–574.
Telford, S. R. (1973a). *J. Protozool.* **20,** 203–207.
Telford, S. R. (1973b). *Int. J. Parasitol.* **3,** 829–842.
Tempelis, G. H. and Galindo, P. (1975). *J. Med. Ent.* **12,** 205–209.
Tesh, R. B., Chaniotis, B. N., Arnonson, M. D. and Johnson, K. M. (1971). *Amer. J. trop. Med. Hyg.* **20,** 150–156.
Thatcher, V. E. and Hertig, M. (1966). *Ann. ent. Soc. Amer.* **59,** 46–52.
Till, W. M. (1957). *J. ent. Soc. sth Afr.* **20,** 120–143.

Vercammen-Grandjean, P. H. (1956). *Arch. Inst. Pasteur Maroc* **5,** 75–86.
Vercammen-Grandjean, P. H. (1965). *Acarologia* **7,** Suppl. 266–274.
Vercammen-Grandjean, P. H. (1968). "The Chigger Mites of the Far East (Acarina: Trombiculidae and Leeuwenhoekiidae). An Illustrated Key and a Synopsis: Some New Tribes, Genera and Subgenera." Publ. U.S. Army Med. Res. Developm. Command, U.S. Government Printing Office, Washington, D.C.
Voss, W. J. (1966). *J. Med. Ent.* **3,** 261–268.
Voss, W. J. (1967). *J. Med. Ent.* **4,** 387–390.
Walker, J. B. and Bezuidenhout, J. D. (1973). *J. S. Afr. vet. med. Ass.* **44,** 381.
Wallach, J. D. (1969). *J. Am. vet. med. Ass.* **155,** 1017–1034.
Walliker, D. (1966). *Parasitology* **56,** 39–44.
Walton, G. A. (1962). *Symp. Zool. Soc. London* **6,** 83–156.
Weitz, B. (1963). *Bull. Wld. Hlth. Org.* **28,** 711–729.
Weitz, B. (1970). *In* "The African Trypanosomiases." (H. W. Mulligan, ed.) pp 416–423. George Allen and Unwin, London.
Wharton, G. W. and Fuller, H. S. (1952). "A Manual of the Chiggers." Entomological Society of Washington Mem. 4.
Will, R. (1977). "Hämatologische und serologische Untersuchungen bei Lacertiden (Reptilia, Squamata)." Thesis, University of Hohenheim.
Womersly, H. (1941). *Trans. R. Soc. S. Aust.* **65,** 323–328.
Yuill, T. M. (1969). *Trans. R. Soc. trop. Med. Hyg.* **63,** 407–408.
Zann, L. P., Cuffey, R. J. and Kropach, C. (1975). *In* "The Biology of Sea Snakes." (W. A. Dunson, ed.). University Park Press, Baltimore, London and Tokyo.
Zumpt, F. (1965). "Myiasis in Man and Animals in the Old World." Butterworth, London.

Index to Volumes 1 and 2

Since this book is intended for use internationally, priority has been given to the scientific nomenclature of animals, and English or popular names have only been used for the most common species.

Likewise trade names of drugs and chemicals have been avoided wherever possible.

Figure numbers are given in italics.

Ablabes (= *Liopeltis*), 242
Ablabophis, 284
Ablepharus boutonii, 366
Abscess, 88, 101, *4·6*, 102, 112, 121, 168–170, 171–174, *6·2, 6·3*, 184, 215, 225, 251, 252, 327, *9·5*, 328, 333, 347, *15·1*, 512, 544, 562
Abscesses, amoebic, 251
Acanthamoeba, 245
Acanthocephala, 339–341
Acanthocephalus anthurus, 340
Acanthocephalus ranae, 340
Acanthodactylus boskianus, 363
Acanthophis antarcticus, 456
Acanthosaura, 236
Acanthotaenia, 303, 315
Acarina (*see* Mites and Ticks)
Accidents (*see* Trauma)
Acclimation (*see* Acclimatization)
Acclimatization, 30, 58, 86, 490
Acrochordus javanicus, 43, 44, 47, *2·10*, 49, 449, 458
Acinetobacter, 115, 116, 124
Actinomycetes, 165, 193–231
Actinomyces bovis, 226
Actinomyces lacertae, 225

Acid-fast organisms (see *Mycobacterium* and Tuberculosis)
Adenophora, 316
Adeleina, 254
Adenoameloblastoma, 458
Adenocarcinoma, 439, 443, 444, 445, 449, 450, 451, 452, 455, 456, 457, 458, 459, 460, 461
Adenoma, 430, 445, 446, 456
Adenoma of thyroid, 438
Adenomatous polyp, 458
Adrenal gland, 66, 400–401, 489–490
Adrenaline, 66, 556, 574, 576
Adrenal weight, 490
Aedes aegyptii, 374
Aedes canadensis, 374
Aeromonas, 115, 124, 168, 176, 180, 181–184, 187, 575
Aeromonas, susceptibility to disinfectants, 532
Aeromoniasis (see *Aeromonas*)
Agama, 236, 237, 245, 256
Agama agama, 213, 322
A. bibroni, 315, 363
A. caucasica, 462
A. erythrogastra, 462

A. sanguinolenta, 462
A. stellio, 363
Agkistrodon bilineatus, 464
A. contortrix, 413
A. halys, 314, 457, 461
A. piscivorus, 248, 284, 457, 461
Ahaetulla, 64
Aids to diagnosis, 514–523
Air sac, 37
Alaeuris, 322
Albinism, 481
Alcohol, 78, 80, 558, 579
Alexeifella, 284
Alimentary tract (*see* Gastro-intestinal tract)
Allergy, 488 (*see also* Immunology)
Alligator (*see* Crocodilia)
Alligator mississippiensis, 166, 7·1, 7·2, 7·4, 7·6, 7·9, 215, 345, 361, 412, 441, 442, 474
Alsophylax, 237
Ambient temperature (*see* Temperature)
Amblyomma aegyptium, 363
A. marmoreum, 363
A. nitidum, 363
A. nuttalli, 363
A. rhinocerotis, 363
A. sylvaticum, 363
A. testudinis, 365
A. tholloni, 363
A. tuberculatum, 364
Amblyrhynchus, 20–21
Amblyrhynchus cristatus, 364, 412
Ambystoma mexicanum (*see* Axolotl)
Ambystoma tigrinum, 432
Ameiva ameiva ameiva, 375
Ameiva lizard rhabdovirus, 156, 160
Aminoglycoside antibiotics, 511, 559
Amoebiasis (see *Entamoeba*)
Amoebida, 244
Amphibians, 4, 5, 6, 10, 15, 28, 34, 37, 62, 135, 141, 157, 158, 172, 197, 206, 244, 281, 295, 296, 303, 306, 312, 324, 331, 344, 369 (*see also* individual species)

Amphibolurus barbatus, 172, 221, 225, 412
Amphibolurus inermis, 412
Amphisbaenids, 23, 26
Amphisbaena manni, 20
Ampicillin, 555, 560
Amplicaecum, 324
Amplicaecum robertsi, 327
Amputation, 545
Amyda spinifera, 304
Amyloidosis, 82, 490
Anaemia, 141, 247, 257, 258, 276, 365, 367
Anaerobic organisms, 167
Anaerobiosis, 59–60 (*see also* Bioenergetics)
Anaesthesia, 391, 491, 499, 500, 522, 535–548
Anaesthetic agents, 536–539, 554, 556–558 (*see also* individual agents)
Anaesthetic chamber, 538, 541–542
Anaesthetic mask, 541
Anaesthetic techniques, 539–542
Analgesia, 535, 538, 539, 556
Anapsida, 9
Anasarca, 418
Anatomy, 4, 9, 73 (*see also* individual organs)
Ankistrodon blomhoffi, 462
Androgens, 66
Angioma, 430
Anguis fragilis, 50, 83, 371, 413, 471, 474
Angusticaecum, 324, 565
Animal models (*see* Biomedical research)
Anole (see *Anolis carolinensis*)
Anolis, 236, 239
Anolis carolinensis, 274, 412, 443, 444, 514
Anolis equestris, 172
Anoplocephalidae, 312
Anorexia, 304, 310, 319, 327, 341, 387, 413, 414, 421, 426, 490, 500, 509, 524, 527, 570, 573–574

Anthrenus, 313
Antibiotics, 118–125, 173, 177, 178, 182, 188, 419, 511, 555–562 (*see also* individual agents)
Antibiotics, suggested doses of, 560–561
Antibiotic sensitivity tests, 118–125, 4·9, 545
Antibody, 167, 169, 340, 347, 488 (*see also* Immunology)
Antimicrobial agents, 554–562 (*see also* Antibiotics)
Antimycotic agents, 564
Antiseptics (*see* Disinfectants)
Antiparasitic agents, 562–570
Antiprotozoal agents (*see* Protozoa, treatment of)
Aphasmida, 361
Aponomma exornatum, 362
A. gervaisi, 363
A. hydrosauri, 362
A. latum, 363
Appendicular skeleton, 23
Appetite (*see* Nutrition)
Aprion virescens, 418
Archosauria, 9
Argas brumpti, 365
Argas persicus (= *Persiargas*) 365–366
Argasidae, 364–368
Arizona, 166
Arizona-elegans occidentalis, 452, 459
Armillifer armillatus, 342, 9·8, 9·9, 351
A. grandis, 350
A. moniliformis, 350
Artefact, 78, 6·3, 285
Arteries (*see* Cardiovascular system)
Arteriosclerosis (*see* Medial calcification)
Arthropoda, 341–350 (*see also* individual species)
Articular gout (*see* Gout)
Ascarid, 291, 323 (*see also* Ascaridida)
Ascaridida, 323–328
Aschelminthes, 315

Ascites, 518
Asepsis, 543 (*see also* Hygiene and Disinfection)
Aspergillus amstelodami, 205, 211
Aspergillus fumigatus, 195, 203, 205, 215, 216
Atheromatosis, 86 (*see also* Cardiovascular disease)
Atropine, 402, 578
Attagenus, 313
Auscultation, 514
Austramphilina elongata, 301
Autolysis, 78, 102
Autopsy (see *Post mortem* examination)
Autotomy, 19 (*see also* Fractures)
Avian (*see* Birds)
Avitaminoses (*see* Vitamins)
Avitaminosis A (*see* Vitamin A deficiency)
Axial bifurcation, 471–476, *14·1*, *14·2*
Axial skeleton, 18
Axolotl, 285

BHC, 579
Babesia, 278, 294
Babesiosoma, 285
Bacillus alvei, 112
Bacteraemia, 165
Bacteria, 84, 125, 165–191, 310, 362, 367 (*see also* Microbiology and individual organisms)
Bacteria, acid-fast organisms (see *Mycobacterium*)
Bacteria, cultivation (culture) of, 107–113, 184, 185
Bacteria, identification of, 113–118
Bacterial disease, types of, 170–187
Bacterial endotoxin, 555
Bacterial infections, 165–191, 208, 449
Bacterial septicaemia, 168
Bacteriological techniques, 93–125, 165
Bacteriology, equipment for, 93–94

Bacterium sauromali, 172
Bacteroides, 115
Baerietta gerrhonobi, 312
Bandages, 389
Barbiturates, 536–537, 554, 556 (*see also* individual agents)
Barium meal, 515, *16·3*, *16·10*, *18·1*, *18·2* (*see also* Radiography)
Bartonella, 373
Basidiobolus meristosporus ranarum, 208
Basiliscus americanus, 221
Beak, 22 (*see also* Mouthparts)
Beauveria bassiana, 204, 211, 215
Behavioural changes, 500
Beneckea (= Bacillus) chitinovora, 175
Bertarellia, 285
Besnoitia (= Globidium) 259, 260, 285, 293
Betadine, 554 (*see also* Povidone-Iodine)
Bible, 5
Bile, 241, 262, 327
Bile-duct, 241, 261, 296, 298
Bile-duct adenoma, 456, 460
Bile-duct infection, 261, 262, 263
Bile salts, 28
Biliary adenocarcinoma, 457, 461
Biliary adenoma, 443, 444, 455, 460
Biochemical techniques (*see* Biochemistry)
Biochemistry, 129–130
Bioenergetics, 50–54, 491
Biomedical research, 5, 6, 76, 140–141, 161, 184, 185, 205, 227, 326, 579
Biopsy, 81, 173, 175, 270, 415, 416, 421, 426, 463, 521–523, 544, 545
Birds, 3, 6, 28, 31, 34, 50, *2·12*, 57, 59, 61, 75, 129, 135, 142, 143, 147, 150, 260, 270, 274, 278, 292, 297, 312, 313, 331, 333, 335, 374, 431, 462
Birds of prey, 331, 344
Bites, 388–390

Bitis arietans, 214, 261, 274, 319, 376, 457, 461
Bitis gabonica, 83, 348–349, 461
Bitis nasicornis, 431, 457, 461
Bladder, 30, 31, 296
Blastomyces dermatidis, 206
Bleeding (*see* Haemorrhage and Cardiac puncture)
Blindness, 87, 223 (*see also* Ocular disease)
Blister disease, 401 (*see also* Integument)
Blood, 43, 44, 45, 141
Blood chemistry, 43 (*see also* Biochemistry)
Blood, composition of, 44
Blood flow, 42
Blood glucose levels, 574
Blood parasites, 235 (*see also* Protozoa and Microfilariae)
Blood sampling (*see* Cardiac puncture and Haematology)
Blood smears (*see* Haematology)
Blow flies (*see* Calliphoridae)
Boa, 242, 333
Boa constrictor, *4·3*, 125, *6·2*, 289, 375, 413, 498 (see also *Constrictor constrictor*)
Boaedon, 242, 284, 295, *16·4*
Boaedon fuliginosus, *16·4*
Boaedon lineatum, 284
Bodo, 237
Body temperature (*see* Thermoregulation)
Bodyweight, *2·11*, *2·12*
Bombyx mori (*see* Silkworm)
Bone, 172, 212, 221
Bone disease (*see* Osteodystrophy)
Bordetella bronchiseptica, 125
Bothridium, 291, 293, 305, *9·10*
Bothridium pithonis, 306, 307, *9·3*
Bothrops, 258
Bothrops atrox, 136, 457
Botulism, 187
Boyle's apparatus, *17·2*
Box turtle (see *Terrapene carolina*)

Brachylophus fasciatus, 323
Brain, 31, *2·9*, 40, 63, 179, 378, 441 (*see also* Nervous system)
Breathing (*see* Respiration)
Breathing movements, *2·8* (*see also* Respiration)
Breeding, captive, 6, 7, 180
Breeding cycles (*see* Reproductive cycles)
Breeding season (*see* Reproductive cycles)
Bromocyclen, 564
Bronchogenic carcinoma, 456, 460
Bronchopneumonia, (*see* Pneumonia)
Brooding, 61
Brood size, 51
Brown and Brenn stain, *6·4*
Brumation (*see* Hibernation)
Bufotoxin, 493
Bugs (*see* Heteroptera)
Bunamidine hydrochloride, 565, 566
Bungarus fasciata, 159
Burkitt's lymphoma, 431
Burns, 184, 396–397
Burns, chemical, 402
Butirosin sulphate, 555

Cachexia, 85–86, 443 (*see also* Inanition)
Caimans (*see* Crocodilia and individual species)
Caiman, 236
Caiman crocodylus, 29, 43, 217
Caiman sclerops, 217
Calcification, 86, 87, 420, *12·5*, 495, 497
Calcium, 48, 49, 66, 129, 410, 422, 496, 501, 572, 577
Calcium borogluconate, 425
Calcium metabolism, 496 (*see also* Osteodystrophy)
Calcium oxalate, 402
Calcium/phosphorus ratio, 423 (*see also* Osteodystrophy)
Calculi, 426 (*see also* Stones)

Calliphoridae, 377–378 (*see also* Myiasis)
Callisaurus draconoides, 412
Callopistes maculatus, 444
Caloglyphus, 371
Calotes, 242, 322
Calotes versicolor, 491
Camallanoidea, 329
Cancer (*see* Neoplasia)
Candidosis (candidiasis) 195, 196, 213
Candida albicans, 195, 213
Canker (*see* Stomatitis)
Cannibalism, 397
Capillaria colubra, 294, 317
Capillaria recurva, 85, 293
Captive breeding (*see* Breeding, captive)
Captivity, effects of, 208, 234, 291, 292, 371, 387 (*see also* Stress and Environment)
Carassius auratus, 418
Carbaryl solutions, 564
Carbenicillin, 182
Carbon dioxide, 547
Carbon monoxide, 547
Carbutamide, 577
Carcinoma (*see* Neoplasia)
Carcinoma of poison gland, 456
Carcinoma of stomach, 437, 438, 439
Carcinoma of thyroid, 438, 439
Carcinoma planocellulare, 444, 447
Cardiac disease (*see* Cardiovascular disease)
Cardiac puncture, 522–523
Cardianema, 335
Cardiovascular disease, 76, 86, 339, 420, *12·5*, 502
Cardiovascular system, 41–45, 85, 336
Caretta, 24, 477, 479
Caretta caretta, 210, 219, 252, 360, 477
Carotid body, 430
Carriers of organisms, 185, 186, 187, 189, 247, 252, 265 (*see also* Latent infection)

Caryospora, 259, 260, 268
Causus, 239, 241, 242, 274
Catheter (*see* Stomach tubing)
Cats, 309
Cell counts (*see* Haematology)
Cellulitis, 555 (*see also* Dermatitis)
Central nervous system (*see* Brain and Nervous system)
Cephalosporium, 206, 217
Ceramodactylus, 237
Ceratopogonidae, 376 (*see also* Midges)
Cerastes, 259
Cerastes aegyptiacus, 20
C. cerastes, 314
C. vipera, 315
Cestodaria, 310
Cestodes, 295, 299, 9·3, 307, 522, 564, 566
Cestodes, treatment of, 564–565
Cestoidea, 299
Cetrimide, 532, 554 (*see also* Disinfectants)
Chaetomium globosum, 203
Chalcides, 245, 322
Chalcides chalcides, 50
Chalcides ocellatus, 263
Chamaeleo, 24, 236, 258
Chamaeleo dilepis, 221, 412, 444, 445
C. fischeri multituberculatus, 272
C. jacksoni, 213
C. lateralis, 213
C. melleri, 221
C. oustaleti, 9·6
C. vulgaris, 213
Chameleon, 5, 2·5, (*see also* individual species)
Chameleon, American (see *Anolis carolinenasis*)
Changes in management, 529–532
Chanos chanos, 418
Cheles fimbriata, 219
Chelodina, 236, 245, 253, 277, 296
Chelodina longicollis, 219, 301
Chelone, 322

Chelonia, 3, 9, 11, 15, 16, 2·3, 18, 2·7, 31, 33, 35, 44, 166, 175, 179, 185, 210, 219, 234, 236, 238, 239, 242, 245, 253, 255, 258, 260 (*see also* individual species and groups)
Chelonia mydas, 139, 210, 219, 252, 437, 440
Chelonians, bacterial infections in, 168 (*see also* Bacteria)
Chelonians, zoonoses from, 187 (*see also* Zoonoses)
Chelus, 16
Chelydra, 245, 255
Chelydra serpentina, 36, 49, 207, 364, 369, 438
Chemotherapy, 523–524
Chicken leukaemia, 434
Chiggers, 369–370
Chill (chilling) (*see* Hypothermia)
Chilodon, 284
Chinemys reevesi, 219
Chigger mites (*see* Trombiculidae)
Chilomastix, 238
Chironius, 274
Chlamydosaurus kingi, 509
Chloramphenicol, 188, 555, 559, 560
Chlorinated hydrocarbons (*see* Insecticides and individual agents)
Chloroform, 547, 558, 579
Chloroma, 430
Chlortetracycline, 560
Cholangioma, 455, 459
Cholecystitis (*see* Bile-duct infection)
Chondroma, 430
Chondro-osteofibroma, 443, 444
Chondrosarcoma, 454, 459
Chordoma, 430
Chorion-epithelioma, 430
Chromaffinoma, 430
Chromatophoroma, 455, 459
Chrysemys, 236, 245, 255, 277, 296, 322, 576
Chrysemys d'orbignyi, 210

C. picta, 361, 369, 377, 412, 436, 439, 492
C. scripta, 492
Chrysomylia megacephala, 377
Chrysopelea ornata, 263
Chrysops callidus, 377
Chrysosporium, 197, 222
Chrysosporium keratinophilum, 213
Ciliates (*see* Ciliophora)
Ciliophora, 283–284
Cingula, 285
Cinixys, 277
Cinosternum (= *Kinosternum*) 255
Citrobacter (= *Escherichia*) *freundii*, 175
Classification (*see* Nomenclature)
Claudius angustatus, 330
Clawed toad (see *Xenopus laevis*)
Cleft lip, 477, 479
Cleft palate, 477
Clemmys spp., 239, 277, 296, 436, 439
Clemmys caspica rivulta, 409, 4·10
C. guttata, 155
C. japonica, 360
C. marmorata, 142, 361
C. mutica, 16·9
Clinical aspects of diagnosis, 507–533
Clinical chemistry (*see* Biochemistry)
Clinical investigation, 508–511
Cloaca, 29, 31, 32, 46, 89, 102, 4·7, 103, 117, 166, 167, 169, 184, 213, 237, 243
Cloaca, diseases of, 170, 177–178, 368, 378, 451, 454, 455
Cloacal carcinoma, 454, 459
Cloacal examination, 513
Cloacal haemangioma, 461
Cloacarus faini, 369
Cloacitis (*see* Cloaca, diseases of)
Clostridia (*Clostridium*) 109, 115, 170, 186
Clostridial infections, 186
Clostridium (*see* Clostridia)
Clostridium nougi, 126
Clupea harengus, 418

Cnemidophorus, 237
Cnemidophorus ceralbensis, 413
Cnemidophorus sexlineatus, 300
Cnidospora, 279–282
Cobra (see *Naja* and individual species)
Cobra, spitting, 28 (see *Naja nigricollis*)
Cobra venom herpesvirus, 159
Coccidia, 259, 263, 368
Coccidiosis, 261–264, 569
Coccidiosis, of chameleons and lizards, 263
Coccidiosis, of gall bladder, 261, 263
Coccidiosis, of intestines, 263, 264
Cockroaches, 168, 245, 249, 345
Coleonyx variegatus, 412
Colitis, 241, 251, 283–285
Colitis, associated with ciliates, 283–285
Colon, 243, 247
Colonic adenocarcinoma, 459
Colonic carcinoma, 445, 449
Coloration, 10
Coluber constrictor, 413, 473, 474
Coluber plagellum testaceus, 455, 459
C. hippocrepis, 314
C. viridflavus, 313
Commensals, 208, 292
Conditions of unknown aetiology, 502
Congenital abnormalities, 469–485, 501
Coniothyrium fuckelianum, 197
Conjunctivitis (*see* Ocular infections)
Conofilaria, 334
Conolophus, 245, 322
Conservation, 6
Constipation, 323, 341
Constrictor constrictor, 45, 84, 2·10, 413, 449, 458, 16·3 (see also *Boa constrictor*)
Convulsions (*see* Nervous diseases)
Copulation, 2·3, 7, 500
Corallus, 274
Cordyceps militaris, 205

Cordylus polyzonus, 445, 448
Coregonus clupeaformis, 418
Corn snake (see *Elaphe*)
Corn snake (*Elaphe*) oncornavirus, 149–150
Coronella austriaca, 214, 413
Corticosteroids, 575, 576, 578
Cortisone (*see* Corticosteroids)
Corynebacterium, 166
Cosmiomma hippopotamensis, 363
Cotylaspis, 296
Coxiella burnetii, 187
Cranium, 20–23
Crepidobothrium gerrardii, 291, 303, 304
Crocodile (*see* Crocodilia)
Crocodilia, 3, 9, 10, 11, 16, 33, 35, 166, 215, 224, 236, 242, 245, 259, 261, 264
Crocodilarus, 278
Crocodylus, 236, 242, 245
Crocodylus acutus, 244, 293, 441, 442
C. niloticus, 112, 218, 7·6, 7·7, 376
C. porosus, 441, 442
Crotalus, 169, 222, 333, 456, 460, 555
Crotalus adamanteus, 222, 555
C. atrox, 456, 460, 537
C. durissus berrificus, 325
C. horridus, 456, 460
C. horridus atricaudatus, 456
C. mitchelli pyrrhus, 457, 461
C. ruber, 457, 461
C. viridis helleri, 456, 461
C. viridis viridis, 261, 456, 461
Crotaphopelbis, 242
Crushing injuries, 390–394, *11·1, 11·2, 16·8*
Crustaceans, 306, 340, 359
Cryosurgery, 177
Ctenosauria, 322
Ctenosaurus hemilopha, 412
C-type virus, 147, 149, 150
Culex, 257
Culex aikeni, 374
C. amazonensis, 374

C. apanastasis, 374
C. decens, 374
C. dunni, 374
C. elevator, 374
C. egcymon, 374
C. gelidus, 374
C. invidiosus, 374
C. pipiens, 375
C. tarsalis, 377
C. tecmarsis, 374
Culicidae, 373–376 (*see also* Mosquitoes)
Culicoides, 376, 377
Culture (*see* Bacteria, Fungi and Viruses)
Cuora, 239, 245, 252
Cuora (= *Cyclemys*) *amboinensis*, 252
Cyclagras, 236
Cyclagras gigas, 136
Cyclophyllidae, 312
Cyclospora, 259, 260, 267
Cyclospora niniae, 267
Cyclops viridis, 304
Cyclops vulgaris, 304
Cyclura cornuta, 443, 444
Cyclura ricordi, 443, 444
Cystic-adenoma of the stomach, 450, 458
Cysticercoid, 312, 313, 314
Cysticercus fasciolaris, 434
Cystic haemangioma, 456
Cystotomy, 545
Cysts, 90, 218, 241, 244, 245, 246, 247, 248, 250, 265, 270, 271, 282, 283
Cytamoeba, 285
Cytology, 463
Cytopathic effect (CPE), 145

d-tubocurarine, 556
DDT, 579
Dactylosoma, 278, 285
Damonia, 236
Dasypeltis, 23
Debility, 125, 184, 196
Decalcification, 80

Deficiency disease (*see* individual vitamins and minerals)
Definitive hosts (*see* Hosts)
Dehydration (*see* Fluid replacement)
Demansia, 236
Dermanyssus natricis (see *Ophionyssus natricis*)
Dermatophilus congolensis, 172, 188, 197, 225
Dermis, 11, 15 (*see also* Skin)
Dermochelys, 16
Dermatitis, 125, 170, 171, 174–175, 222, 555
Development, 44–50
Developmental abnormalities, 7, 48, 89, 179, 469–485, 494, 496
Dexamethasone (*see* Corticosteroids)
Diabetes mellitus, 495, 575, 576 (*see also* Pancreatectomy)
Diagnosis, 507–533
Diaphanocephaloidea, 320
Diaphragm, 24, 37, 38
Diarrhoea, 247, 263, 319 (*see also* Enteritis)
Dichlorophen, 564, 566
Dichlorvos, 562, 563, 566, 568
Diemeria, 236
Diet, 234, 387, 388, 395, 409 (*see also* Nutrition)
Digestion, 26, 30, 411–413 (*see also* Nutrition)
Digestive system (*see* Gastro-intestinal tract)
Digestive tract (*see* Gastro-intestinal tract)
Digits, 220
Diiodohydroxyquin, 253
Dilepididae, 313
Dimetridazole, 240, 243, 249, 567, 569
Di-iodohydroxyquin, 569
Dilepididae, 313
Di-N-butyl-tin oxide, 565
Dinosaurs, 4, *1·1*, 50
Di-phenthane-7-methylbenzene, 566, 568

Diplomonadida, 238–241
Diplopylidium, 313
Dipsosaurus dorsalis, *2·13*, 57, 60, 488
Dipylidium, 313
Discomfort (*see* Pain)
Disinfectants, 117, 183, 530–531, 532, 554 (*see also* Disinfection)
Disinfection, 95–95, 174, 183, 184, 185, 523, 554
Dislocation, 391
Dispholidus, 242
Dispholidus typus, 455, 460
Disposal of waste, 95–96 (*see also* Hygiene)
Dissection (see *Post mortem* examination)
Diuretic, 391, 402, 404, 578
Diving, 41, 42
Dorisiella, 259, 260
Dosages, 551–585
Dracaena, 245
Dracaena guianensis, 36
Dracunculus globocephalus, 330
Dracunculus medinensis, 329
Dracuniculoidea, 329
Dracunculus, 329–330
Drinking, 388
Drowning, 402–404, 578
Drugs, 551–585 (*see also* individual agents)
Drugs, administration of, 523–527, 551–553
Drugs, uptake, 553
Druschia, 27
Drymarchon, 242, 258
Drymarchon corais, 374
Dryophis prasina, 341
Dujardinascaris, 324
Duthersia, 305
Dysecdysis, 389, 397–401, 494 (*see also* Sloughing)
Dysentery (*see* Enteritis and *Entamoeba*)
Dysphagia (*see* Stomatitis)
Dyspnoea (*see* Respiratory disease)
Dystocia, 500 (*see also* Egg-binding)

ECG (*see* Electrocardiography)
EEG (*see* Electroencephalography)
Ear, 2·9, 40, 63, 499
Earthworms, 292, 318
Eastern equine encephalitis virus (EEEV), 154–155, 375
Ecdysis (*see* Sloughing)
Ectoparasites, 85, 275, 359–383, 398 (*see also* individual species and groups)
Ectoparasiticides, 562–564
Ectopic embryos, 482
Ectothermy (*see* Thermoregulation)
Edwardsiella tarda, 166, 187
Egernia, 236, 256
Egernia cunninghami, 413
Egg, 4, 10, 48–49, 54, 180, 500–501, 15·2
Egg-binding, 545, 577 (*see also* Dystocia)
Egg-laying, 500
Egg infection, 169, 203, 501
Eggshell, 48, 49
Eggs, incubation of, 104, 110, 501
Eggs, of endoparasites, 9·10, 349
Eggs, numbers, 51
Egg peritonitis, 578
Egg-tooth, 50
Eimeria, 259, 260
Eimeria bitis, 261
Eimeria cascabeli, 261
Elachistodon, 23
Elaphe, 23
Elaphe climacophora, 222
E. guttata, 142, 149, 222, 225, 434, 452, 459, 481, 16·5
E. longissima, 136
E. obsoleta, 516
E. obsoleta obsoleta, 225, 454, 459
E. obsoleta quadrivittata, 16·6, 304
E. obsoleta rossalleni, 454, 459
E. obsoleta spiloides, 224, 452
E. quadrivirgata, 304
E. radiata, 348–349
E. scalaris, 314
Elaphe oncornavirus, 149

Electro-anaesthesia, 536
Electrocardiography, 520
Electrocution, 396–397
Electroencephalography, 520
Electrolyte balance, 320, 415, 524, 565 (*see also* Fluid replacement)
Electronmicroscopy, 80, 137, 140, 141, 142, 143, 145, 149, 152, 156, 157, 159, 160, 434, 440, 447, 452, 457, 463
Elseya, 255, 277
Emaciation (*see* Inanition)
Embryo, 48, 49, 104, 469–485, 501
Embryonic development, 47–50, 469–485
Embryonic death (*see* Embryonic mortality)
Embryonic mortality, 48, 501
Emetine hydrochloride, 253, 567, 569
Emoia, 236, 256
Emyda, 236, 259, 479
Emydoidea (= *Emys*) 255, 280, 296
Emydoidea blandingi, 374
Emydura, 236, 245, 253
Emys, 16, 277, 239, 245, 253, 322
Emys orbicularis, 361, 436, 438
Enchondroma, 445, 448
Encystation, 239, 246 (*see also* Cyst)
Endocrinal disorders, 493–495
Endocrine system, 61–62, 65–67, 493, 495
Endolimax, 245
Endolymphatic sacs, 496
Endoparasites, 275, 291–358 (*see also* individual species and groups)
Endoparasiticides, 564–570 (*see also* individual agents)
Endoparasiticides, suggested doses of, 566–567
Enema, 266, 402, 578
Energetics (*see* Bio-energetics)
Energy allocation to egg production, 55
Energy budgets (*see* Bioenergetics)

INDEX xi

Energy flow and utilization (*see* Bio-energetics)
Endocarditis, 212
Endothermy (*see* Thermoregulation)
Entamoeba, 89, 251–254, 569
Entamoeba, in chelonians, 251–252
Entamoeba, in crocodiles, 253–254
Entamoeba, in lizards, 252–253
Entamoeba, in marine turtles, 252
Entamoeba, in snakes, 246–251
Entamoeba, in tuatara, 253
Entamoeba invadens, 89, 246, 293
Entamoeba serpentis, 248
Entamoebiasis, pathology of, 246–256
Enteritis, 186, 213, 243, 283–285 (*see also* Diarrhoea)
Enteritis, associated with ciliates, 283–285
Enterobacter, 88, 115, 169
Entomelas, 319
Entomophthora (= *Conidiobolus*) *coronata*, 208
Enucleation, 545
Envenomation (*see* Venom and Poisoning)
Environment, influencing mycotic infections 207, 208 (*see also* Captivity)
Environment, sampling of, 104–105
Enzymes, 29, 159, 411, 414
Epicrates angulifer, 223
E. chenchia maurus, 223
E. stricta, 179
Epidermal papilloma, 458
Epidermis, 4, 11, *6.1*, 330
Epididymis (*see* Reproductive system)
Epithelioma, 448
Epoxy resin, 391, 523, 546, 578
Equipment, for histopathology, 80
Equipment, for microbiology, 93–94
Eremias, 237
Eremias arguta, 243
E. grammica, 462

E. persica, 462
E. velox, 462
Erinaceus europaeus concolor, 363
Erpeton tentaculum, 298, 348
Erythrocyte virus, 141
Erythrocyte (*see* Blood)
Erythrolamprus, 236
Eryx tartaricus, 462
Escherichia coli, 88, 112, 115, 116, 117, 165, 166, 169
Ether, 558, 579
Etorphine hydrochloride, 538
Eublepharis macularius, 501
Eucoccida, 254, 259, 273
Eumeces, 245
Eumeces algeriensis, 363
E. fasciatus, 413, 445, 448
E. obsoletus, 574
E. taeneolatus, 462
Eunectes murinus, 291, 304, 330, 450, 458, 477, *14.4*
European pond tortoise (turtle) (see *Emys orbicularis*)
Euthanasia, 546–547
Eutriatama rubrovaria, 372
Eutrophication, 182, 183
Evolution, 3, 4, 16, 208
Exercise, 86
Excretion, 30–34, (*see also* Faeces and Urates)
Exophthalmia, 477
Experimental infections, 154–156, 206–207, 457–462 (*see also* Biomedical research)
Experimental research (*see* Biomedical research)
Experimental surgery, 546
Exostoses, 498, 515, *16.2*, *16.4* (*see also* Calcification)
Eyes, *2.14*, 63, 64, *6.2*, 171, 178, 214, 219, 221, 222, 223, 368, 499 (*see also* Ocular diseases)
Eyes, opacity of, 398

Faeces, 101, 126, 184, 208, 237, 240, 247, 307

Faeces, eggs in, 297, 303, 304, 307, 313, 316, 318, 321, 332, 333, 344, 348, *9·10*, 349
Faeces, larvae in, 320
Fallisia, 273
Fangs, *2·4*, 22, 83 (*see also* Teeth)
Fat body, 85
Fat storage disease, 441
Fear (*see* Stress)
Feeding (*see* Diet and Nutrition)
Fenbendazole, 566, 568
Fer-de-lance virus (FDLV), 136–139, *5·1, 5·2, 5·3, 5·4, 5·5*, 138, 160
Fertility, 410, 500
Fertilization, 46, 47
Fibre optical instruments (*see* Laparoscopy)
Fibroadenoma, 437, 438
Fibroadenoma of lung, 437, 439
Fibroblastic sarcoma, 459
Fibroepithelial tumours, 440
Fibroma, *5·1*, 139, *5·14*, 151, 430, 435, 437, 440, 451, 452, 458, 459, 460
Fibroma molle, 461
Fibropapillomas, 433, 434, 435, 437, 440, 455, 459
Fibrosarcoma, 90, 445, 449, 456, 457, 458, 460, 461
Fibrosis, 82, 172, 390, 494, 545
Fibrous osteodystrophy (*see* Osteodystrophy)
Filariae (*see* Microfilariae)
Fish, 6, 18, 75, 129, 135, 142, 161, 168, 172, 181, 184, 197, 270, 279, 281, 285, 295, 296, 301, 305, 306, 318, 331, 339, 340, 431
Fixation of fractures, 391 (*see also* Fractures)
Flagellates (*see* Mastigophora)
Flatworms, 295 (*see also* Trematoda and Cestoda)
Fleas (*see* Siphonaptera)
Flesh flies (*see* Sarcophaginae)

Flies, 245, 372–378 (*see also* individual species)
Fluid replacement therapy, 10, 174, 178, 320, 405, 489, 524, 529, 564, 573
Flukes (*see* Trematodes)
Fluoroacetamide (1081), 492
Foleyella furcata, 335, 337
Foleyella philistinae, 335
Follicular adenoma, 449
Food (*see* Diet)
Force-feeding, 177, 491, *16·11*, 524, *16·12*, 525, 526, 527, 528
Formaldehyde, 78, 80, 183
Formalin (*see* Formaldehyde)
Fossils, 4, *1·1*
Fowl sarcoma, 434
Fractures, 5, 391, 409, 423, 426, 448, 497, 515, *16·8*
Free-living reptiles, 6, 171, 182, 195, 234, 246, 315, 373, 440, 455, 479
Freezing of specimens, 78
Frogs, 303, 308, 324 (*see also* Amphibians)
Frostbite (*see* Hypothermia)
Frozen sections, 80
Frusemide, 578
Fungi, 125, 172, 175, 177, 193–231, 463, 501
Fungi, culture of, 125
Fungi, treatment of, 564 (*see also* Antimycotic agents)
Fusarium oxysporum, 203, 206, 212, 221, 222
F. solani, 196
F. urticearum, 194, 222

Gallamine triethiodide, 556
Gall bladder, 213, 261, 263, 280, 296, 298, 299, 300, 434, 440
Gall bladder infection (*see* Bile-duct infection)
Ganglioneuroma, 430
Gangrene, 212, 337 (*see also* Clostridia and Hypothermia)

Garnia, 273, 277
Garter snake (see *Thamnophis* and individual species)
Gas exchange, 34
Gastralia, 19
Gastric lavage, 402
Gastric lesions, 326 (*see also* Enteritis)
Gastroenteritis, 306 (*see also* Enteritis)
Gastro-intestinal tract, 26–30, 196, 213, 219, 245, 253, 277, 280, 552–553, *18·1, 18·2* (*see also* Stomach and intestine)
Gastrotomy, 545
Gecko, 11, 64, 141, 256, 258, 509 (*see also* individual species)
Geckobia, 371
Geckobiella, 370, 371
Geckobiella texana, 260
Gehyra, 256
Gehyra australis, 373
G. punctata, 412
Gekko gecko, 509
Gekkonidae, 11
General adaptation syndrome (*see* Stress)
Genetics, 432, 483, 501–502
Gentamicin, 121, 182, 559, 560
Geochelone, *15·2*
Geochelone carbonaria, 436, 439
G. elephantopus, 439
G. radiata, *16·10*
Geomyda, 239, 255, 296
Geomyda trifuga, 436, 439
Geotrichum candidum, 207, 215, 223
Gerrhonotus, 236
Gerrhonotus multicarinatus, 312
Gerrhonotus validus, 274
Gharial (*see* Crocodilia)
Giant cells, 443, *7·8*
Giant tortoise (see *Geochelone elephantopus*)
Giardia, 238, 241
Glands, 15

Gliomas, 430
Glossina, 257, 376, 377
Glossina brevipalpis, 377
G. fuscipes, 376, 377
G. pallidipes, 377
G. palpalis, 376
G. tachinoides, 376
Glossinidae, 376–377
Glucagon, 575–576
Glucose tolerance curves, 573–574
Glugea, 280
Glugea danilewskyi, 281
Glycerol, 578
Glycosuria, 575–576
Gnathostoma procyonis, 331
Goezia, 324
Gogatea serpentium, *9·10*
Goitre, 493 (*see also* Thyroid gland)
Gonad (*see* Reproductive system)
Gopherus, 16, 322
Gopherus agassizi, Nitrogen metabolism, 33
Gopherus berlandieri, 375; Viral experiments, 156
Gout (articular and/or visceral), 87, 298, 415–416, 496, 559
Gout, false, 416, *12·4*
Graft-versus-host reaction, 488
Gram's stain, 96–97, *6·1, 6·4*
Granulocytic leukaemia, 431, 461
Granulomas, 172, 174, 177, 195, *7·3*, 199, *7·8*, 201, *7·10*, 202, 203, 207, 210, 212, 214, 216, 217, 218, 219, 220, 223, 225, 332, 463
Granulosa cell tumour, 450, 458
Granulosa-theca cell tumour, 457, 461
Graptemys, 255, 277, 296
Graptemys geographica, 492
Grass snake (see *Natrix natrix*)
Graya, 236
Gray-patch disease (*see* Green sea turtle virus)
Greek tortoise (see *Testudo graeca*)
Green lizard (see *Lacerta viridis*)

Green lizard papilloma-associated virus, 152
Green sea turtle virus, 139–141, 160, 361
Growth hormone, 576
Gymnodactylus, 237, 256
Gymnodactylus caspas, 313
Gymnodactylus fedteschenkovi, 462

Haemangioadenocarcinoma, 452
Haemangioendothelioma, 455
Haemangioma, 455, 460
Haemaphysalis otophila, 363, 364
Haematocrit (*see* Haematology)
Haematological techniques (*see* Haematology)
Haematology, 77, 128–129, 181, 182, 235, 237, 247, 256, 276, 522–523
Haematoma, 172
Haementeria, 257
Haemobartonella, 373
Haemocystidium (= *Haemoproteus*), 273
Haemogregarina, 254
Haemogregarina stepanovi, 253, 361
H. mauretanica, 366
H. nicoriae, 361
Haemogregarines, 254–259
Haemogregariniasis (*see* Haemogregarines)
Haemophilus, 109, 115
Haemoproteus gonzalesi, 376
Haemoproteus mesnili, 376
Haemorrhage, 126, 7·3, 389–390, 489 (*see also* Fluid replacement)
Haemosiderin, 181
Haemosporina, 273
Haemostasis (*see* Haemorrhage)
Halothane, 538–539, 554, 558
Hamartoma, 89
Hamster (*see* Rodents)
Handling, 510–512 (*see also* Anaesthesia and Soothing techniques)
Haplotrema constrictum, 440

Harderian gland, 219
Hartmanella, 245
Hartwichia, 324
Hastospiculum, 333
Hatchability, 203
Hazards to man, 538 (*see also* Zoonoses)
Head, 217, 224
Healing of wounds, 175
Hearing (*see* Ear)
Heart, 10, 24, 31, 2·9, 40, 41, 212 (*see also* Cardiovascular disease)
Heart rate, 42
Heatstress (*see* Hyperthermia)
Helicops, 236
Helminths, 85, 295–339 (*see also* individual species and groups)
Heloderma suspectum, 336, 413, 445, 448
Hemidactylus, 236, 237, 245, 266
Hemidactylus angulatus, 346, 347
Hemidactylus flaviviridis, 377
Hemipenis (*see* Penis)
Hemipyrella liguriensis, 377
Henneguya, 279
Hepatic disease, 82, 142, 179, 196, 7·10, 202, 208, 258, 315, 317, (*see also* Liver)
Hepatitis (*see* Hepatic disease)
Hepatoblastoma, 430
Hepatocarcinoma, 445
Hepatomas, 443, 444, 446, 455, 460
Hepatozoon, 254, 259
Hepatozoon domergui, 375
H. mauretanicum, 366
H. rarefaciens, 374, 375
H. triatomae, 372
Hermann's tortoise (see *Testudo hermanni*)
Herpesvirus, 135, 142, 152, 156, 157, 158, 159, 447
Herpetacarus cadignani, 370
Herpetacarus leprochaeta, 370
Herpetomonas, 235
Heterodon nasicus, 455, 460
Heterodon platyrhinus, 455, 460

Heteronota, 256
Heteroptera, 257, 372, 523
Heterotrichida, 284
Hexamastrix, 241
Hexametia, 324
Hexametra quadricornis, 325
Hexamita, 239–241
Hexamita (= *Octamastix*) 238
Hexamita parva, 239
Hexamitiasis (see *Hexamita*)
Hibernation, 47, 58, 155, 178, 489
Hirstiella, 273, 371
Hirudinea, 360–362
Histology (*see* Histopathology)
Histopathological techniques (*see* Histopathology)
Histopathology, 75–91, 84, 169, 172, 210–226, 398, 463
Histopathology, of fungal infections, 210–218, 219–224, 225–226
Histopathology, of bacterial infections, 169, 172, 6·3, 6·4, 6·5, 15·1
Histoplasma capsulatum, 206
Hoarella, 259, 260, 268
Homalopsis buccata, 455, 460
Homoiothermy (*see* Thermoregulation)
Hoplodactylus, 242, 256
Hormones, 574–577
Horseflies (*see* Tabanidae)
Hosts, of parasites (*see* Endoparasites and Ectoparasites)
Housing, 387
Humidity, 174, 319, 370, 374, 398, 401, 470, 500, 501, 529
Humoral antibodies, 340, 347 (*see also* Antibody)
Hunter, John, 5
Hyalomma, 257
Hyalomma aegyptium, 366
H. dromedarii, 363
H. franchinii, 363
H. impeltum, 363
H. syriacum, 366

Hycolin, 554
Hydraspis pilarii, 210
Hydrocortisone (*see* Corticosteroids)
Hydromedusa maximiliani, 359
H. platanensis, 359
H. tectifera, 359
Hydronephrosis, 85
Hydrosaurus amboinensis, 245, 443, 444
Hydroxyapatite, 416
Hygiene, 95–96, 175, 183, 187, 240, 249, 266, 384, 532–533, 543
Hymenolepis, 292
Hyperglycaemia, 574, 575, 576
Hyperkeratosis, 221, 225
Hyperlactaemia, 574
Hyperthermia, 404–406
Hyperimmune sera, 184
Hypocalcaemia, 423
Hypoglycaemia, 489, 576, 577
Hypothermia, 404–406, 536
Hypovitaminoses (*see* Vitamins)
Hypoxia, 539
Hypsirhina, 236

Ichoronyssus serpentium, 366
Iguana (*see* individual species)
Iguana iguana, 76, 86, 4·6, 6·5, 252, 284, 322, 12·5, 12·6, 412, 425, 443, 444, 491, 514, 538, 571
Iguana herpesvirus, 156–159
Iguana sensitivity test, 121, 245
Iguanodon, 5, 1·1
Immune system, 433
Immunofluorescent antibody technique, 249 (*see also* Serology)
Immunization (*see* Vaccination and Preventive Medicine)
Immunological disorders, 488–489
Immunology, 488
Immunosuppression, 433, 575
Impaction, 323, 341
Inanition, 85, 86, 277, 306 (*see also* Anorexia and Cachexia)
Inappetance (*see* Anorexia)
Inbreeding, 502

Incubation of eggs, 470, 501
Infections, generalized, 170, 181–187
Infections, localized, 170, 171–181
Infectious diseases, 4, 84–85, 93, 133–383
Infectious stomatitis (see Stomatitis)
Infertility, 410, 500
Infidum, 9·2
Inflammation, 82, 169, 173, 180
Infra-red radiation, 65, 495
Injection, 524, 527, 540–541
Injections, intramuscular, 524, 527, 16·15, 541
Injections, intraperitoneal, 541
Injections, subcutaneous, 524, 526, 16·14, 541
Injuries (see Trauma)
Insecticides, 471, 491, 492, 498, 562–564, 579 (see also individual chemicals)
Insects, 141, 168, 193, 204, 205, 208, 257, 331, 332, 368, 372–378 (see also individual species and groups)
Insulin, 576–577
Integument, 10–11, 2·1, 82, 98, 4·3, 99, 139–141, 184, 211, 9·4, 310, 317, 367, 10·1, (see also Skin)
Intermediate hosts (see Hosts)
Interstitial cell tumour, 445, 449
Intestinal lesions, 252 (see also Enteritis)
Intestine, 29, 31, 211, 213, 215, 216, 219, 237, 241, 244, 263, 267, 300
Intestine, passage of ingesta through, 552–553, 18·1, 18·2
Intestine, infection of (see Enteritis)
Intoxication (see Poisoning)
Intraheptic duct adenocarcinoma, 457
Intromittent organ (see Penis)
Intubation, 541, 554
Intussusception, 84, 213, 450
Invertebrates, 257, 295, 296, 314, 322, 334, 339, 343, 371 (see also Insects and individual species)

Invertebrates, damage by, 394
Iodine, 425, 426, 572
Iodine tincture, 579
Iodoform, 579
Ionides, C.J.P., 507
Irradiation, 65, 435, 464, 495–496
Isaria farinosa, 205
Islets of Langerhans (see Pancreas)
Islet cell tumour, 445, 449
Isolation (see Quarantine)
Isopora, 259, 260
Isopora naiae, 261, 362
Ixodidae, 362–364
Ixodiderma, 371

Jacobson's organ, 34, 2·8, 36, 62, 2·14, 64
Japanese encephalitis (JE) 154, 376
Jaundice, 299, 327 (see also Gall bladder)
Joyeuxiella echinorhynchoides, 314, 315

Kachuga, 187, 296
Kalicephalus, 122, 293, 320, 565
Kanamycin, 559, 560
Kapsulotaenia, 9·10
Karyolysus, 255, 259
Kenya, 182, 183
Keratin, 11, 12, 15, 166, 167, 168, 174, 197, 209
Kerosene, 579
Ketamine, hydrochloride, 391, 499, 537–538, 554, 557
Ketonaemia, 576, 577
Kidneys, 30, 31, 210, 211, 213, 218, 220, 240, 251 (see also Renal disease)
Killing (see Euthanasia)
Kinetoplastida, 235–237
King snake (see *Lampropeltis*)
Kinixys, 236, 322
Kinosternum scorpioides, 270, 296
Klebsiella, 115, 166
Klossiella, 255, 259
Koch's postulates, 169

Kyphosis, 480–481, 515, *16·5*, *16·6*

Lacerta, 24, 237, 245, 322, 477, *14·4*
Lacerta agilis, 154, 255, 366, 413, 444, 446, 447, *14·1*, 474
L. dugesii, 207, *7·10*
L. lepida, 477, 479
L. muralis, 413, 444, 447
L. saxicola, 470
L. sicula, 89, 445, 447
L. sicula cetti, 447
L. viridis, 152, 154, 194, 213, 222, 366, 445, 446, *17·3*
L. vivipara, 49, 50, 60, 61, 121, 255, 477, 482, *14·4*
Lacertilia (*see* Sauria)
Lachesis, 274
Lachrymal sac, 222
Lampropeltis, 241, 242
Lampropeltis getulus, 413
Lampropeltis californiae, 256, 452, *13·1*, *13·2*, *13·3*, 459
Laparoscopy, 173, 522
Laparotomy, 522, 545–546
Laparotomy, in chelonians, 546
Larvae, fly (*see* Myiasis)
Larvae, helminth (*see* individual species)
Latastia, 237
Latastia longicollis revoili, 373
Latent infection, 158, 160
Latex base, 579
Laticauda colubrina, 364
LD50 values, 495
Leeches, 236, 255, 257, 360, 361 (*see also* Hirudinea)
Leiolopisma delicata, 412
Leimadophis, 284
Leiomyoma, 430
Leiomyosarcoma, 452, 456, 460
Leiperia gehyrae, 350
Leishmania, 234
Leishmania adleri, 237
Lepidodactylus, 256
Lepidosauria, 9
Leptomonas, 235

Leptospira, 115, 116, 170, 186
Leucocytosis, 182 (*see also* Haematology)
Leukaemia, 145, 150, 159
Leukaemic lymphosarcoma, 457, 461
Levamisole, 567, 568
Libido (*see* Fertility)
Lidocaine, 556
Life span (*see* Old age)
Ligation of venom ducts, 545
Lighting, 387 (*see also* Photoperiod and Ultraviolet light)
Lignocaine, 556
Limbs, 23, 220
Lincomycin, 560
Linguatula serrata, 342
Linguatulida (*see* Pentastomida)
Liopeltis, 242
Liopeltis vernalis, 261
Liophis, 284
Liophis merremi, 304
Lipoma, 430, 441
Liponyssus, 257
Liponyssus arabicus, 366
L. natricis, 366
L. serpentium, 366
Liquid paraffin, 426, 499, 578
Lissemys, 294
Liver cell carcinoma, 447, 448
Liver, 31, 85, 86, 181, 210, 211, 212, 213, 214, 216, 217, 218, 219, 221, 251, 252, 262, 263, 277 (*see also* Hepatic disease)
Liver necrosis, 214
Lizards (*see* Sauria)
Local anaesthesia (analgesia) 536, 539, 556 (*see also* Analgesia)
Locomotion, 23–24
London Zoo (*see* Zoological Society of London)
Longevity (*see* Old age)
Lophotoaspis, 296
Loss of blood (*see* Anaemia and Haemorrhage)
Lucilia, 378, *10·2*

Lucké's tumour, 431, 434
Lugol's iodine, 96, 247
Lung, 24, 2·5, 26, 31, 34–41, 65, 7·1, 198, 7·3, 199, 7·5, 200, 7·9, 202, 210, 211, 212, 213, 214, 215, 216, 217, 221, 296, 9·8, 343, (see also Respiratory tract)
Lung lesions (see Respiratory disease)
Lutzomyia, 236, 273
Lutzomyia adleri, 373
L. micropyga, 372
L. trinidadensis, 373
Lygosoma, 236, 256
Lymphatic leukaemia, 430, 449, 458
Lymphatic system, 44
Lymphoblastic leukaemia, 445, 449
Lymphoblastic lymphoma, 437, 444
Lymphoblastic lymphosarcoma, 439
Lymphoid leukaemia, 456, 460
Lymphoid leukosis, 458
Lymphoma, 430, 443, 444, 445, 447
Lymphoreticular neoplasm, 437, 441
Lymphosarcoma, 135, 142, 430, 431, 441, 443, 444, 448, 450, 452, 455, 456, 458, 459, 460, 461
Lyssemysai, 296

M 99, 554, 557
MS222 (see Tricaine methanesulphonate)
Mabuya, 236, 256, 278, 322
Mabuya carcinata, 20
Mabuya quinquetaeniata, 50
Mabuyonyssus, 368
Macdonaldius, 335
Macdonaldius andersoni, 336
M. oschei, 336, 338
M. seetae, 337
Madagascarophis colubrina, 375
Madathamugadia, 335
Magnesium, 129
Malaclemys, 296, 476
Malaclemys terrapin, 153
Malacochesus tornieri, 439
Maladaptation, 490–491

Malaria (see *Plasmodium* and individual species)
Malathion, 564
Malformations, 467–485
Malformations, of the extremities, 479–480
Malformations, of the head, 477–479
Mammals, 34, 37, 43, 50, 2·12, 57, 59, 61, 62, 66, 75, 135, 141, 142, 143, 150, 172, 193, 197, 209, 270, 305, 306, 309, 312, 324, 331, 335, 344, 374, 431, 462 (see also individual species)
Mannitol, 391
Mantonella, 259, 260, 269
Marek's disease, 434
Mastigophora, 235–245
Mastomys natalensis, 346, 9·9
Mating (see Copulation)
Mealworms, 410, 425, 572
Meat, 411
Mebendazole, 567, 568
Media (see Bacteria, cultivation of)
Medial calcification, 86, 87, 495, (see also Calcification)
Medication (see Drugs)
Mehdiella, 322
Melanism, 481
Melanoma, 89, 430, 445, 448, 450, 451, 454, 458, 459
Meningioma, 430
Mephitis mephitis, 332
Meriones unguiculatus, 346
Mesenchymosarcoma, 447
Mesocestoididae, 314
Mesocyclops obsoletus, 304
Metabolic bone disease (see Osteodystrophy)
Metabolic diseases, 87, 496–498
Metabolic rate, 56–61, 2·11
Metabolism, 50–61
Metabolism, anaerobic, 60
Metarhizium anisopliae, 196, 198, 201, 203, 216
Metastases, 438, 439, 446, 452, 455, 464

Metazoan, parasites (*see* Parasites)
Methods of treatment, 523–533
Methohexitone sodium, 557
Methoxyflurane, 539, 558
Methoxymol, 554, 557
Methylcarbonate powder, 564
Metopocercus cornutus, 214
Metronidazole, 244, 253, 567, 569
Mouse (*see* Rodents)
Microabscesses, 174
Microbiological techniques, 78, 93–125
Microbiology, 93–131 (*see also* Bacteria, Fungi and Viruses)
Micrococcus, 166, 172
Microcyclops varians, 304
Microfilariae, 334, 335, 336, 337, *9·6, 9·7*, 338, 339, 366, 375
Microphthalmia, 477
Microsporidia, 280, 281
Microtrombicula chamlongi, 370
Midges, 372, 376 (*see also* Ceratopogonidae)
Miescher's tubes, 272
Mineral deficiencies (*see* individual minerals and calcium/phosphorus ratio)
Minerals, doses of, 572–573, 578
Miscellaneous diseases, 487–502
Mites, 183, 255, 257, 292, 353, 366–371, *10·1*
Mites, control of, 562–564
Moloch horridus, 33, 412
Monitor (see *Varanus* and individual species)
Monkeys (*see* Primates)
Monocercomonas, 241, 242
Monocercomonas filamentum, 243
Monocercomonoides, 241
Monocystis agilis, 292
Morelia argus, 322
Morelia spilotes variegatus, 223, 326
Moridae, 418
Morganella morganii, 166
Mosquitoes, 155, 156, 257, 278, 334, 336, 372, 373–376

Mouth, 214, 219, 220, 221, 223
Mouth lesions, 100, *4·4, 4·5*, 101 (*see also* Stomatitis)
Mouthparts, *11·3*, 395–396, *12·2*
Mouth-rot (*see* Stomatitis)
Mucor, 17·3
Mucor circinelloides, 196, 201, 206, 218, 220
Mugil cephalus, 418
Multicaecum, 324
Multicotyle, 296
Multivitamin/mineral preparations, 573
Mus musculus, 346
Muscles, 23–24, 180, 218, 269, 282
Muscle relaxants, 535, 538, 539, 556
Muscle tone, 511
Muscular degeneration, 365
Muscular lesions, 271, 272
Mycetoma, *7·1*, 198, *7·6*, 200, 203, 210, 214, 216, 219, 220, 223, 226
Mycobacterium, 112, 115, 170, 185 (*see also* Tuberculosis)
Mycobacterium ulcerans, 187
Mycoses (*see* Fungi)
Mycotic infections, 195–203
Myelogenous leukaemia, 430, 436, 437, 438
Myelomatosis, 430
Myeloproliferative disease, 439
Myiasis, 245, 372, 376, 377, *10·2*, 378
Myositis, *6·5*, 180
Myxidium, 279
Myxofibroma, 143, 434, 461
Myxoma, 430
Myxosporidea, 279, 280
Myxosporidiosis, of aquatic chelonians, 280

Naegleria, 245
Nairobi Snake Park, 183 (*see also* Kenya)
Naja, 236, 239, 242, 274, 285, 319
Naja melanolenca, 456, 460
N. naja, 136, 159, 456, 460

N. nigricollis, 28, 376, 456, 460
N. nivea, 456, 460
Naphthalene, 579
Natrix, 236, 239, 259, 297, 304, 319, 365
Natrix cyclopion, 214
N. maura, 480
N. natrix, 20–21, 26, 2·6, 154, 413, 451, 462, 477, 538
N. natrix persa, 348
N. rhombifer, 304
N. sipedon, 223, 304, *14·1*, 480, 481
N. stolata, 455
N. tessellata, 413, 462
N. tigrina, 304
Necropsy (*see* Post mortem examination)
Necrotic dermatitis, 174, 175, 401, 490
Necrotic stomatitis, 419, 490 (*see also* Stomatitis)
Neisseria, 115, 116
Nematodes, 166, 179, 193, 315–339, *9·5*, 328
Nematodes, treatment of, 565–569
Nematotaenia, 312
Nematotaenia tarentolae, 312
N. lopezenyrai, 312
N. mabuiae, 312
Nematotaeniidae, 312
Neodiplostomulum, 297
Neodipsonyssus saurarum, 368
Neoliponyssus, 368
Neoliponyssus saurarum, 255
Neomycin, 179, 182, 184, 186, 559, 560, 562, 564
Neoplasia, 4, 7, 87, 88–89, 160, 172, 197, 206, 211, 220, 221, 222, 224, 361, 429–464, 495, 522
Neoplasia, aetiology of, 142–152, 430–431
Neoplasia, definitions and classifications, 429–430
Neoplasia, diagnosis, 462–464
Neoplasia, in Chelonia, 435–441
Neoplasia in Crocodilia, 441–443

Neoplasia in Squamata: Sauria, 443–449
Neoplasia, in Squamata: Serpentes, 449–457
Neoplasia, treatment of, 464
Neoplasia, viruses associated with, 142–152
Neopolystoma orbiculare, 296
Nephritis, 240 (*see also* Renal disease)
Nephroblastoma, 430
Nephrosis, 211 (*see also* Renal disease)
Nervous disease, 391, 498–499, 559, 576
Nervous system, 62–65, 498–499
Neurilemmoma, 430
Neuro-endocrine control (*see* Endocrine system)
Neuroblastoma, 430
Neurological disturbance (*see* Nervous disease)
Neuromuscular blockade, 559
Niclosamide, 565, 566
Nicoria (= *Geomyda*) 242, 245, 255
Nicotine, 556, 579
Ninia sebae sebae, 267
Nitrofurazone, 569
Nitrogen, 33
Nitrogen metabolism, 33
Nomenclature, of reptiles, 3, 9, 234
Nomenclature, of neoplasms, 429–430
Noradrenaline (*see* Adrenaline)
Normal flora, 165, 168
Nose, 214, 219, 221 (*see also* Rostral abrasions)
Nosema, 281
Notoedres, 292
Nursing, 528–529, 539–540
Nutrition, 409–427, 448, 500 (*see also* Diet)
Nutritional compounds, 570–574
Nutritional secondary hyperparathyroidism (NSH) (*see* Osteodystrophy)

Nuttallia, 278
Nyctotherus, 284
Nystatin, 564

Obesity, 87, 410
Obstruction of gut (*see* Impaction)
Octoporella, 259, 260, 269
Ocular disease, 87, 121, 170, 178–179, 206, 223
Ocular disease, in man (*see* Zoonoses)
Oedema, 220, 511, *16·1*, 578 (*see also* Diuretic)
Oesophagus, 29, 31, 213
Oestrogens, 68
Old age, 7, 87, 433, 435, 438, 441
Olfactory organs, 63–64, 389–390, 500
Onchocerca volvulus, 338
Oncology (*see* Neoplasia)
Oncornavirus, 135, 142, 143, 159
Oochoristica, 312
Oochoristica bivitellobata, 300
Oocysts, 255, 262, 266
Opalinida, 244
Opheodrys, 284
Ophidascaris, 324, *9·10*
Ophidascaris boyli, 324
O. labiatopapillosa, 324
O. sprenti, 324, 348–349
Ophidia (*see* Serpentes)
Ophidiella, 273
Ophidilaelaps, 368
Ophiomegistus, 371
Ophionyssus arabicus, 366
O. lacertinus, 367
O. mabuyae, 367
O. natricis, 183, 366–368, *10·1*
O. serpentium, 366, 367
Ophiotaenia, *9·10*, 565
Ophiotaenia perspicua, 303
O. racemosa, 304
O. testudo, 304, 315
Ophis, 236, 284
Ophthalmic disease (*see* Ocular disease)

Ophthalmoscope, 499, 519
Oplurus sebae, 375
Orbit, 221, 224 (*see also* Enucleation)
Organs (*see* Anatomy and Viscera and individual organs)
Ornithodoros compactus, 365
O. foleyi, 365
O. moubata, 365
O. turicata, 365
O. talaje, 366
Orthopaedic surgery, 545 (*see also* Fractures and Surgery)
Ortleppnema, 322
Osmerus mordax, 418
Osmoregulation, 30–34
Osteitis deformans (Paget's disease) 498
Osteochondroma, 456
Osteochondrosarcoma, 460
Osteoclastoma, 430
Osteodystrophy, 409, *12·2*, 422–426, 481, 496, 497, 545, 572
Osteolaemus tetraspis, 218
Osteoma, 430, 431, 445
Osteomyelitis, 223
Osteoperiostitis, 498
Osteosarcoma, 449, 455
Oswaldofilaria, 334
Oswaldofilaria chlamydosauri, 334, 336
O. belemensis, 336
O. petersi, 336
O. spinosa, 336
Oxyuroidea, 321
Ovarian fibroma, 449, 458
Ovarian haemangioma, 457, 461
Ovarian tumour, 458
Ovary (*see* Reproductive system)
Overfeeding, 86, 410 (*see also* Obesity)
Overgrowth of beak (*see* Mouthparts)
Overheating (*see* Hyperthermia)
Oviduct, *2·5*, 24, 169, 180, 317, 500
Oviductitis, 180, 500
Oviparity, 49, 500

Ovoviviparity, 49, 500
Ovulation, 46
Oxygen consumption, 2·13, 57 (see also Metabolism)
Oxygen dissociation curves, 43, 2·10, 4·4
Oxygen tension, 183, 186
Oxytetracycline, 183, 186, 188, 249, 561, 562
Oxytocin, 577
Oxyurid (see Oxyuridoidea)
Oxyuridoidea, 291, 321–323, 9·10, 568
Ozobranchus, 257
Ozobranchus branchiatus, 440
O. jansenensis, 360
O. margoi, 360
O. shipleyi, 361
Ozolaimus, 322

PCV (see Haematology)
pH, of blood, 38, 40
Package of specimens (see Specimens, carriage of)
Paecilobdella, 236
Paecilomyces farinosus, 195, 199, 200, 216
P. lilacinus, 196, 199, 200, 201, 203, 210, 215, 217
P. viridis, 196, 213
P. fumoso-roseus, 204, 213
Pain, 172, 177, 252, 535, 538, 539, 556, 578
Paint solvents, 579
Palpation, 178, 247, 511–512
Pancreas, 29, 66, 329, 451
Pancreatectomy, 495, 574, 576 (see also Diabetes)
Pancreatic adenocarcinoma, 455, 460
Pancreatic lesions, 82, 455, 460, 495, 574, 576
Panophthalmitis (see Ocular disease)
Papillary carcinoma of the bile-duct, 455, 460

Papilloma, 89, 152, 331, 430, 433, 435, 436, 437, 438, 440, 441, 442, 444, 445, 446, 447, 450, 456, 460, 544
Papovavirus, 152, 447
Paraffin, 579 (see also Liquid paraffin)
Paralysis, 365, 511, 562
Paralaaeuris, 322
Paraechinus ethiopicus, 314
Paramyxovirus, 182
Parasites, 101, 126–128, 172, 175, 195, 440, 463 (see also individual species)
Parasites, in neoplasia, 434, 448
Parasites, sites of, 293–294
Parasitic diseases, 84–85, 234
Parasiticides (see Drugs and Insecticides)
Parasitism, 292
Parasitological techniques, 111, 126–128, 292
Parathyroid adenoma, 437, 439
Parathyroid glands, 66, 439
Parietal eye (see Pineal body)
Paromomycin, 569–570
Parthenogenesis, 44, 470, 474
Pasteurella, 115
Pathogenicity of bacteria, 167–170
Pathological conditions, 83–91
Pathological examination, 77–79, (see also *Post mortem* examination)
Pathological responses, 82
Pathology, 75–91
Pelomedusa subruta, 436, 438
Pelusios subniger, 225, 436, 438
Penicillin, 560, 561
Penis, 29, 2·14, 79, 89, 500
Pentastomida, 293, 9·8, 9·9, 9·10, 341, 346
Pentobarbitone sodium, 536, 547, 556, 557
Pentobarbitone with chloral hydrate, 557
Pentastomes (see Pentastomida)

Percussion, 514
Pericarditis (*see* Cardiovascular disease)
Peritoneal lavage, 578
Peritoneum, 214
Peritonitis, 180, 181, 214, 250, 328
Pesticides (*see* Insecticides)
Pevidine, 554
Pharyngodon, 322, *9·10*
Phasmida, 319
Phelsuma, 496
Phencyclidine hydrochloride, 557
Phaeochromocytoma, 445, 449, 452, 459
Philodrias, 236
Phlebotominae, 372–373 (*see also* individual species)
Phlebotomus californicus, 373
P. caucasicus, 373
P. chinensis, 373
P. cyldei, 373
P. gomezi, 373
P. occidentus, 273
P. ovalesi, 373
P. panamensis, 373
P. papatasii, 373
P. sanguinaria, 373
P. sergenti, 373
P. shannoni, 373
P. stewarti, 373
P. trapidoi, 373
P. vexator, 373
P. vexillarius, 373
P. ylephiletrix, 373
Phosphate (*see* Phosphorus)
Phosphorus, 66, 129, 422 (*see also* Calcium/phosphorus ratio)
Phosphorus aliphatic compounds, 562, 563
Phosphorus heterocyclic compounds, 562–563
Photography, 82
Photoperiod, 46–47
Phrynocephalus, 237
Phrynosoma, 332
Phyllodactylus, 256

Phyllodactylus siamesis, 370
Phyllurus, 236, 256
Physaloptera maxillaris, 332
Physical abrasion (*see* Trauma)
Physical diseases (*see* Trauma)
Physignathus, 245, 256
Physignathus cochinchinus, 252
Physignathus lesueuri, 85, 337, 412
Physiology, 4, 9–73
Pimellaphilus, 371
Pineal body, 63
Pineal eye (*see* Pineal body)
Phyllodactylus, 256
Phyllodactylus siamensis, 370
Pinning (*see* Orthopaedic surgery)
Piperazine, 565, 567
Piratuba, 334
Piratuboides, 334
Pirhemocyton, 285
Pirhemocyton tarntolae, 141
Piroplasmea, 278
Pituitary gland, 47, 67
Pituophis annectens, 452, 479, 473
P. caternifer, 337, 375, 439, 452, 559
P. melanoleucus, 451, 459, *14·2*, 482
P. sayi, 451, 459
Placenta (*see* Placentation)
Placentation, 49, 50
Placobdella, 236, 257
Placobdella catenigera, 255
P. costata, 361
P. papillifera, 361
P. multilineata, 361
P. parasitica, 361
Plasma cell tumour, 445, 449
Plasmacytoma, 430
Plasmodium, 273, 274, 277, 375
Plasmodium (*Simondia*), infection of chelonians, 277
Plasmodium, infection of lizards, 274
Plasmodium floridense, 274
P. mexicanum, 274, 373
P. zonuriae, 274
Plastic media, 80
Plastron, 212, 219
Platemys geoffroyana, 436, 438

Plating (see Orthopaedic surgery)
Pleistophora (= Plistophora) 280
Pleroceroids (see Spargana)
Plica, 236, 278
Platydactylus, 256
Platyhelminthes, 294
Platemys, 236
Platemys radiata, 360
Pneumonia, 181, 194, 196, 7·3, 199, 210, 211, 212, 214, 215, 217, 218, 221, 320, 347 (see also Respiratory disease)
Pneumonitis, 212 (see also Pneumonia)
Podacris hispanica, 55
Podocnemys, 322
Poikilothermy (see Thermoregulation)
Poison gland carcinoma, 460
Poisons, 387, 390, 401–402, 471, 491–493, 579
Pollution, 432
Polydactyly, 480
Polydelphis, 324
Polydelphis quadrangularis, 325
Polymyxin, 179, 559, 561
Polyp, 450 (see also Papilloma)
Polystamoidella, 296
Porocephalus crotali, 342
Portal of entry, of pathogens, 168
Postage of specimens (see Specimens, carriage of)
Post mortem examination, 77, 3·1, 79, 83, 85, 94, 4·1, 95, 100, 102–104, 124, 185, 186, 264
Potassium permanganate, 564
Povidone-iodine compounds, 554, 564
Precardial myxofibroma, 457
Predation, 10, 83
Premedication, 537, 538
Pre-operative care, 539–540 (see also Nursing)
Preventive medicine, 183–184, 533 (see also Hygiene)
Primary polycythaemia, 430

Primates, 325, 347
Probes (see Sexing)
Procaine, 556
Proctitis, 211 (see also Cloaca)
Procyonlotor, 331
Prolapse, 213
Propylthiouracil, 400, 401
Protein deficiency, 413–415
Proteocephalus, 303
Proteromona, 235
Proteus, 112, 115, 118, 166
Proteus mirabilis, 112, 166
P. rettgeri, 112, 118, 187
P. vulgaris, 166
Prototheca, 223
Protozoa, 84, 126, 141, 193, 208, 233–289, 361
Protozoal infections (see Protozoa)
Protozoa, treatment of, 569–570
Providence group, 112
Psammodromus, 259
Psammodromus algiricus, 363, 412
Psammodromus hispanicus, 55
Psammophis, 169, 236, 473
Psammophis punctulatus, 83
Pseudechis, 456, 460
Pseudemys elegans, 239, 245, 255, 277, 296, 436, 439
P. nelsoni, 474, 14·3
P. ornata, 211, 220
P. scripta, 16, 411, 538
P. scripta elegans, 16, 411
Pseudoba, 284
Pseudoboa cloelia, 455, 460
Pseudomonas, 104, 106, 115, 116, 124, 165, 169, 179, 6·5, 181–182, 184, 187, 554, 562, 575
Pseudomonas aeruginosa, 106, 165, 166, 168–169, 176
Pseudomonas pseudomallei, 125
Pseudomonas, susceptibility to disinfectants, 532
Pseudoneoplasms (see Pseudotumours)
Pseudoparasite, 292
Pseudothamugadia, 335

Pseudotumours, 88–89, 463
Pseustes sulphureus, 214
Psylodactylus, 236
Pterygosoma, 371
Ptyas, 259
Public health (*see* Zoonoses)
Pulmonary disease (*see* Respiratory disease and Pneumonia)
Punctoribates, 314
Pus (*see* Abscess)
Pyrantel pamoate, 568
Python, 4·8, 236, 242, 274, 291, 299, 333
Python molurus, 104, 187, 337, 450, 458, 481, *9·1*, *9·3*, *9·7*
P. regius, 180–181, 540, *16·12*, *16·13*, *17·1*
P. reticulatus, 110, 223, *9·1*, *9·3*, *9·7*, 263, 450, 458
P. sebae, 20, 201, 214, 226, 327, 450, 458, 537
P. spilotes, 226, 307
Pythonella, 259, 260, 268

Quarantine, 175, 183, 184, 188

Radiation, 65, 435, 464, 495–496 (*see also* Radiography)
Radiobiology, 579
Radiography, 30, 77, 87, 172, 173, 391, 396, *12·3*, 414, 415, *12·4*, 419, 420, *12·5*, 423, 463, 471, 473, *14·2*, 495, 498, 514–519, *16·2–16·10*, *18·1*, *18·2*
Radiotherapy, 579
Railliettiella, 242
Railliettiella affinis, 346
R. gehyrae, 350
R. hemidactyli, 342, 343
Rana clamitans, 304
R. nigromaculata, 304
R. pipiens, 135, 304, 413
R. ridibunda, 169
Rat (*see* Rodents)
Rat snake (see *Elaphe*)

Rattlesnake (see *Crotalus*)
Reagents, for staining, 96–98
Records, 507–508
Rectum, 31, 211, 213
Red-eared terrapin (turtle) (see *Pseudemys scripta*)
Red blood cell (*see* Blood)
Red leg, in frogs, 184
Reflexes, 499, 513, 540
Regeneration of tail (*see* Autotomy)
Regurgitation, 306, 326, 327, 492, 528
Renal adenocarcinoma, 436, 458
Renal cortical adenoma, 457, 459, 461
Renal disease, 83, 196, 239, 240, 298, *9·1*, 299, 416, 444, 496, 502
Renal neoplasm, 436, 444, 457, 458, 459, 461
Reovirus, 152, 447
Reproduction, 44–50
Reproductive cycles, 46–47
Reproductive disease, 7, 136, 169, 180, 500–502
Reproductive system, 31, 45, 46, 47, 66, 169
Reservoirs, 6, 152, 154, 160, 188, 197, 237
Reservoir hosts, 375
Respiration, 34–41, *2·8*
Respiratory disease, 103, 136–139, 179, 206, 319, 345, 578 (see also *Pneumonia*)
Respiratory signs (*see* Respiratory disease)
Respiratory tract, 34, 195, 209
  mycosis of, 210–218
Restraint (*see* Handling and Anaesthesia)
Reticulum cell sarcoma, 443, 444, 455, 456, 460
Reticulosarcoma, 430
Retortamonadida, 237–238
Retortamonas, 238, 240
Rettgerella rettgeri, 166
Rhabdias, 293, 319

Rhabdias fuscoverosa, 319
Rhabdomyoma, 430, 436, 438, 452, 459
Rhabdomyosarcoma, 150, 434, 450, 454, 458, 459
Rhabdoviruses, 156
Rhamphiophis rostratus, 455
Rhodnius prolixus, 523
Rhynchocephalia (see *Sphenodon punctatus*)
Rhytidoides similis, 440
Ribs, 19–20, *16·2*
Rickets, 419, 448, 496 (*see also* Osteodystrophy)
Rickettsia, 279
Riopa bowringi, 370
Rodents, 125, 292, 308, 421
Rodents, bites from, 389
Rostral abrasions, 388 (*see also* Trauma)
Round cell sarcoma, 441, 442
Roundworms (*see* Nematodes)
Rous sarcoma, 462
Russell's viper oncornaviruses, 143–149

Salmonella, 7, 104, 111, 115, 116, 118, 165, 555, 559, 562, 575
Salmonella marina, 172
Salmonella typhimurium, 165
Salmonellosis, 170, 185–186
Salt (*see* Sodium chloride)
Salt glands, 30, 31
Sand flies (*see* Phlebotominae)
Sand snake (see *Psammophis*)
Saprolegnia, 197, 220
Saprophytes, 195, 197
Sarcocystis, 269, 293
Sarcocystis chamaeleonis, 271–272
S. gracilis, 270
S. kinosterni, 269–271
Sarcoidosis, 90
Sarcoma (*see* Neoplasia)
Sarcoma, of the stomach, 457
Sarcomastigophora, 235–254
Sarcophaga cistudinis, 377

Sarcophaginae, 377
Sarcoptes, 292
Sarcosporidiosis, of chameleons, 271
(see also *Sarcocystis chamaeleonis*)
Sarcosporidiosis, of chelonians, 269
(see also *Sarcocystis kinosterni*)
Sauria, 3, 9, 16, 29, 35, 212–213, 221–222, 225, 444–445 (*see also* individual species and groups)
Saurocytozoon, 273, 294
Saurocytozoon mabuyi, 376
Saurocytozoon tupinambi, 375
Sauromalus obesus, 32, 412
Sauromalus, varius, 172
Sauromella, 285
Sauramoela, 273
Sauroplasma, 278, 285
Saurositis, 335
Scale, 10, 391, *16·14*, (*see also* Shell, Shell defects and Dermatitis)
Scale-rot (*see* Necrotic dermatitis)
Scales, abnormalities of, 481–482
Scaphothrix, 371
Sceloporus, 53, 54, 236, 322
Sceloporus floridianus, 371
S. formosus, 274
S. occidentalis bisetiatus, 314, 274
S. olivaceus, 52
S. undulatus, 371, 374
S. undulatus garmani, 55
Schellakia, 260, 269, 368
Scheloribates, 314
Schistosoma haematobium, 434
Screening, 188
Scurvy, 419
Scute (*see* Scale)
Scyphocephalus, 305
Sebekia oxycephalus, 345
Sections, preparation of, 79–81 (*see also* Histopathology)
Self infection, with parasites, 316
Semen, 47 (*see also* Spermatozoa)
Seminoma, 442, 443
Selection, of animals, 501
Senescence (*see* Old age)

Sensitivity Tests (*see* Antibiotic sensitivity tests)
Septicaemia, 84, 112, 165, 170, 179, 180, 181–185, 186
Septicemic cutaneous ulcerative disease of turtles (SCUD) 175, 185
Sergentomyia, 236
Sergentomyia bedfordi, 372
Serology, 153, 186
Serpentes, 3, 9, 16, 29, 214–215, 222–223, 225–226, 458–461, (*see also* individual species and groups)
Serpenticola easti, 366
Serpenticola serpentium, 366
Serpentoplasma, 285
Serratia anolium, 172
Serratia marcescens, 170, 172
Sertoli cell tumour, 455, 459
Settle plates, 104
Sex hormones, 66–67 (*see also* individual hormones)
Sexing, 30, 44, 177, 500
Sex organs, ducts and products (*see* Reproductive system)
Sex segment (*see* Sexing)
Shamming death, 509
Shell, 18, 31, 48, 100, 175, 181, 197, 219, 220, 391–394, 578 (*see also* Shell defects and lesions)
Shell defects and lesions, 87, 100, 121, 391–394, 578
Shell repair, 391–394, 578
Shield (*see* Scales, Shell and Shell defects)
Shock, 481, 489, 544, 573, 576
Siamese or conjoined twinning, 471–476
Silica gel preparations, 562, 563, 564
Silkworm, 204
Simondia, 273, 277, 377
Siphonaptera, 372
Sistrurus catenatus, 88, 224, 457, 461
Skeleton, 10, 2·2, 15–23

Skin, 10, 11, 2·9, 40, 166, 6·1 167, 209, 215, 219, 220, 221, 222, 223, 224, 225, 226, 297, 377, 378 (*see also* Integument)
Skin, mycosis of, 219–226
Skin allograft rejection, 488
Skin disease, 196–202, 206, 387, 401 (*see also* Integument)
Skin lesions (*see* Integument)
Skin penetration, 320
Skin receptor, 65
Skin shedding (*see* Sloughing)
Skink (*see* individual species)
Skrjabinodon, 321, 322
Skull, 2·2, 14, 2·4, 20–23
Sloughing, 11–15, 2·1, 179, 397 (*see also* Dysecdysis)
Slow-worm (*see Anguis fragilis*)
Snails, 296, 318, 340
Smell (*see* Olfactory organs and Tongue)
Snakes (*see* Serpentes)
Snare wounds, 396
Sodium chloride, 572–573
Sodium iodide, 494
Solafilaria, 334
Somatotrophin (*see* Growth hormone)
Soothing techniques, 514 (*see also* Handling)
Space programmes, reptiles in, 7
Spargana, 306, 308, 9·4, 311
Spargana mansoni, 310
Spargana, in humans (*see* Zoonoses)
Spauligodon, 322
Special senses, diseases of, 499–500
Specimens, carriage of, 78, 105–107
Specimens, collection of, 4·3, 4·4, 4·5, 4·7, 4·8, 98–107
Spectacles, retained, 399, 11·4, 11·5, (*see also* Dysecdysis)
Spermatozoa, 46, 47
Spermatozoa, storage of, 48
Sphaerechinorhynchus, 341

Sphenodon punctatus, 3, 9, 16, 19, 22, 2·5, 31, 33, 47, 75, 166, 234, 245, 255, 280, 281, 282, 412, 435, 448
Sphenomorphus, 236, 256
Spicaria, 204
Spilotes, 274
Spilotes pullatus, 455, 460
Spinal cord, 63, 391, 498 (*see also* Nervous system)
Spinal neurofibrosarcoma, 457, 461
Spindle-cell carcinoma, 459
Spindle-cell sarcoma, 452
Spinicauda freitasi, 322
Spinicauda inglisi, 322
Spiny-headed worms (*see* Acanthocephala)
Spirocerca lupi, 434
Spirometra, 305, 9·4
Spirometra decipiens, 309
Spirometra mansonoides, 308
Spironucleus (= *Hexamita*) 238
Spirotrichia, 284
Spleen, 89, 5·2, 143, 196, 210, 214, 221, 277
Spleen, infections of, 196
Spores of protozoa (*see* Sporozoa or individual species)
Sporozoa, 254–279, 281
Squamata, 3, 9, 11, 33, 221, 222, 225, 234, 236, 237, 239, 241, 242, 245, 254, 255, 258, 259, 260, 264, 267 (*see also* Sauria, Serpentes, Amphisbaenids and individual species)
Squamous cell carcinoma, 437, 444, 445, 446, 448, 452, 455, 457, 459, 461
Staining, of bacteria, 96–98 (*see also* individual stains)
Staining, of blood (*see* Haematology)
Staining, of ova, 127–128
Staining, of protozoa, 247
Staphylococcus, 115, 124, 165, 170
Staphylococcus aureus, 112, 113, 115, 165

Staphylococcus epidermidis, 88, 124, 165
Starvation (*see* Inanition and Cachexia)
Staurotypus, 277
Steatitis, 345, 421, 571 (*see also* Vitamin E)
Steatonyssus arabicus, 366
Sternothaerus (= *Petosios*) 236
Sternotherus carinatus, 220
Stenotherus niger, 436, 438
Stenotherus odoratus, 412, 436, 438
Steroids (*see* Corticosteroids)
Stethoscope (*see* Auscultation)
Stomach, 28, 29, 31, 83, 7·7, 201, 206, 212, 218, 251, 325, 327 (*see also* Gastrointestinal tract)
Stomach tubing, 83, 244, 16·11, 16·12, 16·13, 525, 528, 553, 573–574 (*see also* Force-feeding)
Stomach volume, 552
Stomatitis, 86, 110, 4·8, 110, 121, 170, 171, 175–177, 6·4, 176, 197, 562, 571
Stones, in gastro-intestinal tract, 426, 529 (*see also* Calculi)
Streptococci (*Streptococcus*) 117, 165, 170
Streptococcus faecalis, 165
Streptomycin, 177, 179, 182, 559, 561
Stress, 42, 85–88, 168, 182, 195, 208, 318, 387, 419, 489, 491
Strongyloides, 565
Subspectacle abscess (*see* Ocular disease and Abscess)
Succinylcholine chloride, 556
Sulcascaris, 324
Sulcascaris sulcatum, 327
Sulphadimethoxine, 561
Sulphadimidine, 569
Sulphamethazine, 244, 267, 561, 569
Sulphamethoxydiazone, 266
Sulphonamides, 123, 177, (*see also* individual agents)
Sulphur, lime, 579
Sulphur, powdered, 579

Supplementary nutrition, 573–574
Supportive therapy, 402, 524–529
    (*see also* Nursing)
Surfactant, 209
Surgery, 150, *6·2*, 171, 173, 178, 179,
    180, 181, 182, 426, 451, 452,
    463, 464, 523, 535–548
Surgical adhesive drape, 175, 397
Surgical technique, 543–545
Sutures, 173, 389, 544, 545
Swabs, 98, *4·2*, 99, 100, *4·5*, 101, 103,
    106, *4·8*, 110 (*see also*
    Specimens, collection of)
Symbiosis, 292
Syndactyly, 470
Synovioma, 430
Syphacia, 292

Tabanidae, 377
Tachydromus tachydromoides, 154, 376
Tachygonotria, 322
Tapeworms (*see* Cestodes)
Tarentola, 236, 237, 256, 284, 322
Tarentola mauretanica, 14, 141, 235,
    256
Tarentola platydactyli, 235
Taste, 63 (*see also* Tongue)
Taxonomy (*see* Nomenclature)
Teeth, *2·4*, 22, *2·8*, 83, 89, 169 (*see also*
    Fangs)
Tegu (*see* Teiidae and *Tupinambis*
    and individual species)
Teiidae, 413
Telosporea, 254–279
Temnocephala brevicornis, 259
Temnocephalida, 359
Temperature control (*see*
    Thermoregulation)
Temperature, effect on,
    bacteria, 172, 174, 183
    breeding, 47, 48, 470, 500
    development, 483, 501
    digestion, 411–412
    drugs, 539–553
    incubation, 470, 501
    parasites, 317, 374

pathological processes, 82–83,
    470, 488
protozoa, 234
viruses, 140, 156, 157, 161, 169,
    375
Temperature gradient, 401, 413, 532
Temperature, preferred body (PBT)
    60, 388, 412, *12·3* (*see also*
    Thermoregulation)
Temperature, role in stress, 208
Temperature, voluntary, 412–413
Tenebrio (*see* Mealworms)
Teratoma, 430, 444
Teratoscincus, 237
Terranova, 324
Terrapene, 239, 255, 322
Terrapene carolina, 153, 207, 436, 439,
    459
T. carolina bauri, 377
T. ornata, 377, 412
T. triunguis, 377
Terrapin (*see* Chelonia)
Testis (*see* Reproductive system)
Testosterone, 66
Testudines (*see* Chelonia)
Testudo, 239, 255, 284
Testudo denticulata, 211, 270
T. elegans, 238, 242, 243
T: elephantopus, 211, 220
T. esculenta, 236
T. graeca, *2·7*, 31, 121, *6·3*, *6·4*, 414,
    12·3, 518, 519, 538, 552, 553,
    18·1, *18·2*
T. graeca ibera, 363
T. gigantea elephantina, 211
T. hermanni, 378, *10·2*, 409, *12·2*, 437,
    489, *15·2*
T. horsfieldi, 207, 436, 546
T. illustris, 378
T. nigrita, 212
T. radiata, 212, 221, 315
T. yniphora, 315
Tetrachloroethylene, 568–569
Tetracycline, 183, 561, 562
Tetramisole, 568
Tetrathyridia, 314, 315

Thamnodynastes pallidus, 274
Thamnophis, 155, 236, 238, 242, 259, 292, 319
Thamnophis elegans, 470, 479, 482
T. elegans terrestris, 455, 459
T. sirtalis, 50, 261, 304, 413, 455, 459
Thamugadia, 335
Thaparia, 322
Thecadactylus, 263
Thelandros, 321, 322
Thelonia, 281
Therapeutic agents (*see* Drugs)
Thermoreception, 65
Thermoregulation, 3, 4, 10, 30, 43, 49, 51, 57, 60–61, 63, 167, 209, 539
Thiabendazole, 565, 567
Thiaminase, 418
Thiamine, 499
Thiamine deficiency (*see* Vitamin B$_1$)
Thiopentone sodium, 536–537, 557
Third eye (*see* Pineal body)
Thirst (*see* Drinking and Fluids)
Thrasops jacksoni, 498, 516, *16·2*
Thrombarteritis verminosa (*see* Cardiovascular disease)
Thrombocyte (*see* Haematology)
Thrombocyte, parasites of, 278
Thyroid, 65, 174, 398, 400–401, 493, *15·1*
Thyroid adenoma, 436, 445, 448
Thyroid carcinoma, 436, 437, 445, 448
Thyroid hypoplasia, *12·6*, 425
Thyroxine (*see* Thyroid gland)
Tick-borne encephalitis, 154, 366
Ticks, 255, 257, 278, 334, 336, 362–366, 523 (*see also* individual species)
Tiletamine/zolazepam, 557
Tiligua, 245, 256
Tiligua casuarine, 413
Tilgua scincoides, 252
Toad poisoning (*see* Bufotoxin)
Toddia, 285

Togaviruses, 152–156, 160
Tolbutamide, 577
Tomodan dorsatus, 274
Tong wounds, 396
Tongue, 28, *6·4*, 389, 451 (*see also* Olfactory organs)
Tongue, damage to, *6·4*, 389–390, 500
Tongueworms (*see* Pentastomida)
Tooth tumour, 451
Tortoise (*see* Chelonia)
Toxaemia, 182
Toxic compounds (*see* Poisons)
Toxins (*see* Poisons)
Toxoplasma, 260
Toxoplasma gondii, 272
Trachea, 35, 37, 214, 224, *16·13*
Trachysaurus, 322
Trachysaurus rugosus, 362
Tranquillizers, 537
Transitional cell carcinoma, 451, 458, 461
Transport medium, 106
Trauma, 4, 10, 83–84, 209, 387–407, 435, 499
Treatment, 507–533
Trematodes, 85, 295–299, *9·2*, 300, 434, 440
Trepomonas, 241
Triatoma, 257
Tribolium, 313
Tribromoethanol and amylene hydrate, 558
Tricaine methanesulphonate, 558
Tricercomonas, 285
Trichinella spiralis, 317
Trichlorphon, 183, 563, 564, 578
Trichocercomitus, 285
Trichomonadida, 241–244
Trichomonas, 241
Trichophyton mentagrophytes, 193
T. terrestre, 197
T. verrucosum, 193
Trichoribates, 314
Trichosporon, 197, 215
Trichostomatida, 283

Trimeresurus albolabris, 457, 461
Trimorphodon biscutatus 337
Trionychidae, 39
Trionyx, 245, 255, 277, 280, 296, 322
Trionyx ferox, 361, 441, 476, 479
Tritrichomonas, 241, 243
Trombicula batatas, 369
Trombiculidae, 369–370
Tropidonotus, 236
Tropidonotus natrix, 224
T. platyceps, 314
Tropidurus peruvianus, 256, 412
Trypanosoma, 235
Trypansoma chrysemidis, 361
Tsetse flies (see *Glossina*)
Tuatara (see *Sphenodon punctatus*)
Tuberculosis, 170, 185 (see also *Mycobacterium*)
Tumora calcinosis, 90 (*see also* Neoplasia)
Tumours (*see* Neoplasia)
Tupinambis, 258, 278, 322
Tupinambis nigropunctatus, 214, 375, 444, 446
T. rufescens, 444, 446
T. teguexin, 155, 444, 446
Turpentine, 579
Turtle (*see* Chelonia)
Two-headed reptiles, 416, 471–476 (*see also* Axial bifurcation)
Tylosin, 561, 562
Type-A particles, 149, 5·13
Type-C particles, 5·5, 5·6, 5·7, 5·8, 145, 147, 150
Typhlophorus, 324
Tyzzeria, 259, 260

Ulcers, 196, 7·7, 201, 206, 212, 215, 216, 217, 218, 219, 220, 221, 224, 250, 251, 284, 325, 326, 327, 337
Ulcerative dermal necrosis (*see* Necrotic dermatitis)
Ulcerative stomatitis, 223 (*see also* Stomatitis)
Ultraviolet light, 419, 421, 495

Umbra lima, 304
Underfeeding (*see* Inanition)
Undifferentiated sarcoma, 460, 461
Uranoscodon, 236, 278
Urates, 4, 88, 9·1 (*see also* Gout)
Urethane, 558
Uric acid (*see* Urates and Gout)
Urinary infection, 239 (*see also* Renal disease)
Urine, 239, 240, 255
Urine, parasitic eggs in, 297
Urinogenital system, 2·5, 24
Uromastix, 322, 416, 12·4
Uromastix acanthinurus, 444
Uromastix hardwicki, 33, 315
Uterus, 50, 577 (*see also* Reproductive system)

Vaccines (vaccination), 7, 177, 184, 488, 533, 579
Varanus, 24, 2·8, 236, 245, 256
Varanus bengalensis, 445, 449
V. dracoena, 445, 448
V. gouldii, 413
V. griseus, 462
V. indicus, 187
V. komodoensis, 252, 348, 445, 449
V. salvator, 445
Venezuelan equine encephalitis virus (VEEV) 376
Venom, 26, 28, 159, 169, 176, 182, 579
Venom, bactericidal activity of, 169, 579
Venom ducts, ligation of (*see* Ligation)
Venom fang (*see* Fangs)
Venom glands, infection of, 179
Vent slime, 224
Vermiplex, 568
Verrucal papillomatosis, 437, 439
Vertebral column, 18, 31, 16·4, 16·5 (*see also* Kyphosis)
Veversia, 322
Viper (see *Vipera* and individual species)

Vipera, 242
Vipera aspis, 413, 477, 482
V. berus, 24, 50, 297, 413
V. nurselli, 87, 89, 142, 434, 457, 461
V. palaestinae, 457, 461
Viperidae, 28 (*see also* individual species)
Viruses, 4, 125, 135–164, 197, 208, 285
Viruses, culture of, 135–136
Viruses, in neoplasia, 142–152, 434, 454
Viruses, in papillomata, 152, 447
Viruses, sarcoma associated, 142–151
Virus of Pacific pond turtles, 142
Viscera, 24–26, *2·5*, *2·6*, 26, *2·7*, *3·1*, 79, 194, 196, 207, 213, 215 (*see also* individual organs)
Visceral gout (*see* Gout)
Vision (*see* Ocular disease)
Vitamin deficiencies (*see* individual vitamins)
Vitamin/mineral preparations, 570–573
Vitamins, 81, 416 (*see also* individual vitamins)
Vitamin A, 81, 176, 179, 416–418, 570–573
Vitamin B, 570–571
Vitamin B$_1$, 418
Vitamin B$_{12}$, 525, 528, 570
Vitamin C, 176, 419, 571
Vitamin D, 419, 420, 571 (*see also* Calcium and Osteodystrophy)
Vitamin E, 421, 571
Vitamin K, 570, 571
Vitamin, doses of, 570–572
Viviparity, 49, 500
Vomiting (*see* Regurgitation)
VSW cell line, *5·5*, 144, *5·9*, 149, *5·13*, 151

Warileya nigrosacula, 373
Wart (*see* Papilloma)
Water (*see* Drinking)
Water balance (*see* Osmoregulation)
Weakness (*see* Debility)
Weighing, 540, *17·1*
Weight loss, 528 (*see also* Anorexia)
Welfare, 535, 546–547
Western equine encephalitis virus (WEEV), 154–156, 161, 375
Weyonella, 259, 260, 268
White blood cell (*see* Blood)
White spirit, 579
Whole mounts, 81
Wiring (*see* Orthopaedic surgery)
Wood preservatives, 579
Worm egg counts, 126–128 (*see also* Parasitology)
Worms (*see* Cestodes, Nematodes and Trematodes and individual species)
Wounds, 388–390 (*see also* Trauma)

Xenopus laevis, 135
X-ray (*see* Radiography)
Xiphophorus, 432
Xiphophorus helleri, 432
Xiphophorus maculatus, 432

Yeasts (*see* Fungi)

Ziehl-Neelsen stain, 97
Zonurobia, 371
Zoological Society of London, 194, 195, 203, 208, 209, 235, 251, 261, 265, 443
Zoomastigophorea, 235
Zoonoses, 6, 7, 117, 166, 170, 185, 187–188, 193, 234, 237, 294, 308, 309, 314, 345, 347, 348, 367, 538